Disaster Management and Human Health Risk VI

WITPRESS

WIT Press publishes leading books in Science and Technology.
Visit our website for new and current list of titles.
www.witpress.com

WITeLibrary

Home of the Transactions of the Wessex Institute.
Papers published in this volume are archived in the WIT eLibrary in volume 190 of WIT Transactions on The Built Environment (ISSN 1743-3509).
The WIT eLibrary provides the international scientific community with immediate and permanent access to individual papers presented at WIT conferences.
Visit the WIT eLibrary at www.witpress.com/elibrary.

Sixth International Conference on Disaster Management and Human Health Risk: Reducing Risk, Improving Outcomes

Disaster Management 2019

Conference Chairman

G. Passerini
Marche Polytechnic University, Italy
Member of WIT Board of Directors

International Scientific Advisory Committee

Sponsored by

WIT Transactions on the Built Environment
International Journal of Safety and Security Engineering

Organised by

Wessex Institute, UK
Marche Polytechnic University, Italy

WIT Transactions

Wessex Institute
Ashurst Lodge, Ashurst
Southampton SO40 7AA, UK

Senior Editors

Editorial Board

Disaster Management and Human Health Risk VI

Reducing Risk, Improving Outcomes

Editor

G. Passerini
Marche Polytechnic University, Italy
Member of WIT Board of Directors

WIT*PRESS* Southampton, Boston

Editor:

G. Passerini
Marche Polytechnic University, Italy
Member of WIT Board of Directors

Published by

WIT Press
Ashurst Lodge, Ashurst, Southampton, SO40 7AA, UK
Tel: 44 (0) 238 029 3223; Fax: 44 (0) 238 029 2853
E-Mail: witpress@witpress.com
http://www.witpress.com

For USA, Canada and Mexico

Computational Mechanics International Inc
25 Bridge Street, Billerica, MA 01821, USA
Tel: 978 667 5841; Fax: 978 667 7582
E-Mail: infousa@witpress.com
http://www.witpress.com

British Library Cataloguing-in-Publication Data

A Catalogue record for this book is available
from the British Library

ISBN: 978-1-78466-353-7
eISBN: 978-1-78466-354-4
ISSN: 1746-4498 (print)
ISSN: 1743-3509 (on-line)

The texts of the papers in this volume were set individually by the authors or under their supervision. Only minor corrections to the text may have been carried out by the publisher.

Preface

These Proceedings contain the revised versions of selected papers presented at Disaster Management 2019, the 6th International Conference on Disaster Management and Human Health Risk, held in Ancona, Italy, in September 2019. The conference was jointly organized by Wessex Institute (UK), University of Rome “La Sapienza” (Italy) and Marche Polytechnic University (Italy). The 6th International Conference on Disaster Management was reconvened in Ancona following the success of the previous five meetings, held at Wessex Institute in the New Forest in 2009, the University of Central Florida in Orlando, USA in 2011, A Coruña, Spain in 2013, Istanbul Technical University, Turkey in 2015, and Seville, Spain in 2017.

This series originated with the need for academia, stakeholders and field operators to exchange knowledge and experience required to handle the increasing risk of natural and man-made disasters. Recent major earthquakes, tsunamis, hurricanes, floods and other natural phenomena have resulted in huge losses in terms of human life and property destruction. A new range of human-made disasters have afflicted humanity in modern times; terrorist activities have been added to more classical disasters such as those due to the failure of industrial installations for instance. Finally, Global Warming and the related important alterations in the behaviour of Nature, including the associated extreme events, represent the new spearhead of all such issues.

A full understanding of the nature of these global risks is important to be able to develop models, scenarios, and strategies to prepare for future events and plan effective responses in terms of disaster management. The cooperation between researchers, stakeholders and field operators is essential to achieve such knowledge and fully apply it. Disaster Management offers a great opportunity for gathering, presenting the findings of delegates in form of presentations and papers but also fostering active discussions.

The Editor wishes to acknowledge the authors, the members of the Scientific Committee, the Referees, the Institutional Partners, who supported the Conference, and, in particular, Priscilla Cook, of the Conference Secretariat, who did an outstanding job of coordination together with the WIT Press staff.

Finally, the Editor, the Members of Scientific Committee and of the Conference Secretariat wish to remember the late Professor Carlos Brebbia, founder of Wessex Institute, who foresaw and established this series of meetings.

The Editors
Ancona, 2019

Contents

HURRICANE HARVEY UNSTRAPPED: EXPERIENCING ADAPTIVE TENSIONS ON THE EDGE OF CHAOS

MAGDALENA ANNA DENHAM & NATALIE BAKER
Department of Security Studies, Sam Houston State University, USA

ABSTRACT

This paper is based on the analysis of data collected as part of a research conducted through National Science Foundation (NSF) grant 1760504 – *RAPID: Disaster Preparedness and Response within Communities Affected by Hurricane Harvey*. Our co-autoethnographic study focused on response and short-term recovery in Hurricane Harvey. It consisted of in-depth interviews conducted with emergency management officials, first responders, members of non-governmental organizations, civic leaders, spontaneous volunteers, and flooding victims coupled with an analysis of Crowdsource (spontaneously created virtual platform for citizens' response) data. Our results point to the phenomenon of *unstrapping* identified across standard operating procedures, organizational arrangements, formal communication flows, formal emergency management processes, and resource utilization protocols. While unstrapping has been evidenced in our study to be perceived as threatening by emergency management and response entities, we adapt a complexity-informed worldview to propose unstrapping representing natural processes inherent to complex adaptive systems. Our study highlights unpredictability and change in human and organizational systems and give rise to self-organization, self-regulation that ultimately gives rise to resilience and adaptability. Implications for emergency management and policy are discussed.

Keywords: emergency management, disaster preparedness, complex adaptive systems, response, short-term recovery, resilience, Hurricane Harvey, emergence, self-organization, co-autoethnography.

1 INTRODUCTION

Between 25th and 31st August 2017, the contiguous United States recorded unprecedented total rainfall from the tropical cyclone (TS) formation referred to as Hurricane Harvey (HH). In fact, "Harvey was the most significant tropical cyclone rainfall event in United States history, both in scope and peak rainfall amounts, since reliable rainfall records began around the 1880s" [1]. With the highest peak recoded at 60.58 inches in Nederland, Texas [1], Harvey dumped 1.2 trillion gallons of water on Harris County alone at an average of 40 inches of rain (more than average annual accumulation in the US for the year [2]). The Harris County Flood Control District (HDFCD) estimated 70% of Harris County was flooded by at least 1.5 feet of water as of 31st August. Moreover, of the 154,170 homes flooded, 105,340 (i.e. 68%) were outside the 1% (100 year) floodplain. There were 36 confirmed deaths [3].

Other areas such as Montgomery County (administrative zone north of Houston added to the Presidential Disaster Declaration on 30th August 2017) received an average of 26–30 inches of torrential rain. In low-lying county areas where an average of 100–137 homes have flooded in the past during significant torrential downpours (some of them more than 7 or 8 times), Harvey destroyed hundreds more that never flooded before. Homes in a River Plantation (RP) community received from 12–14 feet of water. "Unfortunately, a lot of those homeowners had no flood insurance because they never had to worry about [flooding] before" [4]. There were five storm-related deaths reported in Montgomery County. In a more rural and isolated Liberty County east of Houston gauges recorded 51 inches of rainfall [5]. The town of Liberty was battered with 32 inches rainfall in a 24 hour period between Saturday 26th August and Sunday 27th August. Resultant record river levels from San Jacinto River tributaries caused flooding in Cleveland, Williams, and Plum Grove; more than 7,000 homes were affected in Liberty County, but no deaths were reported [6].

Research on Texas flooding [7], [8] supports that anthropogenic factors such as urban development, floodplain encroachment, increased impervious cover, reduced overland and channel roughness, decreased storage ability and resource withdrawal have contributed to increasing flooding vulnerabilities. Not surprisingly, the U.S. Army Corps of Engineers predicted on 25th August that Barker and Addicks reservoirs would spill beyond government owned land flooding residential areas. Flooding advisories were not issued in Fort Bend County (south of Houston) until 26th August and Harris County until 27th August when some neighbourhoods were already inundated and reports estimating 4,000 homes and businesses flooded upstream of Barker and 5,000 to 6,000 upstream of Addicks [9]. In Montgomery County San Jacinto River Authority authorized unprecedented amount of water release from lake Conroe to prevent a dam breach. The released water travelled with unparalleled speed of 79,000 cubic feet per second and caused flooding in five large Montgomery County neighbourhoods (McDades Estates, River Plantation, Woodhaven Forste, Artesian Forest, Riverbrook Drive and Riverbrook Circle [10]).

Similarly, when officials opened the gates at Lake Livingston to release into the Trinity River, they unleashed a 5 foot wall of water 15 miles south of Liberty. Mandatory evacuations were ordered in both Montgomery and Liberty Counties on 28th August. Officially, Montgomery Fire Department reported 20 high water rescues in Conroe area and 111 rescues started by emergency responders in tributaries along and near Lake Conroe in Willis were noted [11]. In Harris County alone the government engaged in 60,049 rescues [5]. However, "the widespread flooding necessitated 120,000 rescues exceeding the capacity of formal emergency response organisations and requiring assistance of volunteers with access to boats and large vehicles" [12, p. 2]. In fact, it was the efforts of spontaneous and emergent social rescue activity that served as cues to Harris County fire and rescue officials to switch from emergency modes to disaster operations between Saturday night 26th August and Sunday 27th August. It is noteworthy that Harvey was one of the only flood events where a few people drowned in their home or workplace [3]. It is also important to note that while Harvey was unprecedented, researchers predict large scale weather events to become increasingly frequent and impactful due to anthropogenic changes [12]. It is against the backdrop of a biblical proportions rainfall, catastrophic and/or fast releases of water reservoirs, challenges of build urban environment (Houston), chronic flooding vulnerabilities and isolation of rural communities (Montgomery and Liberty Counties), that we have conducted this research. Our experiences come from those three counties where we were personally involved in disaster response and short-term recovery.

As natural, technological and manmade disasters continue to affect modern society, response systems and networks involved in crisis management have grown in complexity as well. Within those systems there exist actions and interactions of local, state, and federal agencies, private and nonprofit organizations, faith groups, unincorporated groups of local actors connected by tight and loose relationships [13]. Uscher-Pines et al. [14] noted 75 Federal Emergency Management Agency (FEMA)-declared major disasters in the United States in 2008 while globally natural disasters alone affected over two billion people in 2000s. In the United States, since 9/11 and Hurricane Katrina, the Homeland Security and Emergency Management complex spurred national directives, policies, and frameworks aimed at improvement of crisis management processes. Of those, planning and preparedness have taken center stage. Concurrently, communities and households – a local bedrock of emergency management system have been called upon to become more prepared for emergencies and purportedly more resilient. Ironically, initiatives for citizens' preparedness through campaigns such as Ready.gov, America's PrepareAthon, or National Preparedness Month among others have generally found little endorsement by Americans at large. Moreover, research has not offered compelling evidence for those programs to be generally effective even though "Emergency managers assume that encouraging citizens to prepare is constructive because preparing requires little time and effort and has no obvious downside... families whose daily lives are dominated by concerns about poverty, unemployment, and violence may consider government exhortations to prepare for an earthquake or terrorist attack as misguided at best, and out of touch at worst" [14, pp. 171–172]. FEMA's [15] 2009 Citizen Corps National Survey results revealed public outreach and education campaigns were ineffective with respect to local preparedness. The most recent FEMA report [16] represents grim preparedness profile based on 2014 records: 14% of the publics endorsed disaster preparedness activities; 21% were working on it, 18% had it on their mind, and 46% did not even consider it. Meanwhile, the disaster response system albeit robust, follows bureaucratic patterns thus grounding response in traditional norms [17]. Its components exhibit rigid structures and vertical hierarchies of authority, yet routine preplanning activities are inadequate in non-routine situations [18], [19]. Extreme, unprecedented events like HH defy predefined directives, routines, and worst-case scenario contingencies [20], [21]. While the premise is that government can plan for disasters [22], [23], some (for example [24]) have considered such plans persuasive, illusory, and informed by political ends. In this study we endeavored to explore through our own crisis response and short-term recovery immersion experiences in HH, how despite low community preparedness levels coupled with breakdowns in bureaucratic disaster management structures, communities persevered, people got saved, and the response was generally considered effective. In other words, we looked for illumination what processes contributed to the system not collapsing into chaos.

2 METHODOLOGY AND ANALYSIS

We selected autoethnography "a methodology that allows us examine how the private troubles of individuals are connected to public issues and to public responses to these troubles" [25, p. vii] as design. Autoethnographic (AE) inquiry allows for the dual role of participant and researcher [26], interpretation of connectivity between self and others [27], [28], and reflexivity [29]. Even though AE has been popularized as individual, evocative methodology, collaborative approaches have emerged favouring multi-researcher designs (duo ethnography, co-ethnography, collective AE, co-autoethnographic, co-autoethnography (CAE), community autoethnography, and community-based ethnography); researchers [26] note that in spite of nuances in labels, "CAE is emerging as a pragmatic application of the autoethnographic approach to social inquiry" [26, p. 21]. We have adopted the CAE term because our HH investigations adhered to the tenets of the method being (a) self-focused; (b) researcher-visible; (c) context-conscious; and (d) critically dialogic [26]. We were particularly attentive to the critically dialogic [30] aspects of our journey because it strengthened the need for ongoing negotiations between our own differing approaches to the field of disaster studies (pragmatic vs critical theory). The dialogic aspect of CAE forced us through difficult conversations, self-disclosure, and conflict often putting us at the boundaries of testing our own assumptions, with areas of convergence and divergence. Inarguably, as advocated by [26] dialogic iterative analysis of self and both led to mitigation of (a) researcher subjectivity; (b) balance in power-sharing; (c) enrichment of the research process; (d) deeper learning of self and both; and (e) community building.

As volunteers in HH, our direct experiences were separate (both spatially and temporally). Moreover, as prosocial responding is dissipative [31], we had to rely predominantly on evocative anchoring (relying on emotional self-reflexivity [32]). Further, engagement in the community at sensitive and emotionally charged intervals prevented us from traditional data collection such as note-taking, image artefacts, or structured debriefings. The analysis of those experiences progressed post-facto and sequentially (contributing to the pool of data one person at a time). However, as we expanded our CAE to associated interviews, classroom practice and exchanges with students, participation in community meetings, brown bags, after action reviews, joint conferences and meetings, our experiences and CAE conversations became more aligned, concurrent, and "akin to more conventional ethnography, grounded on ethnographic data collection, analysis, and interpretation" [26, p. 19]. This is not to say however that the analytical dimension superseded the evocative one; in fact, our iterative CAE always resonated back to our specific crisis and personal epiphanies of direct experiences in the evaluation on new data intersubjectively. Epiphany can be described as "singular, unique experience" [33, p. 173] that illuminates larger understanding of underlying phenomena. Moreover, epiphanies are characterized by deep revelations during events, leave lasting impact through which "interpretative researchers attempt to secure self and personal experience stories that deal with events …that leave effects at the deep level of a person's life" [34, p. 130]. Whereas we discussed general epiphanies experienced during HH within the concept of an ideal community elsewhere [35], the specific contribution of this study lies in the interweaving and distilling of our own response and short-recovery tension trough groups of others immersed in the context of HH.

We used QDA Miner [36] for data management, coding, and analysis. First, we extracted a priori four figures from our field research. We agreed each was symbolic and symptomatic of (a) how planning/preparedness processes fail to address complex crises marked by unprecedented unpredictability (as in HH); and (b) how the analysis of mechanistic and linear processes alone does not capture the nuance of individual and group actions in dynamic contexts. Figs 1–3 depict revelations of shortcomings in planning processes we identified during our engagement while Fig. 4 represents emergent outcome of nonlinear individual and group actions.

The assistance request process depicted in Fig. 1 has been described as "a fast and simple process flow designed to empower local municipalities with ability to request resources, information and mission assignments with less board setup time and more visibility from state level down" [37, para. 1]. It is noteworthy that areas symbolized by a hand icon denote formal approvals by qualified officials in order to push the order down the path. In clear skies (absence of an emergency or disaster) the process might take approximately 20 minutes when all authorized personnel are in one location and available to make request decisions. The use of the State of Texas Assistance Request (STAR) system during HH was not optimized. In our analysis of data, the STAR process pictogram served as an exemplar of constraining forces among emergency management professionals involved in Harvey response and short-term recovery in Texas.

Fig. 2 represents qualitative assessment of the effectiveness of communication protocols during HH by the American Red Cross (ARC) disaster managers (on a scale of 1 = Poor to 10 = Excellent). Due to regionalized structure of the organization there was a clear disconnect with volunteer base at local levels. This manifested itself by inability of drivers with logistical support to access community areas unfamiliar to them topographically, timely processing and communication of resource needs, proper allocation of resources to areas most affected by the storm, tracking of resources, effective use and activation of existing local volunteer base (the ARC volunteer management platform called Volunteer Connection collapsed shortly after the rainfall), and lack of interoperability with other agencies and sheltering and feeding

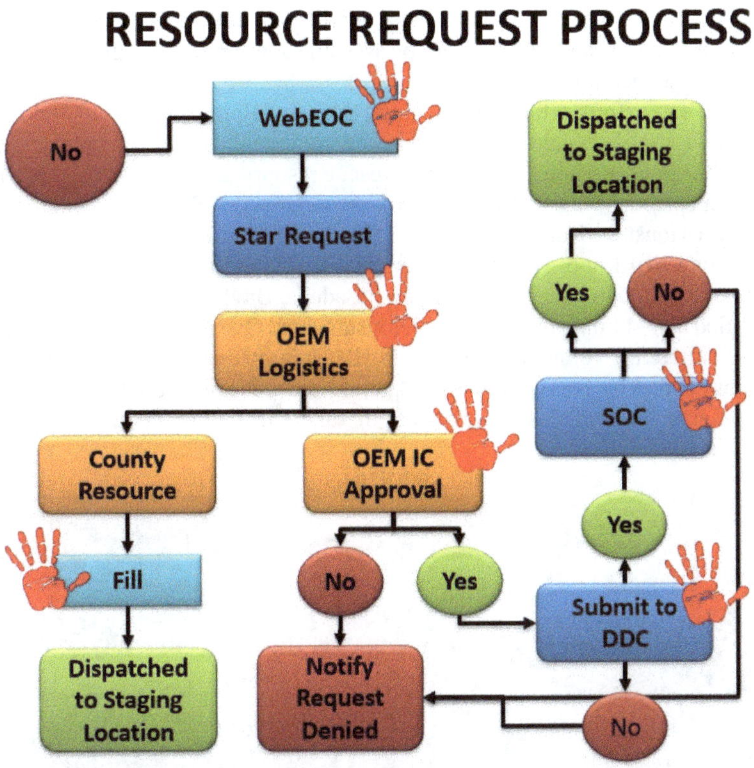

Figure 1: Standardized STAR adopted by governmental crisis management in the state of Texas. *(Source: Authors.)*

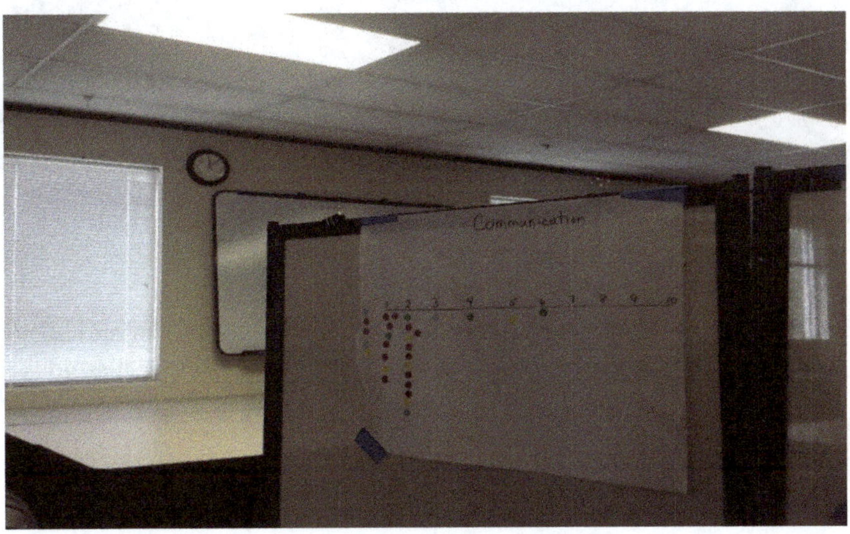

Figure 2: Assessment of the effectiveness of communication protocols by the ARC management in HH after action review briefing. *(Source: Authors.)*

facilities. In our analysis of data, this figure grounded our field experiences and observations in both Liberty County and Harris County as well as interviews with credentialled NGO volunteers at those locations.

Fig. 3 represents efforts at the Harris County Office of Homeland Security and Emergency Management to establish volunteer database of credentialled boat operators with eligible equipment who could augment limited water rescue resources in HH. Overall, the final record in a form of a spreadsheet listed 237 records across areas of Spring, Tomball, North West Houston, West Houston, Katy, Interstate 45 South and Southeast Houston, Houston inside 610 Loop, along 610 Loop, Northwest Houston, Sugarland and Richmond and Southwest side, Humble, Kingwood, and East Houston, Pasadena, Baytown, Montgomery County, and those identified as 1–4 hours outside of the Houston area. Overall, those records do not reflect the scope of watercraft volunteer response in HH. It is noteworthy that volunteer reception points recommended by best practice in planning did not operationalize in the hours after HH. This figure grounded our analysis of uncredentialled spontaneous volunteers' experiences in HH.

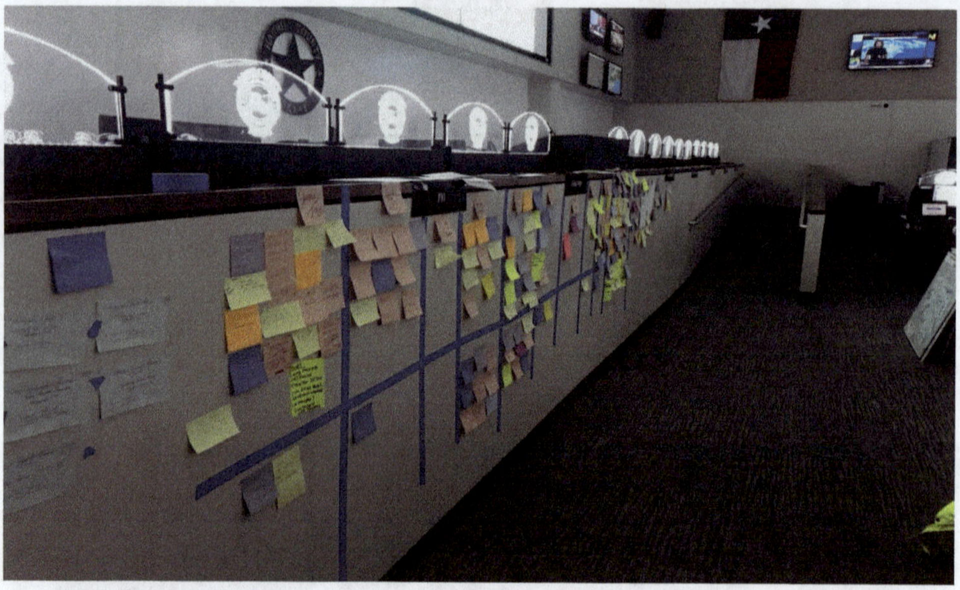

Figure 3: Volunteer tracking system at the Harris County Office of Homeland Security and Emergency Management.

Fig. 4 represents a website mapping platform created amid HH to alleviate challenges in communication of rescue needs. It linked spontaneous volunteers with citizens asking for help in their respective geographical areas. It evolved into a crowdsourcing tool and ultimately into a not-for-profit disaster relief organization. Fig. 4 grounded our coding related to self-organization and emergence.

Subsequently, for this study we used the corpus of 40 hours of structured interviews, shorter ad hoc interviews with 30 individuals, 100 hours of immersive field-experience by researchers, 40 hours of observations and engagement in community events and post-HH

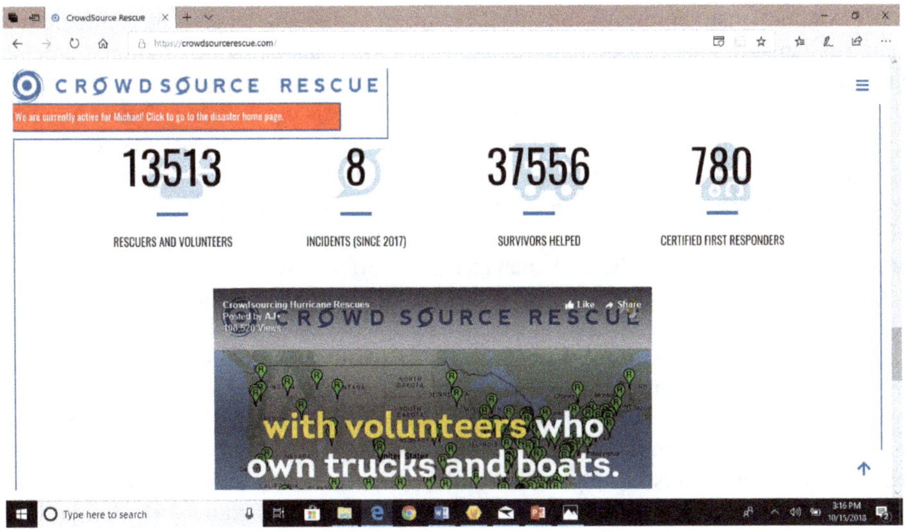

Figure 4: Crowdsource rescue application used by spontaneous volunteers in HH. *(Source Crowdsource Rescue Services.)*

panel sessions as well as selected analysis of Crowdsource rescue data (total 7,700 records) and archival documents. We coded, linked, and interpreted data that were directly associated with behaviors, decisions, and actions of individuals in our study (to include ourselves) who engaged in response and short-term recovery during HH. Next, we attempted to discern an overarching tension identified across all groups of respondents, shared by both of us and offering deepest and most impactful revelation when interpreted within the rest of the data and with respect to the research question.

3 RESULTS

3.1 Unstrapping

The first author's previous experience in emergency management (e.g. staffing an emergency operation center during hurricanes and special events, volunteer work for the ARC, and teaching practice among others) instilled in her the obligation to follow procedure and process against self-dispatching, deviance from existing protocols, or acceptance of uncredentialled volunteers in disaster. In HH she consciously broke all those rules. She did not heed recommended evacuation orders for her residence, she circumvented ARC processes she found ineffective in shelter management, pet-care and donation management; she communicated outside of formal protocols and advised others – to include spontaneous volunteers – to take actions inconsistent with official messaging. The concern about her actions being deviant and misguided coupled with reflexivity on exemplars (Figs 1–4) about structured planning processes and spontaneous action guided our data analysis process. In negotiating our data against our own lived experiences during HH, the *Unstrapping* became focal because it was revealed across all groups represented in our research which was the purpose of our current study. Specifically, professional emergency responders, elected public officials, citizens affected by the flood, faith group leaders, as well as formal and informal volunteers knowingly and independently engaged in the practice we termed Unstrapping. We came to define Unstrapping as individual or group action undertaken in contradiction to existing standard operating procedures (SOPs), standardized formal processes, organizational communication protocols, or public warnings occurring as a normal human response to conditions constraining sense-making in large scale events. Our data allowed us to discern Unstrapping occurred along three major categories: (a) backchannel communications; (b) circumvention; and (c) violation. Each of those categories was characteristic to different respondent groups in our study albeit some overlapped.

Backchannel communications occurred predominantly among professionals in emergency management, elected officials, and management staff of NGOs (paid positions). It was displayed among personnel at mid to mid-upper level of management who had domain knowledge, subject matter expertise and established networking relationships allowing them to access alternative openings and connections to overcome process or system inertia or failure. Backchannel communications were consistently discovered in after action reports (AARs), personal interviews and unstructured field-work debriefings. Many responders who engaged in backchannel communications in our study stressed high levels of risk associated with their decisions to unstrap. Specifically, decisions to use backchannel communications were accompanied by fear of termination of employment, reassignment, demotion, loss of political appointment, organizational ostracism, and loss of esprit de corps within the agency/organization or professional community. Perceived risks associated with backchannel communication unstrapping cannot be underestimated as we found evidence unstrapping in Harvey was perceived as threatening to emergency management and response institutions. Specifically, official AARs we analysed stressed backchannel communications were needed to be eliminated "the availability of resources during HH was a significant issue for the initial 72 hours of Harris County's impact. Automatic and mutual aid response assets were unavailable due to the widespread geographic impact of the region. Along with local resource availability issues, the State was receiving requests for resources all along the Texas Gulf Coast. Each jurisdiction was experiencing their own internal disaster and those who were minimally affected were unable to provide resources due to mobility issues. These issues created an environment where the prescribed processes for resource requests were being circumnavigated by local responders via back channels to various State and Federal officials. The process for resource allocation through 'back channel' communications greatly reduced the ability of personnel, at the local level, who were involved in determining the operational priority of resources. However, back channel communications outperformed formal prescribed methods for resource requests. Recommendation: Local response agencies should follow local basic plans and the State's plan for resource requests. State and Federal Officials should enforce plans for resource ordering". In addition, few responders in our study who engaged in backchannel communications reported early retirement, reassignment, or loss of position within an agency post Harvey. In juxtaposition, we interpreted the *Unstrapping by Backchannel Communications* as a successfully adaptive behaviour underlying the phenomenon of sense-making in high consequence-high risk events.

Circumvention consisted of modifying, altering, or sabotaging established routines, processes, or guidelines and manifested itself among formal volunteers as well as spontaneous responders who sought ways to solve challenges. Unlike backchannel communications, those respondents who engaged in unstrapping by circumventing relied on common, everyday knowledge and optimal solutions available to them without a vast network of connections or specialized domain expertise. Concurrently, because of their lower degree of emergency response or political affiliation (e.g. credentialed volunteers) they reported lower levels of anxiety when assessing risk and consequences of their actions. As one of the ARC volunteers confided "yes, I know I am not supposed to be taking the shelter resident into my car to get their medications; what are you going to do? Fire me from volunteering?" Examples of circumventing included abandoning posts in which they were assigned in place and not utilized, re-emerging at different locations when told to go home and stay there until needed, switching officially assigned duties to attend to staffing gaps identified ad hoc, rearranging resource pathways, altering ways and routes of distribution, modifying established processes, or engaging in activities beyond the scope of the suggested protocols. Unstrapping by circumvention was the most pervasive which we attribute it to lower levels of perceived distributed risks and vast numbers of credentialled volunteers and spontaneous responder-citizens we met in our study.

Violation or direct rule-breaking occurred mostly among spontaneous, unaffiliated citizen responders and flood victims. It manifested itself in disregard to SOPs, organizational arrangements, formal communication flows, emergency management processes, and resource use protocols. Those engaged in unstrapping by violation rejected warnings, defied existing authorities (intentionally breaking road blockade to access event site, wading in toxic waters in spite of risk communications to avoid those areas), or sought untested solutions (e.g. attempting kayak rescues in swift waters) in the absence of formal response. As echoed by one of the citizens those unstrapping by violation represented the extreme urgency of action in the absence of imminent actionable plans "they don't know enough in the aspect of is this safe, is this right, do I have to have a permit, do I have to apply for this particular funding grant…they don't wanna wait for someone else, they don't wanna wait for government to help them, so they out of the sudden build this sense of resiliency as well. That is the majority of the population. Resilience is not something you build – it's when crisis happens people just do things". Indubitably, the unstrapping by violation category was most threatening to official emergency management structures. Our data suggested most of emergency management professionals (albeit not all of them overtly) decried unstrapping by violation as irresponsible, high-risk behaviours detrimental to official response and short-term recovery efforts (e.g. liabilities). In fact, many used the term "evacuations by convenience" explaining that many residents who did not need to evacuate did so because of opportunity rather than need. Our analysis of Crowdsource Rescue data of residents requesting rescues did not confirm that. Conversely, spontaneous action during HH has been concurrently depicted as transformative "considering the disaster magnitude the death toll in Harris County was mercifully low, in large part due to the bravery and generosity of Houstonians: people who launched their fishing boats to rescue strangers trapped in their homes, or on their roofs…the surgeon who canoed to is hospital to perform emergency surgery on a teenager, a midwife who paddled an inflatable swan to help a patient in labour" [2, p. 87]. Considering inherent issues of planning and preparedness that do not translate well on the ground in response and short-term recovery in unprecedented catastrophic events (Figs 1–3), judgements such as un-preparedness and the idea publics are threatening in disaster situations allow institutions to pass responsibility of poor response to vulnerable communities. They might also foster the illusion that strong planning as well as command and control approaches to disaster response are fundamental when it could be that underlying phenomena such as unstrapping are equally important. For each of the types of Unstrapping we discovered, we created representative storyline narratives whose elements we found useful to then link the *Unstrapping* to theoretical lens, namely the complex adaptive system's (CAS) framework. The vignettes portray selected examples of real HH contexts that led to unstrapping and underscore that actions taken by those involved in response and short-term recovery were short of chaotic, but deeply purposeful. Most importantly, those narrative write into our lives [38], [39] because we crystalized our own experiences through becoming more aware of our identity development as disaster researchers.

3.2 Unstrapping vignettes

3.2.1 Rheba: The backchannel communicator (professional emergency responder)

Rheba had more than 20 years of experience in Fire Response and Homeland Security at the time of HH. She had attended many FEMA programs and was an ardent advocate for simulated forecasting of flood impacts in the city of Houston. In 2016 with new governance for the city (new mayor, new fire chief, new police chief), she lost political clout in a new system. On the eve of Harvey, watching National Weather Service forecasts she knew the hurricane would be devastating. "We were going to be trapped in small islands in the city" she thought and shared her predictions with superiors. Meanwhile, management was thinking business as usual "Even on the eve of the rains on Saturday morning they were still managing everything as business as usual" she recalled. Even though the fire department had a plan for activation, the new administration had not read it "it is a very large document and often boring". It did not help that the new fire chief during non-existent transition (in the middle of the hurricane season in July 2017) kept only three of the ten of his executives. In August when Harvey struck, they were still trying to figure out the layout and parking spots in the new building. In absence of pre-activation Rheba watched first as the city flooded, then as people moved around in boats, jeeps with snorkels, and semi-organized groups she referred to as swamp people. Meanwhile, her and her crew had absolutely nothing to do but watch it rain. By Sunday, the decision was made to open the dams to prevent potential catastrophic failures; thus, entire neighbourhoods were purposefully flooded. A year earlier catastrophic failure of Addick's and Barker reservoirs was considered. Rheba herself delivered a briefing with simulations suggesting in 90 minutes after dams' failure 100,000 people would be lost in Houston's chemical junk mudslide travelling into the Bayou. She suggested officials consider those zones for pre-evacuations. No evacuation orders were ever considered during Harvey in Houston. By Sunday Rheba assessed data and predicted continued deterioration, extreme flooding, and a total shutdown of the region for at least a week. She was further worried that even if the dams were open, they were still vulnerable to breaking. Concurrently, the mayor did not want to call in state or federal resources out of fear for losing jurisdiction over the city. Despite being told by many public safety officials that is was time to call for aid, he remained unwilling to do it.

Due to her years of professional experience, Rheba possessed deep connections at the state level. She knew a lot of people and navigated back channels very well, so she decided to make inquiries about reaching state help without formal request for help. On Sunday morning she reached out to risk management for the state of Texas, presenting intelligence and assessment contrary to her chain of command and beyond the scope of authority. Upon her alarming reports state representatives started exerting pressure on Houston Emergency Center and within an hour Rheba got confirmation from the state that the aid will be coming. Indeed, because state resources were pre-staged, help to Houstonians started flowing within 3–4 hours "floodgates of help opened up" Rheba reminisces with a smile. By Monday the management got tired of Rheba sending updates and she was asked to report to George R. Brown Convention Center to Unified Command – they were multiple commands; in fact, Rheba suggested none of the command structures mirrored textbook prescriptions of Unified Command or Area Command. It was very messy. Rheba continued her work straight to attend to medical emergencies such as Ben Taub and St Joseph's hospitals. She took early retirement from her agency a year after the hurricane.

3.2.2 Margaret: The circumventer (credentialled volunteer)
Margaret had been an ARC volunteer for 5 years by the time HH hit. She had previous law enforcement and educational background and on the eve of Harvey's landfall she tried to obtain her assignment to assist with shelter operations in Montgomery County; unfortunately, she was unable to register because the Volunteer Connection platform for assignments and scheduling collapsed. It was not until later in September when she was finally able to reconnect and reengage (by then the organization was much beleaguered by criticism of ineptitude in HH direct aftermath particularly with deployment of sheltering plans). By the second week of September the ARC was organizing to help phase out various sheltering operations particularly those housed in smaller faith centers, or civic centers that needed to resume their regular services to communities. Part of that initiative was the activation and dissemination of the Immediate Assistance Program (IAP) – a $400 cash stipend for individuals from 39 Harvey affected counties based on the following criteria: (a) primary residence was severely impacted by the hurricane; (b) household became displaced because of the hurricane; (c) household needed emergency assistance; and (d) residence could be verified in one of the 39 counties. Margaret was asked to oversee the launching of the IAP in several shelters in Liberty County. She received a brief just-in-time training for the IAP and participated in three initial days of its roll-out. The components of the operationalization of the IAP consisted of a Tablet used by ARC volunteer to gather pertinent data and application details. ARC volunteers were to assist applicants to (a) create an online ARC account; and (b) receive a code via email or text message that would then be used in Walmart or MoneyGram International to collect cash. ARC volunteers were advised that they could only guide applicants through answers to the questions and were instructed to not record or retain any identifying information; in case of language needs they were to switch applications on the Tablet to another language for the applicant.

Several things became immediately apparent to Margaret, who was not a resident of Liberty County herself, nor had she ever before visited the area. First, neither Walmart or MoneyGram locations were accessible to persons without transportation or with mobility issues in shelters she worked. Second, many elderly in the shelters did not have smart phones to retrieve their emails (most of the did not own email accounts); many still used landlines in homes they vacated and many of those who owned flip-phones did not have chargers and had not had access to phone communications for days (shelters generally could not provide chargers for old models of phones). Thirdly, many Latino shelter visitors and residents did not have email accounts or felt extremely apprehensive about using them in the application process; it was evident many of the applicants did not have a documented status. Finally, the language switch interface used google translation which prevented recorded data to be integrated properly because in Spanish language dates are spelled in reverse of English standards. Thus, the system would automatically deny those who used Spanish interface because of its inability to execute verification. "I had a choice of going through the motions, knowing that many applications will be denied, rejected, or simply impossible to operationalize. I realized IAP inadvertently discriminated and marginalized just by its design. But I also believed in the Red Cross, after all it tracked my relatives after WWII. I decided to get creative and go on a limb".

For three consecutive days Margaret circumvented formal IAP roll-out processes in order to secure as many approvals as possible. After all, everyone housed in those shelters (often called shelters of last resort) was eligible. If it was to her, she would be distributing cash to every individual asking for it. First, in spite of strong policies against driving disaster victims in personal vehicles, she personally escorted several elderly individuals and mothers with children to Walmart and MoneyGram locations to pick up their cash – "You know I was a cop – I can do my risk assessment fairly well" she noted. She established on her own electronic devices numerous email accounts where applicants could receive emails with their passcodes; at times she was concurrently establishing email accounts on her cell phone, iPad, and laptop she brought in on a third day. She encouraged Latino applicants not to use their native tongue and trust her with data input in the English version of the IAP; she gathered dozens of notes with personal identifying information so that she could ascertain which accounts and codes belonged to whom. In short, she ran a circumvention enterprise within the ARC with numbers of rejections declining by day 3. "We tried to fix and alter everything that seemed to be wrong with the system but thinking back the system was total crap and people deserved better". Margaret continued to work in shelters and remained involved with the ARC at the time of our study.

3.2.3 Matt: The circumventer (spontaneous citizen responder)

For Matt thinking about Harvey started "unceremoniously" – planning was not on his mind. He remembered people overreacting after hurricane Katrina and evacuating Houston needlessly for Rita. On Saturday night his thoughts were on a televised fight. He woke up to flooding in Houston area of Memorial City/Memorial Villages, so he jumped on his bicycle to take stock. Realizing that some areas received more than 10 feet of water, he estimated his Emergency Medical Technician credentialing (albeit by then expired) could make him useful in disaster. However, when he approached formal responders offering help, they sent him to report to staging area at a fire station 3 miles away. Had Matt driven a car, he might have reported there, and he would have been turned away as many others were, he reminisced. However, Matt assessed biking 3 miles in high waters was a waste of precious time. Instead, he folded himself into uncoordinated, private boat operator rescues and made seven trips in 6 hours on Sunday afternoon; all residents reached by boats (as well as their cats and dogs) wanted to be rescued.

Matt absorbed details of spontaneous actions taken, listened, took pictures, memorized streets and topographical markers. Later that night when official responders could not come up with a plan to rescue isolated residents of the community hit by lingering water bands, Matt's local church was in desperate need of solutions beyond official help. Matt and his business partner decided to use some of the information gathered by Matt and launch a website – matching people who want rescues with those who wanted to help. They put it up in a matter of hours, though Matt remembered thinking late Sunday night newspaper headlines might read "idiot develops a rescue site" on Monday. On Monday, however, there were hundreds of people weaving through the site and incident numbers started to grow exponentially as the site became what is known today as Crowdsource Rescue Services (CRS). By the end of 28th August, the application Zello – a free walkie-talkie app – became spontaneously adapted to dispatch service matching those being rescued with the rescuers; Cajun Navy (volunteer group of boat operators from Louisiana) among others merged into the rescue effort as well. Matt focused on short phone calls conceptualizing the platform for its users, troubleshooting, and advising people not to use 9/11 system which by then was generally overwhelmed and ineffective. He realized circumventing 9/11 communications was the best course of immediate action even though he admits he realized some redundancy of effort would become an issue later; wading in a new territory, he was concerned that is platform might spiral into "Wild West" as spontaneous response tends to be depicted by emergency management officials. He spent 20 hour days providing training to dispatchers and managing the companion Facebook site.

Over time immediate rescue connectivity of the CRS became augmented by folding into it a hotline sex trafficking center. Specifically, the center with professional crisis counselors shifted their operations to Harvey using 150 call takers and adapting existing scripts and templates to provide rescue wellbeing follow-up services. The number of volunteers in Matt's and his partner's office swell as well. Self-organizing complementarity of emerging services was hardly managed at all. Matt recalls one of the proudest moments – a local news anchor reached to Houston police to help rescue her friend trapped in a car and lodged in swift waters. However, Houston police did not have boats available, so CRS disseminated its number to match anyone who would geographically fit the area; the communication conducted over Zello was captured by the coastguard who leveraged the crowdsourcing and sent a unit to the location. Overall, during its 3 day rescue operation in Houston alone (it was ultimately leveraged for Beaumont, Port Arthur, Louisiana and even Puerto Rico response to Maria) CRS Houston housed a repository of 7,700 records of households that were evacuated during Harvey. Low estimates indicate 25,000 individuals were reached. Today CRS is a nonprofit disaster rescue organization while Matt remains actively engaged in Texas disaster legislature as well as networking with researchers as well as professional and spontaneous disaster communities.

3.2.4 Andrew: The violator (spontaneous citizen responder)

Andrew was a Texas University student at the time of HH. On 26th August, a friend from Minnesota arrived with a boat to lend hand in imminent rescues. Andrew contacted the local emergency operation center (it took him 30 attempts to get through on volunteer hotline) and was told help was not needed. However, technologically savvy young man could not be deterred. On 27th August Andrew and friend loaded the boat and decided to follow the I-45 Interstate South until the road would be impassable despite warnings to stay off the roadways because of the risk of closures; he used Zello that connected him to rescue communications traffic. In his assessment, where the road would end, people would be flooded and needing help. Indeed, in Cypress Wood they ran into the Spring Branch fire department who desperately needed help and did not have a boat so they followed them around in a low income community moving people out of trailer homes "So we both had our water gear on and then we went out there and physically grab like help people you know get into boats, assist in any way we could get them to a little higher ground"; their depth finder was reading 37 feet of water in some areas. On the 28th Andrew communicated via Zello with Cajun Navy who instructed them to go to Port Arthur (LA) because they needed people with boats there. On a way to Port Arthur they were driving with her life jackets on is a very large four-wheel drive, lifted-up SUV. Even though they operated in risky environment, they followed an 18-wheeler that pushed water away. Finally, when they got to the last stretch of freeway into Port Arthur, the two-lane road was packed with a mile-long stretch of vehicles and boats. When they were finally out of the flooded stretch there was a sheriff standing in the middle ordering all to turn around denying access.

It took 5 hours for the mile of cars with boats to get turned around back towards flooded highway, but Andrew and hundreds of others found a blocked offramp on the other side of the road where the sheriff wasn't and made it through anyway. Past that point they passed various units of coastguard, Cajun Navy, dozens of volunteer organizations, and citizens active in response. Andrew commented that the only time he came across first responders it was the fire department in Spring on the 27th and the sheriff in the middle of the road. There was no centralized command at any point in Port Arthur, yet things were moving. After numerous rescues and navigation help from local resident, they came across a nursing home where the manager did not allow anyone to be removed; the policy was to wait for coastguard helicopters. Andrew and friend looked at the people in wheelchairs water reaching their stomachs, oxygen tanks getting to empty and started triaging of bedridden and wheelchair bound who needed to get out first. The told the manager they were sending pictures of the facility to the Media. They generally took control over and dispatched for help from one official coastguard member; soon after, they initiated moving people out of the nursing facility onto the boats (by then they had a chain of them and hundreds of volunteers to help) and to the bowling alley area which served as medical point and from where they eventually would be airlifted to another city (Conroe). The area swarmed with nurses and medics. Each trip from the nursing home lasted 20–25 minutes and Andrew recalled grabbing medical records "You know we have huge bags of medicines. The entire medical history and records for the entire nursing home everything in a trash bag multiple trash bags that were in the boat". He had to for the first time in his life change an oxygen tank – the patient was put on their boat with 5 minutes supply for a 20 minute ride. Andrew remained in Port Arthur performing rescues and merging with Cajun Navy volunteers while his friend flew with rescued patients to Conroe. Andrew graduated and currently works for local emergency management.

3.2.5 Jenny: The violator (engaged citizen in a community affected by floods)

Jenny was instructed to evacuate her home in an established retiree golfing community when water was suddenly released from lake Conroe. The local fire department knocked on doors urging people to leave. She briefly considered a hotel, but ones in the proximity were full. She was not willing to drive 200 miles to Dallas. She knew there were others in the area who would stay – they had nowhere to go, no finances to pay for hotels, or no mobility. Among those were the bedridden, the elderly, the widowed, the undocumented – she directly knew many and knew of the most. Moreover, she had political connections with an elective county official and sensed she might be needed to get some strings pulled. Even though she never really looked at the flood zones' map that hang on the community wall office where she volunteered for years, it did not matter much she recalled – she knew they were flooding and that it would be bad.

Thus, Jenny violated the evacuation order and immediately went into action; she helped people move selves and belongings to higher floors in their homes, she kept notifying those who evacuated about the status of water levels, she provided information to citizen boat operators who came to rescue those stranded (some of the homes in her community were flooded up to 12 feet high). She coordinated with the official she knew to secure waste zones and debris removal services immediately after the storm. All the while, she was able to weather the storm in her home. Immediately after waters started receding, Jenny realized the speed of short-term recovery was critical. She set up a community center which in the following 14 days swarmed with hundreds of volunteers who came to mock flooded homes from areas as far as Nebraska. The center took form and was the hotbed on local grassroot activity before any official external aid, before her county emergency management services, before ARC (whose substandard food consisting of cold hot dogs and canned green peas Jenny refused to accept; grassroots efforts in her community provided nutritious, healthy, wholesome and efficient food service and ingenious golf cart delivery by youth for all victims and spontaneous volunteers), or before FEMA. After the storm Jenny became an ardent advocate against the planned sale and subsequent urban development of the golf course (the only natural watershed in the community). She is leading citizens' efforts of the community to purchase the land and turn the area into the green belt in order to mitigate future catastrophic floods.

4 DISCUSSION AND IMPLICATIONS

Unprecedented catastrophic events like HH create a state of disequilibrium. In such a state, systems involved such as response organizations, volunteers, NGOs, and victims are moved away from their routines. A CAS displays adaptive tension which triggers emergent self-organization, spontaneous yet purposive rearrangement of components without central control [40]. Evidently, complexity seems to be an important concept for understanding modern government and governance processes. Nevertheless, the domain of emergency management (and in the US associated homeland security studies) have not yet made extensive use of the concepts and ideas of complexity theorists. CAS concepts have had limited influence on theories of emergency management with some exceptions noted in resiliency and disaster risk reduction, e.g. [41]. Recently, [42] defined the following five characteristics of CAS: (a) network of many differentiated agents; (b) emergent quality; (c) no central control; (d) multiplicity of interconnections, integrations, associative behaviour; and (e) evidence of system learning [42, pp. 1093–1094]. We propose that the Unstrapping we discerned through our study is one representation of adaptive tensions experienced throughout the response and short-term recovery system during the hurricane. Such tensions triggered repairs (through back channel communications, circumventing, and violation) and emergent self-organization serving as catalyst to counterbalance processes working during periods of stability and characteristic of mechanistic systems.

Specifically, unstrapping might help account for how systems during response and short-term recovery did not fail given purported 84% of population in the US does not prepare for disasters and indications of government inadequacy or NGO planning revealed through our research. There are several implications of our findings. First, in order for a system to be considered a CAS, there has to be evidence of system learning [42]. Therefore, emergency management governance requires an understanding that nuanced unintended/unanticipated patterns of behaviours that emerge in catastrophic events are a norm rather than deviation. Echoing [43] "the complexity and the multiple, emergent properties of complex systems will make these systems unmanageable… The argument is that since dynamics, self-organization and emergence are the norm, adjusting to these changes is often a wiser strategy than trying to get a grip on them. In this situation, a manager adjusts and adapts to developments rather than directing them" [43, p. 313]. In other words, emergency management governance will continue to run on what researchers [44], [45] labelled *the edge of chaos.* Admittedly, in Harvey the biggest factor of system learning was ultimate realization that efforts to direct or "manage" or direct spontaneous force were futile. Ultimately, "ad hoc civilian responders turned out to be a huge asset.… Instead of turning them away, Texas and Florida welcomed them and helped coordinate their efforts. It was a necessary element in the field" [46]. For the ARC, the experience with Mega Shelters altered their philosophy on sheltering with stronger focus on including community centres, or faith and Samaritan groups that repaired ARC breaks in sheltering plans during Harvey.

Second, social research tends to consider social dynamics through the lens of society or community as a heterogeneous set of individuals and ensuing policies and plans (e.g. evacuation planning, sheltering, IAP roll-out) generally reflect that view. Under CAS lens social dynamics play out through non-linear interactions [44], [47] of diverse sets of individuals (e.g. crowdsourcing) and studying those could contribute significantly to our understanding of how micro-level decision-making influence larger social dynamics. For example, Unstrapping and launching of Crowdsource Rescue in Harvey did not only change the context of response in time of the hurricane, but also caused changes at regional and state level (i.e. Texas 86th legislation 2019 unanimously passed House Bill 3365. It provides immunity from civil liability for a person who gives care, aid, and advice with respect to the management of an incident during a natural disaster). This in turn would affect various communities in the future and would support evidence of system's learning. Finally, the anatomy of Unstrapping allowed us the view Harvey response and short-term recovery through a range of tight and loose coupling patterns exhibited. According to CAS researchers [44], [45] resilient CAS displays the range of coupling patterns from loose to tight. Complex interactions of loose and tight systems in turn serve as creative pathways of adaptation under a range of conditions. In HH tightly coupled systems (e.g. governmental organizations, emergency response agencies, and NGOs) shared situational space with diverse communities and households affected as well as with dispersed spontaneous citizen responders operating in loose-coupled systems. The anatomy of Unstrapping revealed to us interdependence and complementarity. For example, spontaneous volunteers performing rescues were not constrained by thinking about liability even though formal responders were. In the words of an emergency management official: "they were in a way more resilient than us". Indeed, we met several respondents at field level who wished they could "do something" but instead were assigned "to watch it rain". One important implication for emergency management is the understanding of a shared situational space in a CAS. Only then, non-linear, emergent actions could be understood as a behavioural norm versus hindrance in critical events.

REFERENCES

[1] Blake, E.S. & Zelinsky, D.A., National hurricane center tropical cyclone report: Hurricane Harvey. Report AL092017, 2018. www.nhc.noaa.gov/data/tcr/AL092017_Harvey.pdf. Accessed 15 Jul. 2019.

[2] Swartz, M., Troubled waters: A year after Harvey, has Houston learned anything? *Texas Monthly*, pp. 84–93, 22 Aug. 2018.

[3] Harris County Flood Control District, Immediate report: Final, Hurricane Harvey: Storm and flood information, 2018. www.hcfcd.org/media/2678/immediate-flood-report-final-hurricane-harvey-2017.pdf. Accessed 5 Jun. 2018.

[4] Schafler, K., Montgomery County homes vulnerable to flooding issues, community impact. *Community Impact Newspaper*, Conroe Montgomery Edition, 19 Apr. 2018.

[5] Snyder, M., Final report: Harvey's impact on Houston area laid out in grim detail. *Houston Chronicle*, 5 Jun. 2018. www.chron.com/news/houston-texas/houston/article/Harvey-s-impact-on-Houston-area-in-grim-detail-12969537.php. Accessed 4 Jun. 2019.

[6] Harden, J.D., Harvey recovery continues in parts of flooded Liberty County. *Seattle Times, Nation & World*, 2017. www.seattletimes.com/nation-world/harvey-recovery-continues-in-parts-of-flooded-liberty-county/. Accessed 5 Jul. 2019.

[7] Brody, S.D., Blessing, R., Sebastian, A. & Bedient, P., Examining the impact of land use/land cover characteristics on flood losses. *Journal of Environmental Planning Management*, **57**, pp. 1252–1265, 2011.

[8] Brody, S.D., Zahran, S., Highfield, W.E., Grover, H. & Vedlitz, A., Identifying the impact of the built environment on flood damage in Texas. *Disasters*, **32**, pp. 1–8, 2008.

[9] Olsen, L., Flood threat known early: Corps predicted the reservoir spill before Harvey hit. *Houston Chronicle*, 2018. www.houstonchronicle.com/news/houston-texas/houston/article/barker-addicks-dams-flooding-predicted-army-corps-12632041.php. Accessed 5 Jul. 2019.

[10] Conroe Community Development Department, 2017.

[11] Schafler, K., Homes, businesses rebuild after Hurricane Harvey: Montgomery County residents help neighbors together to restore communities. *Community Impact Newspaper*, Conroe Montgomery Edition, 23 Oct. 2017.
[12] Van Oldenborgh, G.J. et al., Corrigendum: Attribution of extreme rainfall from Hurricane Harvey, August 2017. *Environmental Research Letters*, **13**, pp. 1–11, 2018. DOI: 10.1088/1748-9326/aaa343.
[13] Nowell, B. & Steelman, T., The role of responder networks in promoting community resilience. *Disaster Resiliency: Interdisciplinary Perspectives*, eds N. Kapucu, C.V. Hawkins & F.I. Rivera, Routledge, pp. 232–257, 2013.
[14] Uscher-Pines, L., Chandra, A., Acosta, J. & Kellermann, A., Citizen preparedness for disasters: Are current assumptions valid? *Disaster Medical Public Health Preparedness*, **6**(2), pp. 170–173, 2012. www.cambridge.org/core/services/aop-cambridge-core/content/view/C3BB34848AAA4CE0A24A5B4352A28DC9/S193578930000471 7a.pdf/citizen_preparedness_for_disasters_are_current_assumptions_valid.pdf. Accessed 5 Jul. 2019.
[15] Federal Emergency Management Agency (FEMA), Personal preparedness in America: Findings from the 2009 Citizen Corps National Survey, Report, 2012. www.fema.gov/media-library/assets/documents/29972. Accessed 5 Jul. 2019.
[16] Federal Emergency Management Agency (FEMA), Building cultures of preparedness: A report for the emergency management higher education community, Washington, 2019. https://training.fema.gov/hiedu/docs/latest/2019_cultures_of_preparedness_report_10.22.18%20final.pdf. Accessed on 10 Jul. 2019.
[17] Schneider, S.K., Governmental response to disasters: The conflict between bureaucratic procedures and emergent norms. *Public Administration Review,* **52**, pp. 135–145, 1992.
[18] Kendra, J.M. & Wachtendorf, T., Creativity in emergency response after the World Trade Center attack. *Beyond September 11th: An Account of Post-Disaster Research*, Special Publication No. 39, Natural Hazards Research and Applications Information Center, University of Colorado: Boulder, CO, pp. 121–146, 2003.
[19] Morgan, G., *Images of Organization*, SAGE: Beverly Hills, CA, 1986.
[20] McConnell, A. & Drennan, L., Mission impossible? Planning and preparing for crisis. *Journal of Contingencies and Crisis Management*, **14**(2), pp. 59–70, 2006.
[21] Kapucu, N., Interagency communication networks during emergencies: Boundary spanners in multiagency coordination. *American Review of Public Administration*, **36**(2), pp. 207–225, 2006.
[22] McLoughlin, D., A framework for integrated emergency management. *Public Administration Review*, **45**, pp. 165–172, 1985. DOI: 10.2307/3135011.
[23] Petak, W.J., Emergency management: A challenge for public administration. *Public Administration Review*, **45**(2), pp. 3–7, 1985. DOI: 10.2307/3134992.
[24] Bissell, W.C., From Iraq to Katrina and back: Bureaucratic planning as strategic failure, fiction, and fantasy. *Sociology Compass*, **2**, pp. 1431–1461, 2008. DOI: 10.1111/j.1751-9020.2008.00139.x.
[25] Denzin, N.K., *Interpretive Autoethnography*, 2nd ed., SAGE: Los Angeles, 2014.
[26] Chang, H., Ngunjiri, F.W. & Hernandez, K.A., *Collaborative Autoethnography (Developing Qualitative Inquiry)*, Routledge: New York, 2016.
[27] Bochner, A.P. & Ellis, C. (eds), *Ethnographically Speaking: Autoethnography, Literature, and Aesthetics*, Alta Mira: Walnut Creek, 2002.
[28] Ellis, C., *The Ethnographic I: A Methodological Novel About Autoethnography*, Alta Mira: Walnut Creek, 2004.

[29] Adams, T., Ellis, C. & Holman Jones, S., *Autoethnography: Understanding Qualitative Research*, Oxford University Press: New York, 2015.
[30] Bakhtin, M.M., *Toward a Philosophy of the Act*, trans. V. Liapunov, eds V. Liapunov & M. Holquist, University of Texas Press: Austin, 1993.
[31] Perry, R.W. & Lindell, M.K., Understanding citizens repose to disasters with implications for terrorism. *Journal of Contingencies and Crisis Management*, **11**, pp. 46–90, 2003.
[32] Ellis, C., Evocative autoethnography: Writing emotionally about our lives. *Representation and the Text: Re-Framing the Narrative Voice*, eds W. Tierney & Y.S. Lincoln, State University of New York Press: Albany, pp. 116–139, 1997.
[33] Craig, G., Everyday epiphanies: Environmental networks in eco-makeover lifestyle television. *Environmental Communication*, **4**, pp. 172–189, 2010. DOI: 10.1080/17524031003775620.
[34] Denzin, N.K., Interpretative autoethnography. *Handbook of Autoethnography*, eds S.H. Jones, T.E. Adams & C. Ellis, Routledge: New York, pp. 123–142, 2010.
[35] Baker, N. & Denham, M.A., For a short time we were the best version of ourselves: Hurricane Harvey and the ideal of community. *International Journal of Emergency Services*, 2019. DOI: 10.1108/IJES-12-2018-0066.
[36] Provalis Research, QDA Miner, computer software, Version 5.0.5, Montreal, 2017.
[37] Texas Interagency Coordination Center (TICC), State of Texas Assistance Request, 2019. https://ticc.tamu.edu/Response/STAR.htm. Accessed 5 Jul. 2019.
[38] Coia, L. & Taylor M., Moving closer: Approaching educational research through a co/autoethnographic lens. *Proceedings of the Sixth International Conference on Self-Study of Teacher Education Practices. Collaboration and Community: Pushing Boundaries Through Self-Study*, East Sussex, pp. 59–62, 2006.
[39] Convery, I. & O'Brien, V., Traveller narratives: Making sense of place – A co-ethnography. *Narrative Inquiry*, **22**(2), pp. 332–347, 2012. DOI: 10.1075/ni.22.2.07cpn.
[40] Capra, F., *The Web of Life: A New Scientific Understanding of Living Systems*, Anchor Books Doubleday: New York, 1996.
[41] Coetzee, C., Van Niekerk, D. & Raju, E., Disaster resilience and complex adaptive systems theory: Finding common grounds for risk reduction. *Disaster Prevention and Management*, **25**, pp. 196–211, 2016. DOI: 101108.DPM-07-2015-0153.
[42] Meek, J.W. & Marshall, K.S., Cultivating resiliency through system shock: The southern California metropolitan water management system as a complex adaptive system. *Public Management Review*, **20**, pp. 1088–1104, 2018. DOI: 10.1080/14719037.2017.1364408.
[43] Klijn, E.H., Complexity theory and public administration: What is new? *Public Management Review*, **10**, pp. 299–318, 2008. DOI: 10.1080/14719030802002675.
[44] Marion, R. & Bacon, J., Organizational extinction and complex systems. *Emergence*, **1**(4), pp. 71–96, 2000.
[45] Marion, R., *The Edge of Organization: Chaos and Complexity Theories of Formal Social Systems*, SAGE: London, 1999.
[46] Inserra, D. et al., After the storms: Lessons from hurricane response and recovery in 2017. Special Report No. 201, Heritage Foundation, Washington, DC. www.heritage.org/sites/default/files/2018-04/SR-201.pdf. Accessed 15 Jul. 2019.
[47] Begun, J.W., Zimmerman, B. & Dooley, K., Health care organizations as complex adaptive systems. *Advances in Health Care Organization Theory*, eds S.M. Mick & M. Wyttenbach, Jossey-Bass: San Francisco, pp. 253–288, 2003.

INFORMATION SYSTEMS SUPPORTING DISASTER MANAGEMENT OF DROUGHTS

MARIJA TRAUT[1], ANDREA HOELTL[2] & ROMAN BRANDTWEINER[1]
[1]Vienna University of Economics and Business, Austria
[2]Danube University Krems, Austria

ABSTRACT

In the context of disaster management, drought may seem a relatively harmless natural hazard, but according to the Food and Agricultural Organization (FAO) more than 2 billion people have been affected by drought since 1900 and more than 11 million people died because of it since 1900. These alarming numbers show quite clearly that information concerning droughts needs to be gathered and analyzed in a structured manner by using advanced technologies, so the effects of droughts can be minimized. Our research has its focus on the usage of information systems in the management of droughts in South Asia. It is designed as desk research. We concentrate on documents released by institutions such as International Water Management Institute and apply the method of document analysis. First, the paper defines disaster management and its different stages, then the natural hazard drought itself, followed by the state of the art of existing information systems. The conclusion provides improvement proposals for the usage of information systems in the field of disaster management.
Keywords: information systems for disaster management, disaster management cycle, drought management, drought indicators, South Asian Drought Monitoring System (SADMS), Global Integrated Drought Monitoring And Prediction System (GIDMaPS).

1 INTRODUCTION

The Red Cross and the Red Crescent societies define disaster management, as "the organization and management of resources and responsibilities for dealing with all humanitarian aspects of emergencies, in particular preparedness, response and recovery in order to lessen the impact of disasters" [1]. It's a complex set of parallel activities and processes which need to be structured, organized, supervised, continually assessed and improved. Key challenges are linking the different activities to each other in an effective and efficient manner, making sure information is always passed on to the right person or team, raising awareness among the population especially in developing countries and learning from previous events in order to improve the whole process of disaster management. The literature defines the cycle of disaster management consisting of four distinct components: mitigation, preparedness, response, recovery [2]:

1. Mitigation: This phase of disaster management is focused on reducing or eliminating the likelihood or the impact of a hazard, or both.
2. Preparedness: During this phase it's important to assess all possible risks, to develop preparedness plans, train staff, develop awareness among society and implement early-warning systems.
3. Response: Involves activities during a disaster in order to reduce the current impact of it. (Delivering food, provide medical assistance, establishing temporary housing.)
4. Recovery: Returning the victims' lives to a normal stage following the impacts of disaster consequences. This phase usually begins right after the immediate response and can continue for months and years.

WIT Transactions on The Built Environment, Vol 190, © 2019 WIT Press
www.witpress.com, ISSN 1743-3509 (on-line)
doi:10.2495/DMAN190021

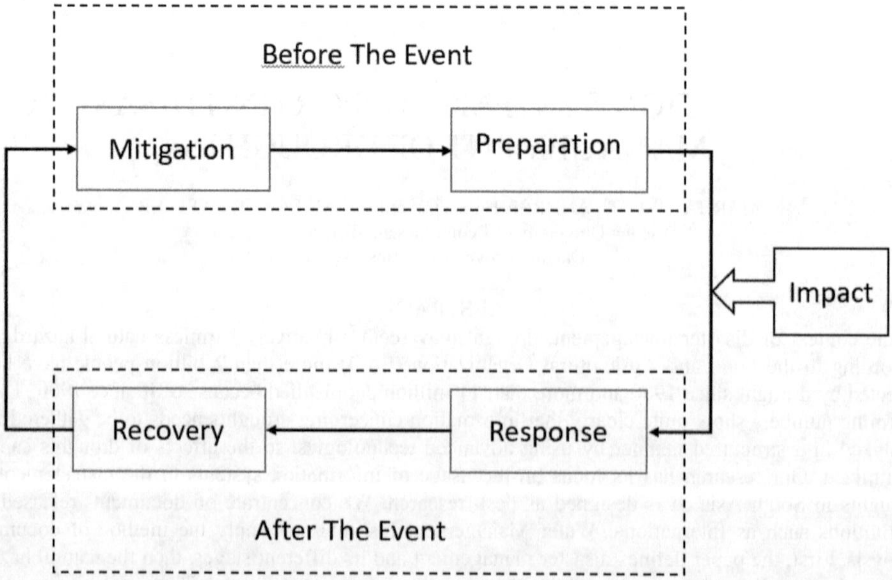

Figure 1: The disaster management cycle [3].

This sure visualizes the different stages of disaster management. This linear model is very popular among institutions and governments for it simplifies the delegation of different tasks [3].

2 THE NATURAL HAZARD "DROUGHT"

In the context of disaster management, drought may seem as a relatively harmless natural hazard. By investigating this topic closer it becomes evident that droughts belong to the most devastating natural disasters with the tremendous effects such as loss of harvest, the deaths of livestock, food insecurity for the people resulting in human deaths. According to the Food and Agricultural Organization (FAO) more than 2 billion people have been affected by drought since 1900 and more than 11 million people died because of it since 1900. Moreover, droughts arise more frequently causing widespread human and animal deaths [4].

There is a series of different definitions for drought, focusing on different aspects of the phenomenon. Almost all definitions agree on the fact, that drought is the result of the reduction or absence of precipitation over some period of time, usually a season or more. It's a slow-onset or "creeping" hazard that receives little attention at the beginning, but causes serious problems over time [5]. It differs from other natural hazards since it's very difficult to determine the onset and the end of drought and its impacts are non-structural because they are spread over a much bigger geographical area, compared to other disasters such as floods and hurricanes. Droughts can be distinguished by three essential attributes: intensity, duration and spatial coverage. The intensity is quantified by the degree of the precipitation shortage and by the severity of the impacts of that shortage on society. The duration of drought must be at least two months and can last for years. Droughts also differ from each other in their geographical characteristics because drought-prone areas usually trespass national boarders [6]. Obviously, it's not facile to identify droughts from the beginning on, because many drought-affected regions are usually zones with ongoing high temperatures. It's also difficult to estimate its regional spread and consequences.

For all these reasons, people are dependent on the usage of information systems for drought assessment and monitoring. Therefore the main research question of the paper is: How do current information systems support the disaster management of droughts?

3 THE TYPES OF INFORMATION SYSTEMS IN THE MANAGEMENT OF DROUGHTS

We differentiate between two types of information systems in the management of droughts. First, there are the data collecting technologies, such as satellites equipped with sensors, and second, information systems that process the data and establish through different algorithms the so-called drought indicators. With the help of these indicators, it's possible to give an early warning to the affected people. On these grounds, they are called early-warning systems (EWS). Both of the IS types refer to the stage preparedness. Due to the little attention that droughts have received, in contrast to other hazards like hurricanes, the research for the management of droughts has not been fully developed [5]. There is no all-embracing information system at this moment that is able to capture all activities and to interconnect all involved stakeholders accurately. We focus on the two types of IS that support the processes of the preparedness phase.

3.1 Sensors

"A sensor is a mechanical device sensitive to light, temperature, radiation level or the like, that transmits a signal to a measuring or control instrument" [7]. The device in this context is the Moderate Resolution Imaging Spectroradiometer (MODIS) aboard the TERRA and AQUA satellites of the NASA. The two satellites cover the Earth every one to two days, acquiring data in 36 spectral bands or groups of wavelengths, thus creating data bases for research fields like the atmosphere, ocean, land etc. [8]. Some of the 36 spectral bands are relevant for drought assessment [9]. These remote sensing data can be downloaded from the NASA website and utilized for different purposes. MODIS is the fundamental instrument for gathering and aggregating data about our earth system. Sensors might not seem important but MODIS plays an important role in the drought assessment process.

3.2 Early warning systems

Early warning (EW) is "the provision of timely and effective information, through identified institutions, that allows individuals exposed to hazard to take action to avoid or reduce their risk and prepare for effective response" [10]. Early warning is based on the idea that the earlier and more accurately risks associated with disasters can be predicted, the more likely the impacts of the disasters on society, economy and environment can be mitigated and managed. Furthermore, it's important that the early warning systems (EWS) are people and location oriented by incorporating the following principles: (1) knowledge of the risks faced; (2) technical monitoring and warning service; (3) dissemination of meaningful warnings to the affected people; and (4) public awareness and preparedness to act [5]. But the natural hazard drought itself has not received that much attention such as other disasters like hurricanes or floods. That's the reason why most countries and governments in drought prone regions apply reactive and crisis-driven approaches [11]. Nevertheless, after hundreds of droughts hitting Asia and the other parts of the world since the midst of the 20th century [12], the governments, international organizations and NPOs are now aware of the importance of EWS.

3.3 Drought indicators

In this section the authors will describe and explain the most common international drought indicators, which are used by the information systems (IS) described later in this paper.

The Standardized Precipitation Index (SPI), developed by McKee et al., is "the" index concerning the measurements of droughts. It measures the observed rainfall as a derivation from a certain probability distribution function (e.g. gamma distribution) that represents the empirical data concerning precipitation over a long period of time. This probability distribution function has to be transformed to a normal distribution and the SPI conforms the standard deviation by which the currently collected data diverges from the long term mean. The drought intensity is reflected in the SPI values. Drought starts as soon as the SPI falls below zero. 0 to -0.99 stands for mild drought whereas -1.0 to -1.49 represents moderate drought and -1.50 to -1.99 already for severe drought. All values below -2.0 stand for extreme drought. Through the SPI a quantitative and functional definition of drought can be created for each period of time. The only requirement for the calculation of the SPI are historic records, which are not always available especially in developing countries [6].

The second indicator we want to introduce is the Normalized Difference Vegetation Index (NDVI). It was first suggested by Tucker in 1979 as an index of vegetation health and density and is the most commonly used vegetation index [13]. For the calculation of the NDVI, you need data from MODIS which is the "primary sensor for monitoring the terrestrial ecosystem in the NASA Earth Observing System (EOS) programme" [14]. The data are radiometric measures of the vegetation constitution and health, profiting from the unique spectral signals of canopy elements, particularly in the red and near-infrared (NIR) portions of the spectrum. The NDVI itself does not reflect drought or non-drought conditions. But the severity of drought or the extent of wetness can be defined as the NDVI deviation from its long-term mean. You can calculate it by measuring the difference between the NDVI for the current point of time (e.g. August 2019) and a long term mean of that month (e.g. the NDVI for all Augusts between 1999–2019). When the deviation is negative it indicates a vegetation condition that is below normal levels and therefore suggests drought conditions. The bigger the negative result the greater the magnitude of the drought [9].

The Vegetation Condition Index (VCI) shows how the NDVI of a current point of time differs to the long term $NDVI_{min}$ and was first suggested by Kogan [15]. The long term index is calculated by using the $NDVI_{max}$ and the $NDVI_{min}$ of a long period of time for a specific month, e.g. the February of 18 years. The values are measured in percent where 50% means fair vegetation conditions whereas 50–100% indicates an optimal constitution of the flora. At the VCI value of 100%, the NDVI value of that month is equal to the $NDVI_{max}$. Percentages below 50% represent different stages of drought severity [9], [16].

The Temperature Condition Index (TCI) also recommended by Kogan [15] is calculated similarly to the VCI, except its equation was adjusted in order to display the vegetation's response to temperature (the higher the temperature, the more severe the drought). This index is also displayed in percent, values below the 50% suggest drought conditions, the lower the value the more extreme the drought. In combination to other indices, the TCI plays a significant role in the prediction of droughts [9].

The Precipitation Condition Index (PCI), is an index based on the data provided by the Tropical Rainfall Measuring Mission (TRMM). The tropical rainfall measuring mission (TRMM) is a cooperation between the NASA and the National Space Development Agency (NASDA) of Japan. The PCI stands for the ratio of $(TRMM–TRMM_{MIN})/(TRMM_{MAX}–TRMM_{MIN})$. TRMM represents a concrete amount of rainfall and $TRMM_{MIN}$ and $TRMM_{MAX}$

the minimum respectively maximum of it, in same month during a specific period of time e.g. 2009–2019 [17].

The Integrated Drought Severity Index (IDSI) is an integrated indicator used in South Asia and has been developed by the International Water Management Institute [18]. The approach to calculate this index is based on using different remote sensing data (observations of vegetation conditions, climate data and other biophysical information such as land cover/land use type, topography and river basin details) and develop through them individual indicators such as the NDVI, the Vegetation Condition Index (VCI), the Temperature Condition Index (TCI) and the Precipitation Condition Index (PCI). The result of the composition of the former mentioned indicators is the IDSI. The values of the IDSI are then visualized on a map application on the website of the South Asian Drought Monitoring System (SADMS) and can be downloaded and viewed weekly. The description and explanation of the SADMS can be found in the next section [18], [19].

4 SOUTH ASIAN DROUGHT MONITORING SYSTEMS (SADMS)

Asia is the biggest continent with the highest population density, being the home of 4.4 billion people. That represents 62% of the world's population [20]. But the Asian continent is also very vulnerable for all kinds of natural disasters such as tsunamis, floods, cyclones and droughts as well. Asia has suffered a lot from droughts, 345 million people were affected by droughts in the years 2015 and 2016 [21]. The need for efficient drought assessment has never been bigger before.

The South Asian Drought Monitoring System (SADMS) was implemented in 2014 by the International Water Management Institute. It covers the countries Afghanistan, Bangladesh, Bhutan, India, Nepal, Pakistan and Sri Lanka. The system uses remote sensing data, which is derived from sensors such as the Moderate-Resolution Imaging Spectro-Radiometer (MODIS) that are provided from the NASA and other metrics like the Tropical Rainfall Measuring Mission (TRMM), Land Use and Land Cover (LULC), Land Surface Temperature (LST), Globeland and Waterbody Mask [18], [19].

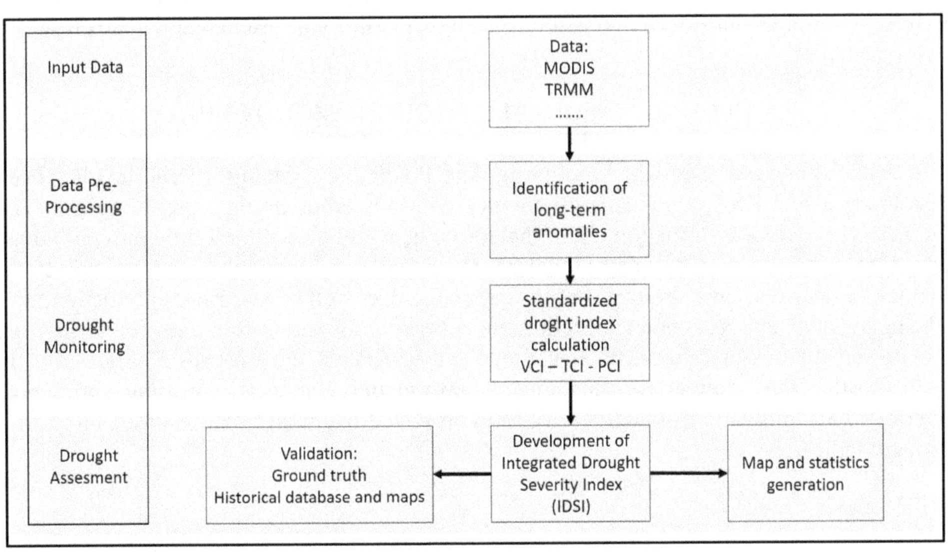

Figure 2: The drought monitoring approach of the South Asian Drought Monitoring System [18], [19].

The developed ISDI is being validated with the ground truth values and historical data maps [18], [19]. Ground truth values are physically proven facts, that have been checked locally [22]. In this process the remote sensing images are being compared to the proven facts. After that, it's being integrated on maps of the user application which can be accessed online and statistics are generated too. Through the weekly update of the maps, governments, farmers and the affected people can stay up-to-date and determine actions if needed. The SADMS does not include a specific alerting tool that gives warnings to decision-makers or others. In order to receive a warning, one must access the website and use the application "drought viewer". As the SADMS only replays the current status of drought conditions and does not forecast, we suggest to call it a "real time warning system". The nature of drought is slow and "creeping". Hence there is no requirement for fast, immediate actions. The SADMS visualization makes it easier to gain a better understanding of the drought dimensions and its severity.

4.1 The application "drought viewer" (User Interface of the Drought Monitoring System)

The user interface of the viewer is clear to understand, it includes the map with the covering countries (India, Bangladesh etc.), a legend for the drought severity, e.g. dark red stands for extreme drought whereas green means healthy vegetation conditions. The map offers three different layers: (1) the standard precipitation index; (2) an eight-day drought extent; and (3) the monthly drought extent. The two latter are understandable due to the drought severity legend. The SPI is not explained and has no legend, but based on logical thinking one can assume, that areas marked dark blue, are areas with strong rainfalls to this current point of time. In contrast to those, are the yellow/red marked areas, which represent regions with currently little or scarce precipitation.

The integrated player in the application allows it to replay past years by choosing different time intervals, although it only begins from 2001. Other tools like zoom in and out and the appearance/disappearance of the legend are incorporated too. The discussion of the SADMS will follow after the introduction of another drought monitoring system that will be presented in the next part.

5 GLOBAL INTEGRATED DROUGHT MONITORING AND PREDICTION SYSTEM

The Global Integrated Drought Monitoring And Prediction System (GIDMaPS) has been developed in the USA, another large country with numerous drought-prone regions. The GIDMaPS provides information about meteorological and agricultural drought conditions, based on numerous satellite- and model-based precipitation and soil moisture data sets. It includes a near-real time drought monitoring element as well as a seasonal prediction tool. The aggregated data sets contain past drought severity information from the monitoring tool and presumable seasonal forecasts. In contrast to the SADMS, the forecasts of GIDMaPS are probabilistic, thus delivering fundamental information for early warning, protective operations and mitigation strategies [23]. Both provide drought information based on several drought indicators.

5.1 Methods

The GIDMaPS applies a similar algorithm calculation as the SADMS using remote sensing data from the Modern-Era Retrospective analysis for Research and Applications

(MERRALand), the North American Land Data Assimilation System (NLDAS), the Global Land Data Assimilation System (GLDAS) and the Global Drought Climate Data Record (GDCDR). The results generated by the algorithm are the following three indicators: The Standardized Precipitation Index (SPI), the Standardized Soil Moisture Index (SSI) and the Multivariate Standardized Drought Index (MSDI) [23], [24]. The SPI and the SSI refer to meteorological and agricultural droughts and are acquired through a nonparametric method [25]. The probabilities of soil moisture and precipitation are computed based on empirical data.

As you can see in Fig. 3, there is a monitoring component as well as a prediction component which is based on the theory of the Ensemble Streamflow Prediction (ESP) method that has been the foundation for several other hydrological and climate studies. The concept of this method suggests that historical data can represent probable future conditions. The prediction component broadens the duration-based drought prediction to a multi-index scheme by integrating different variables, thus providing short-time forecasts for the univariate (SPI, SSI) and the multivariate index (MSDI) [23], [24].

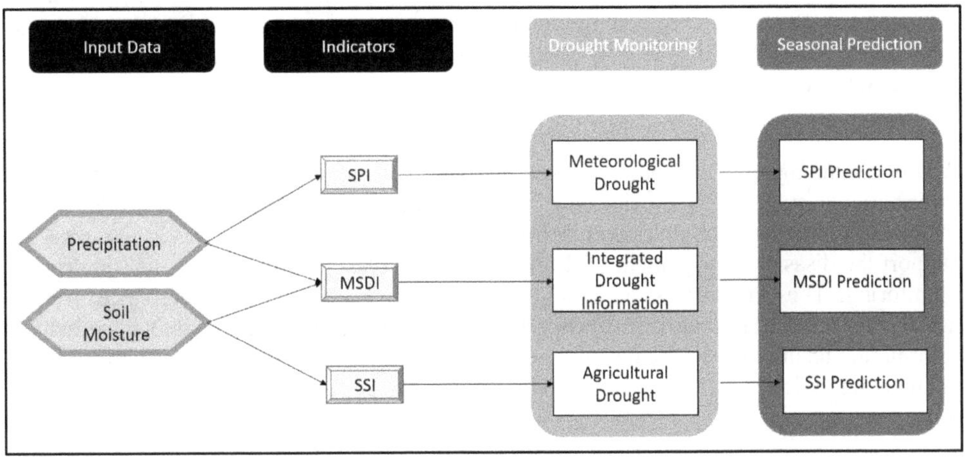

Figure 3: The schematic view of the GIDMaPS' algorithm (SPI, SSI and MSDI) [23].

5.2 The application of GIDMaPS/user interface

Unlike the SADMS, the GIDMaPS covers the entire globe and shows dry and wet conditions at the same time. You can choose between the three indicators and between drought monitoring as well as the predictions. The legend is explained below the user interface. At this moment, one can find the application on a sub-website of the University of California, Irvine (UCI) [23]–[25]. But, as it seems, the GIDMaPS is currently not operating.

6 ANALYSIS OF THE SADMS AND THE GIDMAPS

The information systems SADMS and GIDMaPS are both sophisticated instruments for the assessment of drought conditions. The two rely on remote sensing data from which they derive their chosen drought indicators. The calculation of those is based on algorithms that generally compare historical data of factors such as precipitation, with current measures of that factor. Furthermore, one and the other have developed integrated drought indices, the SADMS the Integrated Drought Severity Index (IDSI), the GIDMaPS the Multivariate

Drought Severity Index (MDSI). These indices are the results of the composition of the other indices (SPI, TCI, VCI; SPI, SSI). In contrast to the SADMS, the developers of the GIDMaPS claim to have included a prediction tool. The authors were not able to verify how far the prediction tool works, because it has not been updated since May 2016. The calculation of the forecasts was not fully replicable due to lack of information. However, the approach to implement a risk variable seems to be reasonable and more advanced, compared to the SADMS. After the establishment of the drought indicators, they are integrated and visualized on maps, so affected people and decision-makers are able to see and catch the extent of the droughts. Both tools of both systems are comprehensible and self-explaining, so local people like farmers, can access them online and monitor their region comfortably. The monitoring application is a big advancement for the developing countries in the management of droughts in South Asia. Farmers can extract data from the tool and turn to the government for help. The application makes droughts tangible for the locals as well as for the authorities. Although the SADMS has not a distinct early warning component, the real-time warning is already a progress and sufficient for reactive measures. It is needless to say, that the two scrutinized information systems only cover the stage of preparedness in the cycle of disaster management. But due to the complex nature of droughts, research heavily focused on the assessment process, which is why the other phases of disaster management have been neglected more or less.

7 RESULTS

At the beginning of our drought related studies, the authors had the ideal of a holistic information system that interconnects all stages in the management of droughts. However, the results of our research revealed that information systems like the SADMS in South Asia, support the disaster management of droughts in the assessment of droughts and in drought monitoring. These processes are crucial for the management of droughts since drought assessment is such a complicated task which cannot be accomplished without the help of information technologies. The development of a reliable drought assessment instrument is a challenging assignment, which is why research heavily concentrated on this part of disaster management.

8 CONCLUSIONS

Droughts are still the least understood of all natural hazards [11], causing significant water deficits, economic losses and food insecurity [9]. Even though it has received less attention than other natural hazards like earthquakes or hurricanes, functional drought assessment methods have been developed all over the globe, setting a milestone for further research and development potential. The recommendations of the authors for the SADMS are, the integration of a prediction/forecasting component that also considers the factor risk similarly to the GIDMaPS. Furthermore, we recommend to implement an alerting/communicating unit, that sends automatic notifications to authorities and decision-makers, e.g. a specific region in Pakistan is suffering due to very high temperatures and no rain for the last three months. The alerting unit, recognizes the current problem and notifies the regional government of that affected area by sending emails to assigned persons whose email addresses are deposited in the SADMS. An analysing instrument must be established and integrated in order to achieve this goal. But the alerting tool won't solve the problem of droughts, of course. Many drought researchers criticize the fact that governments operate responsively rather than preventively. For the effective management of droughts, it's important that governments and authorities develop a plan what to do when a drought strikes, assign and train staff for the emergency case, raise funds for droughts and implement profound strategies for the efficient mitigation of future events. It's substantial that all activities and processes of disaster management have been carefully considered, process owners assigned and resources made available.

REFERENCES

[1] International Red Cross and Red Crescent, National Societies about disaster management. www.ifrc.org/en/what-we-do/disaster-management/about-disaster-management/. Accessed on: 22 May 2017.

[2] Coppola, D.P., *Introduction to International Disaster Management*, Elsevier/Butterworth-Heinemann: Amsterdam, Boston, Heidelberg, London, New York, Oxford, Paris, San Diego, San Francisco, Singapore, Sydney, Tokyo, 2006.

[3] Wilhite, D., Sivakumar, S.V.D. & Wood, D.A., *Early Warning Systems for Drought Preparedness*, World Meteorological Organization, 2000.

[4] Food and Agricultural Organization (FAO), About droughts. www.fao.org/emergencies/emergency-types/drought/en/. Accessed on: 20 May 2017.

[5] Grasso, V.F., *Early Warning Systems: State-of-Art Analysis and Future Directions*, United Nations, 2012.

[6] McKee, T.D., Doesken, N.J. & Kleist, J., The relationship of drought frequency and duration to time scales. *Eighth Conference on Applied Climatology*, Anaheim, California, 1993.

[7] www.dictionary.com/browse/sensor. Accessed on: 20 Jun. 2017.

[8] NASA, The Moderate Resolution Imaging Spectroradiometor (MODIS). https://modis.gsfc.nasa.gov/about/. Accessed on: 29 May 2017.

[9] Thenkabail, P., Gamage, M. & Smakhtin, V., *The Use of Remote Sensing Data for Drought Assessment and Monitoring in Southwest Asia*, 1st ed., International Water Management Institute: Colombo, Sri Lanka, 2004.

[10] UNISDR, Terminology: Basic terms of disaster risk reduction, 2006. www.unisdr.org/files/7817_7819isdrterminology11.pdf. Accessed on: 29 May 2017.

[11] Pulwarty, R.S. & Sivakumar, M.N.V., Information systems in a changing climate: Early warnings and drought risk management. *Weather and Climate Extremes*, **3**, pp. 14–21, 2014.

[12] Spinoni, J. et al., A new global database of meteorological drought events from 1951 to 2016. *Journal of Hydrology: Regional Studies*, **22**(2019), 100593.

[13] Jensen, J.R., *Introductory Digital Image Processing: A Remote Sensing Perspective*, Prentice Hall: Saddle River, NJ, 1996.

[14] Justice, C.O. et al., The MODIS fire products. *Remote Sensing Environments*, **83**(1–2), pp. 244–262, 2002.

[15] Kogan, F.N., Application of vegetation index and brightness temperature for drought detection. *Advances in Space Research*, **15**(11), pp. 91–100, 1995.

[16] Jiao, W., Zhang, L., Chang, Q., Fu, D., Cen, Y. & Tong, Q., Evaluating an enhanced Vegetation Condition Index (VCI) based on VIUPD for drought monitoring in the Continental United States. *Remote Sens.*, **224**, 2016. www.researchgate.net/publication/297754967_Evaluating_an_Enhanced_Vegetation_Condition_Index_VCI_Based_on_VIUPD_for_Drought_Monitoring_in_the_Continental_United_States. Accessed on: 19 May 2019.

[17] Du, L. et al., A comprehensive drought monitoring method integrating MODIS and TRMM data. *International Journal of Applied Earth Observation and Geoinformation*, **23**(2013), pp. 245–253, 2013.

[18] International Water Management Institute, The South Asian Drought Monitoring System, 2014. http://dms.iwmi.org/index.php. Accessed on: 29 May 2017.

[19] SADMS Drought Monitoring System. http://dms.iwmi.org/app/. Accessed on: 29 May 2017.
[20] World Atlas, www.worldatlas.com/webimage/countrys/as.htm. Accessed on: 19 May 2019.
[21] Guha-Sapir, D., Hoyois, P., Wallemacq, P. & Below, R., *Annual Disaster Statistical Review 2016: The Numbers and Trends*, 2016. https://reliefweb.int/report/world/annual-disaster-statistical-review-2016-numbers-and-trends. Accessed on: 19 May 2019.
[22] www.dictionary.com/browse/ground-truth. Accessed on: 21 Jun. 2017.
[23] Hao, Z., AghaKouchak, A., Nakhjiri, N. & Farahmand, F., Global integrated drought monitoring system. *Scientific Data 1*, 140001, 2014. www.nature.com/articles/sdata20141.pdf.
[24] GIDMaPS Drought Viewer, http://drought.eng.uci.edu/. Accessed on: 29 May 2017.
[25] Hao, Z. & Agha Kouchak, A., Multivariate standardized drought index: A parametric multi-index model. *Adv. Water Resour.*, **57**, pp. 12–18, 2013.

ROAD TRAFFIC ACCIDENTS: REVIEWING THE EFFICACY OF ROAD SAFETY MEASURES IN NEW SOUTH WALES, AUSTRALIA

PETER J. KAVALAMTHARA[1], SAJAN CYRIL[2], YIYANG LIU[1] & VIVIENNE SAVERIMUTTU[1]
[1]School of Business, Western Sydney University, Australia
[2]Australian Institute of Higher Education, Australia

ABSTRACT

Road traffic accidents are a major cause for concern worldwide. The World Health Organisation, in its 2018 report, estimates that approximately 1.35 million fatalities occurred on the roads in 2016. In 2009, this statistic was 1.22 million deaths per year resulting from a road accident. This steady growth has occurred despite an increasing number of countries introducing laws to promote best practice in reducing road accidents that could lead to fatalities on the road. Australia has been no exception in introducing laws targeting a reduction in accidents over the years and has been relatively successful compared to some Asian countries, for example India or China. There is a wide variation in the traffic death toll adjusted for number of vehicles or population across countries. The effectiveness of strategies adopted to manage this problem over the years also varies significantly across countries. Within Australia, New South Wales (NSW) is the most populous state and has the highest share of total vehicles in the country. Yet, the number of road traffic fatalities per 100,000 of population, in NSW, is less than the national average. This study is a review of the efficacy of road safety measures undertaken by the NSW Centre for Road Safety between 2010 and 2016 to improve road safety and reduce fatalities related to speeding. Data for the review is based on statistical reports and other studies issued by the NSW Centre for Road Safety and the Australian Bureau of Statistics. This review highlights lessons learned from the NSW experience that may be adopted by other countries in addressing this man-made disaster.

Keywords: road transport, fatalities, speeding, safety measures, lessons learned.

1 INTRODUCTION

In 2010, when the UN General Assembly [1] announced the "Decade of Action for Road Safety 2011–2020", the purpose was to assist countries to improve their management of this man-made hazard on various fronts and thereby save approximately five million lives. The World Health Organisation (WHO) [2], in its 2018 report, estimated that approximately 1.35 million fatalities occurred on the roads in 2016, with the number of deaths rising steadily over the years from 1.22 million in 2009. Despite this alarming statistic, the report concluded that a constant fatality rate prevailed over the timeframe, within the context of the growth in population and the rapidity of motorisation, pointing to the success of road safety measures that have been introduced over the years by many countries.

However, concern still remains as, apart from the human and social costs of road traffic accidents, the resulting trauma and injuries from an accident have lingering consequences for families, governments and associated health care systems. Further, an increasing number of countries have been introducing laws to promote best practice with the expectation of reducing motor vehicle accidents that could lead to fatalities and injuries on the road. According to the WHO [2] report, the average fatality rates differ significantly across the world between its regions and countries. Among the regions, the highest estimated average fatality rates were in Africa and South East Asia whereas Europe had the lowest rate. In low income countries, fatalities were estimated to be three times as high as in high income countries.

WIT Transactions on The Built Environment, Vol 190, © 2019 WIT Press
www.witpress.com, ISSN 1743-3509 (on-line)
doi:10.2495/DMAN190031

Australia was no exception in introducing laws and adopting best practices targeting a reduction in accidents over the years and has been relatively successful compared to some Asian countries. Fig. 1 compares road fatalities per 100,000 of population in Australia and selected neighbouring countries [2]. Since the 1970s, Australia has been introducing initiatives to improve road safety that have steadily decreased road fatalities. Over 30 years, between 1980 and 2010, despite a 50% growth in population and a two-fold increase in registered vehicles, road fatality rates in Australia decreased from 22.3 to 6.1 deaths per 100,000 people [3]. In 2018, the reported number of road deaths during the calendar year was estimated at 1137 [4]. The estimated annual cost of road fatalities and injuries to the Australian economy is $27 billion based on valuing human life on the "willingness to pay" method. Using the "human capital approach", the estimate would be $18 billion [3].

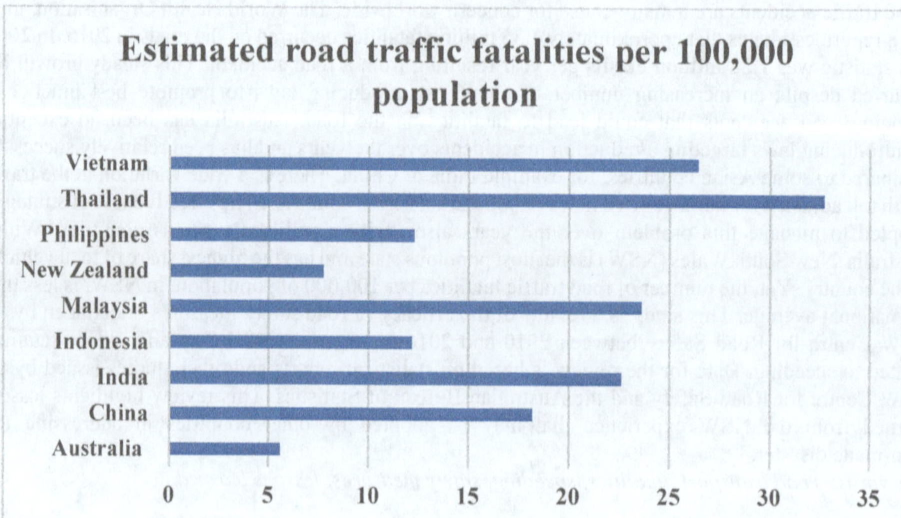

Figure 1: Comparison of road traffic fatality rates in Australia with selected Asian countries in 2016 [2].

When Australia adopted the National Road Safety Strategy 2011–2020, it was with a vision to embrace a safe system approach to reducing fatalities. This strategy is aligned with the global plan that provides direction on safe system principles. The objective is to educate road users and enforce road rules so that safety is paramount. Essentially, the adoption of this strategy is a commitment by "federal, state and territory governments", and not an implementation plan, thus requiring continued "financial, legal and administrative support" from "individual jurisdictions" [3].

Within Australia, New South Wales (NSW) is the most populous state and has the highest share of total vehicles in the country. For the year ending 30th June 2019, the number of motor vehicles in Australia was estimated at 19 million. NSW represented the highest proportion – 29% – of the national fleet as well as the highest proportion – 29% – of kilometres travelled [5]. Yet, the number of road traffic fatalities per 100,000 of population, in NSW, has consistently been less than the national average. The NSW Government plans to reduce the number of fatalities by 30% from the 2008–2009 levels by 2021 [6]. Table 1 [7] compares the road traffic fatalities per 100,000 of population of NSW with that of the national average between 2010 and 2017.

Table 1: A comparison of road traffic fatalities per 100,000 of the population in NSW and the national average [7].

Year	NSW	Australia
2010	5.6	6.1
2011	5	5.7
2012	5.1	5.7
2013	4.5	5.1
2014	4.1	5.7
2015	4.6	5.1
2016	4.9	5.3
2017	4.9	5

This study is a review of the efficacy of road safety measures undertaken by the NSW Centre for Road Safety (CSR) between 2010 and 2016 to improve road safety and reduce fatalities related to speeding. Data for the review is based on statistical reports and other studies issued by the NSW Department of Transport and the Australian Bureau of Statistics. Simple statistical analysis reveals that the three major causes of fatalities in NSW are speeding, driving under the influence of alcohol and driver fatigue. Speeding remains the major cause of death and injuries on roads in NSW despite successes in reducing fatalities. Installation of speed cameras, red light cameras and mobile speed cameras are seen as effective in reducing fatalities on roads. Application of fines and demerit points on breaching speed limits generates revenue for the State and also represses incongruent behaviour. This review highlights lessons learned from the NSW experience that may be adopted by other countries in effectively addressing this man-made disaster.

2 ROAD FATALITIES IN NEW SOUTH WALES

New South Wales is the most populous state in Australia with an estimated population of 7.992 million and an average growth rate of approximately 1.3% between 2011 and 2019. This movement in population is mostly due to the job opportunities available in Sydney, the capital city of NSW and the most populated in Australia [8]. According to the vehicle registration census data NSW also has the highest number of passenger vehicles on the roads at approximately 4.3 million. However, the number of all motor vehicles including buses on NSW roads is approximately 6 million [9].

Fatalities on NSW roads have been steadily declining over the past decades. In 1970 the number of fatalities per 100,000 of population was approximately 28.9 and had declined to 4.1 per 100,000 of population by 2014, despite the increase in the number of motor vehicles on the roads [10]. Road fatalities occur mainly due to human errors such as speeding, driving under the influence of alcohol or drugs, ignoring the use of legally enforced safety measures and succumbing to distractions such as using mobile phones while driving. Fatalities from road accidents can also occur due to unsafe roads and vehicles, inadequate post-crash care and inadequate enforcement of traffic laws [11]. Despite all the improvements, fatal crashes do still occur. An analysis of the number of fatalities that occurred on the roads in NSW between 2010 and 2017 shows that the three major reasons for fatal crashes on the roads are speeding, driving under the influence of alcohol and driver fatigue.

Speeding proved to be by far the most dominant contributor to fatal crashes. Descriptive statistics based on data gathered over the eight-year period are given in Table 2. A one-sample t-test (Table 3) was carried out to test the hypothesis at 95% confidence level, which confirmed that speeding was involved in at least 35% of the fatal crashes.

Table 2: Descriptive statistics: proportion of fatal crashes in NSW involving speeding, alcohol and fatigue [7].

Variable	Total count	Mean	SE mean	Std. dev.	Minimum	Maximum
Fatal crash (speeding)	8	0.3753	0.0111	0.0313	0.3178	0.4164
Fatal crash (alcohol)	8	0.1411	0.0063	0.01782	0.11781	0.1726
Fatal crash (fatigue)	8	0.15925	0.00765	0.02164	0.12877	0.19178

Table 3: One-sample t-test (proportion of fatal crashes involving speeding.

Null hypothesis	H_0: $\mu = 0.35$
Alternative hypothesis	H_1: $\mu > 0.35$
t-value	p-value
2.29	0.028

3 SPEEDING AS A RISK FACTOR IN FATALITIES

The WHO, in its Global Status Report, identifies five key behavioural risk factors, such as driving over the speed limit, driving under the influence of alcohol or drugs and failing to use seat belts, motorcycle helmets or child restraints, all of which could potentially result in fatalities. Only six billion people from 123 countries have the benefit of laws enacted that promote best practice in at least one or more of these factors. Though all five risk factors are potential threats individually, the risk of speeding leading to a fatality is vastly enhanced if combined with driving under the influence of alcohol or drugs and the absence of seatbelts or child restraints. Thus speeding as a threat is in a category of its own. Only approximately three billion people from 46 countries have the protection of national laws meeting best practice in addressing speeding on roads in both urban and rural areas [1].

In 1970, Australia experienced its first sustained reduction in fatalities after the State of Victoria introduced laws requiring the use of seatbelts for both drivers and passengers, though not for children under the age of eight years. This was soon followed by the other States. Subsequently, there was a significant reduction in fatality rates resulting from an accident except for children under the age of eight years [12]. Currently laws enacted to meet best practice in 105 countries protect approximately 5.3 billion people in the world [1]. The compulsory use of restraints for children under the age of eight was not introduced until 1974, followed by continued legislation on improvements to child seats and harnesses in 1988 [13]. National child restraint laws applying to all children under the age of seven were introduced in NSW in 2010 requiring age-appropriate seating in cars [14]. A study by Brown et al. [15] found that there was improper use of child restraints among non-English speaking families of low socioeconomic status in urban Sydney after the legislation was introduced. However, it was observed that overall there was an increase in best practice use.

Random breath testing (RBT) targeting driving under the influence of alcohol was another initiative that resulted in a sustained reduction in the number of people killed or injured on the roads. After RBT was first introduced in NSW in 1982, the number of people that were charged in 1983 fell from 5,348 to 5,096 in 1984 emphasising the increase in community awareness as a result of the extensive publicity and the intensity of the enforcement. The savings arising from the reduced number of fatalities and changes in community behaviour were considered to be well worth the cost of the initial exercise, even though subsequently the charges laid reduced despite increased testing [16].

Speeding habits can be classified according to driver demographics. Driving above the speed limit is seen as a common trait among younger drivers than in those above 55 years of age [17]–[19]. There appears to be a difference in opinion in academic literature whether gender is a factor in speeding [17], though evidence has been presented that male drivers are more likely to crash and have higher fatality rates than females. Young male drivers were also found to be more likely to speed under the influence of alcohol. Thus according to these studies gender is crucial when it comes to speed-related crashes [17], [19], [20]. Overall, a study in NSW from 1997 to 2007 found that speed-related crashes among male drivers declined over the 10-year period [19].

Young rural drivers were also seen as more likely to be involved in speed-related crashes than young urban drivers [19], [21]. Speeding was perceived by rural drivers as inevitable and therefore acceptable. The general perception was that speeding on less dense country roads was not comparable to driving under the influence of alcohol and that it was safe to exceed the speed limit by five to ten kilometres per hour. Evidence from rural Northern Queensland also found that males were more likely to be involved in speed-related fatalities [21]. Speeding was also a risk factor among learner drivers within any age group in NSW. Distractions from outside of the vehicle posed a risk for those above 25 as well as 16-year olds. Driving at night was a risk for those aged between 20 and 25. The risk of fatalities were higher for females than males, though crash rates for males in general were higher except for those aged 25 and above [22]. Under the Graduated Licensing Scheme (GLS) introduced in 2000, learning to drive is spread over four years to promote safer drivers. One graduates from learner to P1, then P2 before earning an unrestricted licence [23].

Other solutions to curb speeding and reduce serious injury or fatalities include speed limits in school zones with and without flashing lights. In NSW, speed is limited to 40 km/hr with the expectation that a vehicle will travel at reduced speed prior to entering the school zone. However, more often than not, cars will slow down, whether there is a speed camera or not, only after entering the school zone. When a vehicle travelling at 50 km/hr collides with a pedestrian the probability of a fatality doubles compared with travelling at 40 km/hr. By reducing the speed limit in NSW school zones, pedestrian casualties decreased by 45% [24], [25]. Speed limits in combination with warning signs were found to be much more effective in road work zones than speed limits alone [26]. However, excessive speeds combined with driver inattention have resulted in roadwork zone crashes [27]. One of the most effective ways of controlling speed is police presence implying a high probability of being charged [28].

4 EFFECTIVENESS OF NSW SPEED CAMERA STRATEGY

Vehicles travelling above the speed limit or at inappropriate levels of speed during risky conditions increase the likelihood of fatalities or at the very least serious injury. The strategy for speed enforcement in NSW is based on an integrated framework that conforms to universal best practice in improving road safety. Fixed and red-light speed cameras that are signposted and clearly marked mobile speed cameras are listed such that the public are clearly warned of their locations. The aim of the speed camera enforcement program is to change behaviour patterns through promoting the perception of punishment if an infringement occurs and thus reducing fatalities and injuries [29].

The program is reviewed periodically to assess the safety benefit of cameras and requires a minimum of five years of post-installation data to assess the reduction in casualty crashes, casualties and infringement rates. A camera location is included in the review only if the required data is available. Recommendations are made for each camera location based on the findings [30]. A fatality is said to have occurred if a person dies within 30 days of a crash. A casualty crash refers to death occurring immediately as a result of the crash. To measure the reduction in fatalities at camera locations, which is a part of the overall review of the program, fatalities at each location over five years prior to the installation of a camera are compared to fatalities in each current five-year analysis period [31].

4.1 Fixed speed camera program

The fixed speed camera program commenced in NSW in 1997. Most of the fixed speed cameras have been installed for at least for five years now. The purpose was to address problem areas (black spots) with a history of crashes by locating cameras at road lengths such that they deter speeding [30]. At the end of 2016, there were 138 cameras at 109 locations however only 94 locations were reviewed for the purpose of recommendations [29].

Using the methodology described in Section 3, the annual reductions in fatalities, as a result of the installed fixed speed cameras were calculated and reported by the CRS in their annual reviews. For the year ended 2016, the reduction in fatalities due to fixed speed cameras was 85% [29]. Descriptive statistics based on reductions in fatalities over a seven-year period (2010–2016) are reported in Table 4.

A one-sample t-test (Table 4) was carried out to test the hypothesis at 95% confidence level which confirmed fixed speed cameras contributed to a reduction in fatalities by at least 75% in locations where they were installed.

Table 4: Descriptive statistics and one sample t-test: reduction in fatalities at fixed speed camera locations.

Descriptive statistics				
Fixed speed camera locations				95% Lower bound
N	Mean	Std. dev	SE mean	for μ
7	0.86	0.0872	0.033	0.796
μ: mean of reduction in fatalities				
t-test				
Null hypothesis	H_0: $\mu = 0.75$			
Alternative hypothesis	H_1: $\mu > 0.75$			
t-value	p-value			
3.34	0.008			

4.2 Red-light speed camera program

The red-light speed camera program was introduced in 2009. The cameras are installed at high risk intersections with signals where the driver is at risk of a right-angle crash or a pedestrian is at risk of being killed. The cameras are designed to deter both speeding and running a red-light. Intersections are high risk as fatalities can occur even at low speeds, given the unexpectedness of a car running a red light [31].

At the end of 2016, there were 191 cameras at 171 locations, however, only 91 locations were reviewed for the purpose of recommendations as data was not available. The five-year post-installation requirement was not met at 80 locations [29].

Using the same methodology as for fixed speed cameras, the annual reductions in fatalities resulting from the installed red-light speed cameras were calculated and reported by the CRS in their annual reviews. At least half of the red-light cameras meet the post installation requirement of a minimum of five years. For the year ended 2016, a reduction in fatalities due to red-light speed cameras was 54% [29].

Descriptive statistics based on reductions in fatalities over a 7-year period (2010–2016) are reported in Table 5. A one-sample t-test (Table 5) was carried out to test the hypothesis at 95% confidence level which confirmed that red-light speed cameras have contributed to a reduction in fatalities by at least 40% during that period in locations where they were installed.

Table 5: Descriptive statistics and one-sample t-test: reduction in fatalities at red-light camera locations.

<table>
<tr><td colspan="5">Descriptive statistics</td></tr>
<tr><td colspan="4">Red light speed camera program</td><td rowspan="2">95% Lower bound for μ</td></tr>
<tr><td>N</td><td>Mean</td><td>Std. dev</td><td>SE mean</td></tr>
<tr><td>7</td><td>0.86</td><td>0.0872</td><td>0.033</td><td>0.796</td></tr>
<tr><td colspan="5">μ: mean of reduction in fatalities</td></tr>
<tr><td colspan="3">t-test</td><td colspan="2" rowspan="5"></td></tr>
<tr><td>Null hypothesis</td><td colspan="2">H_0: $\mu = 0.75$</td></tr>
<tr><td>Alternative hypothesis</td><td colspan="2">H_1: $\mu > 0.75$</td></tr>
<tr><td>t-value</td><td colspan="2">p-value</td></tr>
<tr><td>3.34</td><td colspan="2">0.008</td></tr>
</table>

4.3 Mobile speed camera program

Mobile speed cameras were originally introduced in 1991 and ceased operations in 2008. In 2009, speed-related crashes increased by 36% and the death toll increased by 20% compared to the categories in 2008. Consequently, mobile speed cameras were reintroduced 2010. Thus they are considered highly effective in producing a sustained change in speeding behaviour as they may be located anywhere along the road network and drivers are unable to predict where or when they could be caught speeding [32]. As with the other two speed camera programs, warning signs display the speed limit as the driver approaches and the mobile speed camera vehicles are highly visible. In this program speed and crash data are collected across NSW and not at any specific mobile speed camera location [31]. Table 6 shows the total number of traffic fatalities and fatalities related only to speed [7]. The data suggests a decrease in fatalities for both categories from 2010 to 2016 in comparison with 2009. The statistical significance of the percentage decrease in total and speed-related fatalities is tested further.

Descriptive statistics are given for total road traffic fatalities in Table 7 and speed related fatalities in Table 8. One sample t-tests carried out at 95% confidence levels confirm that the decrease in total traffic fatalities is at least 15% in comparison with total fatalities in 2009, while the decrease in speed related fatalities is at least 20% in comparison with speed related fatalities in 2009.

Table 6: Road-traffic fatalities in NSW 2009–2016: total and speed-related.

Year	Number of road traffic fatalities	
	Total	Speed-related
2009	453	207
2010	357	161
2011	364	152
2012	364	146
2013	309	140
2014	307	127
2015	350	146
2016	380	159

Table 7: Descriptive statistics and one-sample t-test: A decrease in total traffic fatalities 2010–2016 in comparison with total traffic fatalities in 2009.

Descriptive statistics				
N	Mean	Std. dev	SE mean	95% Lower bound for μ
7	0.2336	0.0628	0.0237	0.1875
μ: Mean of % decrease (total) traffic fatalities				
t-test				
Null hypothesis	H_0: μ = 0.15			
Alternative hypothesis	H_1: μ > 0.15			
t-value	p-value			
3.52	0.006			

Table 8: Descriptive statistics and one-sample t-test: a decrease in speed-related fatalities 2010–2016 in comparison with speed-related fatalities in 2009.

Descriptive statistics				
Speed related fatalities				95% Lower bound
N	Mean	Std. dev	SE mean	for μ
7	0.288	0.0576	0.0218	0.2457
μ: mean of % decrease (Speed-related) fatalities				
t-test				
Null hypothesis	H_0: μ = 0.2			
Alternative hypothesis	H_1: μ > 0.2			
t-value	p-value			
4.04	0.003			

5 CONCLUSION, RECOMMENDATIONS AND LIMITATIONS

Australia's record in best practice traffic law enforcement over the years has resulted in a lower road traffic fatality rate in comparison with neighbouring countries (Fig. 1). The performance of NSW, the most populous state with 29% of the national fleet (the highest proportion in comparison with other states), in lowering its traffic fatalities per 100,000 of population has been consistently better than the national average between 2010 and 2017

(Table 1). This is clearly due to law enforcement of best practice that has been gradually introduced since the 1970s. In 1970 the road fatality rate in NSW was 28.9 per 100,000 of population and it fell to 4.1 per 100,000 of population. Since then the fatality rate has steadily risen to 4.9 per 100,000 of population in 2017. Speeding has been identified as the main reason for the increase in road fatalities. The speed camera programs are still effective and of the three programs, mobile speed cameras are the most effective. This was proven when the fatality rates rose in 2009 after the cessation of the program in 2008, and a decrease was experienced after its reintroduction.

The CRS has reported that data on fatalities related to driving under the influence of illicit substances is available only for fatal crashes and for the financial years ending 2010–2011 to 2015–2016. Data for non-fatal crashes are not available. Thus a limitation of this paper is that driving under the influence of drugs may not have been excluded from the speed related data though speeding was a factor in the fatal crash. A probable explanation for the increase in fatalities since 2014 is the increased use of illicit drugs while driving. The information available shows that the percentage of total fatalities involving a motor vehicle controller with an illicit drug was 15.7% in the 2013–2014 financial year and rose sharply to 20.6% by the 2015–2016 financial year [33].

However, based on the NSW experience up to 2014 it is still possible to make recommendations on how to manage this man-made disaster. There are many lessons to be learned from the NSW experience by developing countries where road traffic fatalities are high. Strategies that benefitted NSW include the following. The introduction of the compulsory use of seatbelts in 1971 though children under 8 were excluded until legislation was introduced in 1974. This was followed by the introduction of RBT in 1982. National child legislation on improvement to child seats and harnesses was adopted in 1988. In 1990, the Road Safety (RS) 2000 strategy was adopted. During this period fixed speed cameras and mobile speed cameras were introduced [10]. Also in 1995, the then premier of NSW committed his government to reducing deaths by 500 and serious injuries by 5,500 as part of the RS 2000 strategy [34]. The "National Walk Safely to School Day" was introduced and is now in its 20th year [35]. Consequent to all these traffic law enforcements and the steady decline in road fatalities, in 2000 the trend began to reverse [36] and in the same year the 2000 Graduated Licensing Scheme was introduced.

In 2012 the Road Safety Strategy 2012 to 2021 was adopted. This strategy emphasises a safe system approach following Scandinavian best practice. The underlying elements are safer people, safer roads, safer speeds and safer vehicles [37]. A topic for future research is the innovative road safety initiatives that are now being pursued in earnest by the CRS with full support from all levels of Government to reverse the increasing trend in fatalities that has occurred since 2014.

REFERENCES

[1] WHO & UN Road Safety Collaboration, Decade of Action for Road Safety 2011–2020. www.who.int/roadsafety/decade_of_action/en/. Accessed on: 30 Aug. 2019.

[2] WHO, Global Status Report on Road Safety. 2018. www.who.int/violence_injury_prevention/road_safety_status/2018/en/. Accessed on: 24 Jul. 2019.

[3] Australian Transport Council, National Road Safety Strategy 2011–2020. www.roadsafety.gov.au/nrss/files/NRSS_2011_2020.pdf. Accessed on: 30 Aug. 2019.

[4] Department of Infrastructure, Transport, Cities and Regional Development, BITRE. www.bitre.gov.au/statistics/safety/. Accessed on: 30 Aug. 2019.

[5] Australian Bureau of Statistics, Survey of motor vehicle use, Australia. www.abs.gov.au/ausstats/abs@.nsf/mf/9208.0. Accessed on: 30 Aug. 2019.

[6] NSW Government, Road Safety Plan 2021. Towards Zero. https://towardszero.nsw.gov.au/sites/default/files/2018-02/road-safety-plan.pdf. Accessed on: 30 Aug. 2019.

[7] Centre for Road Safety, Road traffic casualty crashes in New South Wales. Statistical Statements for Years ended 2010 to 2017. https://roadsafety.transport.nsw.gov.au/downloads/crashstats2017.pdf. Accessed on: 24 Jul. 2019.

[8] Population Australia, NSW population, 2019. www.population.net.au/population-of-new-south-wales/. Accessed on: 20 Aug. 2019.

[9] Motor Vehicle registration slowdown. www.abs.gov.au/ausstats/abs@.nsf/lookup/9309.0Media%20Release131%20Jan%202019.

[10] Transport NSW, Centre for Road Safety. https://roadsafety.transport.nsw.gov.au/statistics/fatalitytrends.html. Accessed on: 20 Aug. 2019.

[11] WHO, Road traffic injuries. www.who.int/news-room/fact-sheets/detail/road-traffic-injuries. Accessed on: 20 Aug. 2019.

[12] McDermott, F.T. & Hough, D.E., Reduction in road fatalities and injuries after legislation for compulsory wearing of seat belts: experience in Victoria and the rest of Australia. *British Journal of Surgery*, **66**(7), pp. 518–521, 1979.

[13] Department of Infrastructure, Transport, Cities and Regional Development, Vehicle occupant protection in Australia. www.infrastructure.gov.au/roads/safety/publications/1988/pdf/Prot_Aust_1.pdf. Accessed on: 31 Aug. 2019.

[14] Child Restraint Laws in NSW, www.repcoservice.com/car-care-advice/child-car-seat-laws/child-restraint-laws-nsw. Accessed on: 31 Aug. 2019.

[15] Brown, J., Keay, L., Hunter, K., Bilston, L.E., Simpson, J.M. & Ivers, R., Increase in best practice child car restraint use for children aged 2–5 years in low socioeconomic areas after introduction of mandatory child restraint laws. *Australian and New Zealand Journal of Public Health*, **37**(3), pp. 272–277, 2013.

[16] TRID, The National Academies of Sciences Engineering Medicine. The impact of random breath testing in New South Wales. https://trid.trb.org/view/1194447. Accessed on: 31 Aug. 2019.

[17] Ellison, A.B. & Greaves, S., Driver characteristics and speeding behaviour. *Proceedings of the 33rd Australasian Transport Research Forum (ATRF'10)*, 2010.

[18] Ogle, J.H., *Quantitative Assessment of Driver Speeding Behaviour using Instrumented Vehicles*. Doctoral dissertation, Georgia Institute of Technology.

[19] Chen, H.Y. et al., Road crash trends for young drivers in New South Wales, Australia, from 1997 to 2007. *Traffic Injury Prevention*, **11**(1), pp. 8–15, 2010.

[20] Wundersitz, L., Hiranandani, K. & Baldock, M., *Annual Performance Indicators of Enforced Driver Behaviours in South Australia, 2007,* Centre for Automotive Safety Research, 2009.

[21] Knight, P.J., Iverson, D. & Harris, M.F., Early driving experience and influence on risk perception in young rural people. *Accident Analysis & Prevention*, **1**(45), pp. 775–781, 2012.

[22] Lam, L.T., Factors associated with young drivers' car crash injury: comparisons among learner, provisional, and full licensees. *Accident Analysis & Prevention*, **35**(6), pp. 913–920, 2003.

[23] Centre for Road Safety, Australian graduated licensing scheme. Policy framework. https://roadsafety.transport.nsw.gov.au/downloads/gls.pdf. Accessed on: 2 Sep. 2019.

[24] Ellison, A.B., Greaves, S.P. & Daniels, R., Speeding behaviour in school zones. *Proceedings of the Australasian College of Road Safety National Conference*, 2011.

[25] Peden, M. et al., *World Report on Road Traffic Injury Prevention*, World Health Organization, 2004.
[26] Haworth, N., Symmons, M. & Mulvihill, C., *Safety of Small Workgroups on Roadways*, 2002.
[27] Garber, N.J. & Patel, S.T., Control of vehicle speeds in temporary traffic control zones (work zones) using changeable message signs with radar. *Transportation Research Record*, 1995.
[28] Arnold, E.D., *Use of Police in Work Zones on Highways in Virginia*, Virginia Transportation Research Council, 2003.
[29] Centre for Road Safety, Speed camera programs: Annual Review 2017. https://roadsafety.transport.nsw.gov.au/downloads/2017-speed-camera-review-appendices.pdf. Accessed on: 1 Sep. 2019.
[30] Carseldine, D., RTA: Fixed, digital speed cameras in NSW – Impacts on vehicle speeds and crashes. https://acrs.org.au/files/arsrpe/RS030027.pdf. Accessed on: 1 Sep. 2019.
[31] Centre for Road Safety, Speed camera programs: Annual Review 2015. https://roadsafety.transport.nsw.gov.au/downloads/2015-speed-camera-review.pdf. Accessed on: 1 Sep. 2019.
[32] NSW Government, Transport for NSW, NSW speed camera strategy 2012. www.rms.nsw.gov.au/roadsafety/downloads/nsw_speed_camera_strategy.pdf. Accessed on: 3 Sep. 2019.
[33] Centre for Road Safety, Drug driving trauma trends: Report. https://roadsafety.transport.nsw.gov.au/downloads/trauma-trends-drug-driving.pdf. Accessed on: 2 Sep. 2019.
[34] Pedestrian Council of Australia, Excerpt from the Foreword to STAYSAFE 47, 1998. www.walk.com.au/pedestriancouncil/Page.asp?PageID=573. Accessed on: 2 Sep. 2019.
[35] WSTSD, www.walk.com.au/WSTSD/. Accessed on: 2 Sep. 2019.
[36] Road Transport Authority, Road traffic accidents NSW, 2000. Statistical statement. https://roadsafety.transport.nsw.gov.au/downloads/accidentstats2000.pdf. Accessed on: 2 Sep. 2019.
[37] Centre for Road Safety, Towards zero a safe system approach. https://roadsafety.transport.nsw.gov.au/aboutthecentre/safe-system/index.html. Accessed on: 3 Sep. 2019.

BUILDING BACK BETTER WITH VULNERABILITY: POST-HAIYAN REFLECTIONS ON RISK PERCEPTION

MICHIKO BANBA[1], MARIA MAKABENTA IKEDA[2], MAYUMI SAKAMOTO[1] & YOSHIKI TOMINAGA[1]
[1]University of Hyogo, Japan
[2]Kyoto Sangyo University, Japan

ABSTRACT

Several studies show that the lack of information about the scale of disaster risks contributed to the increased vulnerability of many people affected by Typhoon Haiyan in 2013. A conceptual framework based on the behavioural intention model is used to examine how demographic attributes, experience of disaster occurrence, knowledge about natural hazards and community-based disaster risk reduction efforts affect disaster risk perception. We analyse how effective disaster knowledge and community efforts are in raising risk awareness and influencing risk reduction behaviour. A questionnaire survey is conducted among households living in the cities of Tacloban, Palo and Tanauan, located along the north-eastern coast of Leyte, Philippines. Using structural equation modelling (SEM), we empirically test hypotheses on risk perception and behavioural intention to reduce disaster risk using data from 282 households. We attempt to investigate how risk perception and risk reduction behaviour are affected by two elements that we think can be potentially harnessed for sustainability of the build-back-better process: (a) knowledge about disasters and (b) community efforts. Our results show model compatibility for the variables (1) disaster experience, (2) risk perception and (3) knowledge about natural hazards. On the other hand, we find weak model compatibility for the variables (1) disaster education and (2) community efforts.

Keywords: disaster risk reduction, knowledge, risk perception, behavioural intention model, adaptive behaviour, intention, disaster education, community, vulnerability, resilience.

1 INTRODUCTION

Typhoon Haiyan in 2013 exacted a severe toll both in economic damages and human lives throughout Leyte Island in the Philippines (Table 1).

The possibility of recurrence of strong typhoons like Typhoon Haiyan is more likely than estimates of once in 100 years due to climate change. Thus, people should not underestimate extreme weather and potential disaster impacts. In order to reduce disaster risks, building capacities of people and resilient communities through modules of self-help, mutual assistance and public-private partnership initiatives is essential.

Even after a major disaster like Haiyan, it is not easy to raise the disaster risk awareness of people and conduct community efforts for disaster risk reduction during normal or calm conditions. Although preparation for disaster should be made before another serious disaster occurs, people need constant reminders to engage in protective behaviour. Essential to an ideal disaster preparedness program as well as the build-back-better reconstruction of post-Haiyan Leyte is the regular dissemination of disaster awareness information and conduct of community disaster drills. This study focuses on the importance of understanding the factors affecting risk perception or psychological mechanisms that influence the performance or non-performance of broad-based disaster preparedness and risk reduction efforts by people living in post-Haiyan Leyte.

Quite a few studies have analysed the differences of psychological mechanisms affecting risk perception and disaster risk reduction. In particular, we studied concepts related to the Theory of Planned Behaviour and Theory of Reasoned Action [2], [3]. According to these

www.witpress.com, ISSN 1743-3509 (on-line)
doi:10.2495/DMAN190041

Table 1: Top 10 natural disasters and number of deaths, Philippines 1970–2018. *(Source: EM-DAT [1].)*

Popular name/Type of Hazard	Date of event	Total number of deaths
Typhoon Yolanda (Haiyan)	8-Nov-2013	7,354
1976 Mindanao earthquake	17-Aug-1976	6,000
Typhoon Uring (Thelma)	5-Nov-1991	5,956
1990 Luzon earthquake	16-Jul-1990	2,412
Typhoon Pablo (Bopha)	4-Dec-2012	1,901
Tropical Depression Winnie	29-Nov-2004	1,619
Typhoon Titang (Kate)	13-Oct-1970	1,551
Typhoon Sendong (Washi)	15-Dec-2011	1,439
Typhoon Nitang (Ike)	1-Sep-1984	1,422
Typhoon Reming (Durian)	30-Nov-2006	1,399

models individuals make logical, reasoned decisions to engage in specific behaviours by evaluating the information available to them. In addition, the performance of a *behaviour is determined by the individual's intention*, which in turn is affected by one's attitude or value placed on the behaviour and subjective norms or views of other people in a family or community) and the perceived ease with which one can act on one's intentions or perception that the behaviour is within one's control. In a study which analysed the mechanism of risk perception and behaviour towards disaster risk of residents in Metro Manila, it was found that intention was predicted by attitude, subjective norms and risk perception, and risk aversive behaviour was predicted by intention [4]. Fishbein's theory of planned behaviour was followed by many studies also in the field of disaster research.

There are some studies based on Leyte related to risk perception and disaster risk reduction after Typhoon Haiyan. Lejano et al. [5] discussed about the risk perception through investigation of the role of risk communication. Tuhkanen et al. [6] discussed the risk perception of people after Haiyan in terms of trade-offs in development and disaster risk reduction. However, there are very few studies which have attempted to analyse the mechanisms involving risk perception, intention and structurally targeted risk reduction behaviour in post-Haiyan Leyte. Thus, this study aims to formulate a conceptual framework and then empirically investigate the interrelated nature of these mechanisms to understand the factors that affect risk perception of people after a major disaster like Typhoon Haiyan.

The importance of enhancing the resilience of communities vulnerable to natural hazards cannot be emphasized more in countries like the Philippines with limited resources for construction of state-of-the-art infrastructure or technology for disaster prevention. A possible approach towards community resilience is to foster each resident's adaptive behaviour towards natural hazards. In so doing, the capacity of each member of the community to engage in self-help and mutual help initiatives can potentially be increased. Adaptive behaviour is expressed as preparation for potential disasters by reducing identifiable risks. Individual or community-initiated risk reduction behaviour is assumed to be related to how people perceive disaster risks. Risk perception and engagement in risk reduction behaviour are affected by factors including *disaster experiences, information, disaster knowledge and community coping as well as the capability to implement build-back better strategies*. In this study, we clarify important factors affecting how people perceive disaster risks and conduct risk reduction behaviour. By doing so, we can ascertain whether current grassroots initiatives related to disaster education and community activities are effective in raising risk awareness and influencing risk-reduction behaviour of people to support the build-back-better process of their communities.

In this study, a behavioural intention model is developed to analyse factors of risk perception and disaster risk-reducing behaviour in high-risk areas (that is, natural hazards frequency of at least once in every 10-year cycle). A questionnaire survey was conducted in communities in Leyte to collect data to be used for the empirical analysis.

2 CONCEPTUAL FRAMEWORK: BEHAVIOURAL INTENTION MODEL FOR DISASTER REDUCTION

In this study, a behavioural intention model is conceptualized to analyse important factors affecting how people perceive disaster risks and intend to conduct adaptive behaviour to reduce disaster risks. Adaptive behaviour is defined as disaster risk reduction behaviour, such as preparing goods for emergency, planning for evacuation or building strong structure houses. We focus on two critical elements of (a) knowledge about disaster and (b) community efforts for disaster risk reduction in analysing how risk perception is related to risk reduction behaviour. Observed variables for disaster experiences and Demographic characteristics are included in the empirical analysis of factors that influence risk perception and preparedness through engaging in risk reduction behaviour.

2.1 Factors affecting disaster preparedness and risk perception

In developing the empirical model, we needed to identify the factors to be analysed. In the discussion with the local partner who helped conduct this survey, it was decided not to use the concept of subjective norms or normative beliefs in the questionnaire due to the potential implementation drawbacks and communication gaps between the enumerators and respondents. Thus, the model and factors were simplified to avoid misinterpretation of survey questions. Six factors are identified, which are "experiences of disaster", "Demographic characteristics", "risk perception", "knowledge", "intention for disaster preparedness" and "community efforts". In this study, risk perception is considered an important factor to link other factors in the model. Those factors are expressed as follows.

1) Disaster experience: Whether the respondent has previously experienced the occurrence of a natural disaster;
2) Demographic attributes: Age, sex, education, income;
3) Risk perception: The way one perceives risk of a natural disaster;
4) Intention: Behavioural intention of an individual's readiness to perform disaster risk reduction activities or behaviour;
5) Knowledge: Knowledge about natural hazards, disaster, or countermeasures related to natural hazard;
6) Community: Community efforts for disaster risk reduction.

2.2 Hypothesis building and model formulation

Previous disaster experiences are considered the most effective factor to affect risk perception of people according to recent studies by Bustillos Ardaya et al. [7], Lechowska [8]. It is postulated that risk perception is different depending on the degree or extent of damages or costs people incur. Risk perception is defined as how serious people understand and perceive

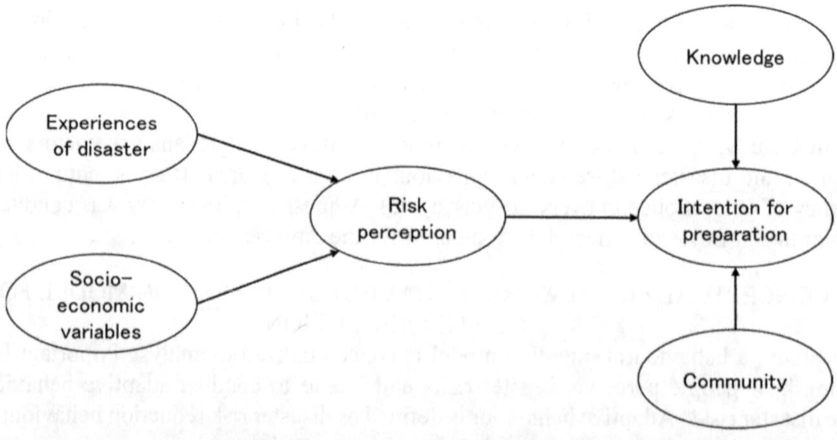

Figure 1: Behavioural intention model.

disaster risks in both positive and negative ways. Thus, it is expected to affect intention to conduct disaster risk reduction behaviour. Our study considers factors related to community initiatives based on behavioural intention model analysis of Paton [9]. Paton and Tedim [10] indicated community engagement affects intention to prepare for disaster risk reduction, which affects behaviour. In our study, the intention to conduct disaster risk reduction is also postulated to be affected by the level of knowledge about natural hazards of individuals and commitment to engage in efforts for disaster risk reduction as a community.

Hypotheses are formulated based on the assumption of reciprocal relations of factors as follows and the conceptual model of behavioural intention model is shown in Fig. 1.

1) Previous experience of disaster affects risk perception;
2) Demographic attributes of respondents affect risk perception;
3) Risk perception affects intention to engage in disaster risk reduction behaviour;
4) Community efforts to conduct disaster management affects individual disaster risk reduction behaviour;
5) Knowledge level of natural hazards affects disaster risk reduction behaviour.

3 QUESTIONNAIRE SURVEY

Questionnaire survey was conducted to collect data to analyse risk perception, intention for disaster risk reduction and related factors. Locations of barangays or communities were chosen from affected communities according to the degree of community-based commitment towards disaster risk reduction according to authors' evaluation and/or observation of community activities as well as upon consultation with barangay or local community leaders. Barangay is the "primary planning and implementing unit of government policies, plans, programs, projects, and activities in the community" located in contiguous territory of at least 2,000 inhabitants who elect the following officials (one barangay captain or "punong barangay", seven (7) sangguniang barangay members (barangay advisory council members), and one sangguniang kabataan (youth advisory council) chairman. There are also two appointive officials (secretary and treasurer). The sangguniang barangay council is tasked with forming the peace and order brigade or "lupong tagapamayapa" as well as other community brigades "deemed necessary to carry out the purposes of the Barangay government in accordance with the needs of public service" [11].

3.1 Sampling areas

Three heavily damaged communities in the cities of Tacloban, Palo and Tanauan located in the eastern coast of Leyte, Philippines are chosen as sampling areas. (See Fig. 2). More specifically, respondents in Tacloban are located in the district of Anibong (or Barangay 69); while those in Palo are residents of Barangay San Joaquin, and finally, respondents from Barangay Bislig in Tanauan comprise the sample of this survey.

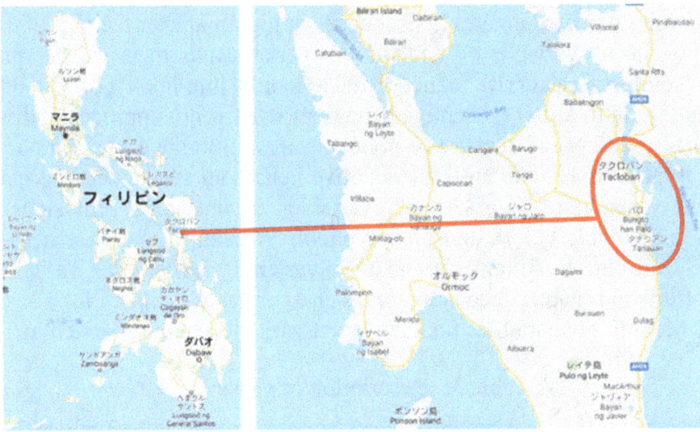

Figure 2: Geographic location of sampling areas. *(Source: Google).*

The sampling areas are categorized based on the level of disaster risk reduction commitment: (1) Anibong (Barangay 69), relatively high; (2) Barangay San Joaquin, moderate; and Barangay Bislig, relatively low. Sampling areas level of community-based commitment towards disaster risk reduction are summarized in Table 2.

Table 2: Characteristics of sampling areas.

Level of DRR community commitment/ description	Relatively high	Moderate	Relatively low
Community	Brgy. 69 Anibong	Brgy. San Joaquin	Brgy. Bislig
Municipality	Tacloban	Palo	Tanauan
Main natural hazards	Storm surge	Storm surge	Flooding
Drill pre-Haiyan	Drills for various hazards	No drills	No drills
Drill post-Haiyan	Quarterly drills for various hazards	Once a year	Being planned
DRR Program developments	Community hazard map, Community prioritization gas provision for emergency	Construction of evacuation center	Expansion of Barangay hall (Budget on request)

3.2 Survey method

Questionnaires were prepared to collect data pertaining to the hypotheses formulated in Section 2.2. For the latent variable of "*demographic attributes*", "sex", "age", and "education" were chosen as measurable variables. For the latent variable of "disaster experiences", we asked respondents whether they or their families incurred damages to properties and/or injuries. For latent variable of "*risk perception*", we asked how likely they think a strong typhoon like Haiyan will happen again in the future and psychological factors such as recurring memories or visual images in flashbacks or nightmares or feelings of trauma related to Haiyan. For latent variable of "*intention*", variables to measure the intention of a respondent to conduct disaster risk reduction behaviour by him/herself or with other members of the community. In this study, adaptive behaviour itself is not approached directly, but the intention is measured instead because respondents are still in the early years of the recovery process, and it takes more time until the adaptive behaviour is planned and put into action. For the latent variable of "*knowledge*", variables to measures provisions for disaster education by individuals before and after typhoon Yolanda", and awareness of the word "storm surge" were chosen. Finally, for the latent variable "*community*", variables measuring community efforts to practice evacuation drills and construct facilities for disaster reduction were chosen. Measurable variables for each latent variable are summarized in Table 3.

Table 3: Description of variables.

Latent variables	Measurable variables	Description
Disaster experience	Injury	Whether respondent was injured by typhoon Haiyan
	Loss of family members	Whether respondent lost families by typhoon Haiyan
Demographic attributes	Sex	Sex of respondent
	Age	Age of respondent
	Education	Highest education a respondent has
Risk perception	Perceived likelihood of recurrence	The extent a respondent thinks a strong typhoon will happen again
	Flashback	A respondent remembers images (in flashbacks and/or nightmares) of the typhoon
	Stress/trauma	Whether a respondent feel trauma when he/she thinks about the typhoon
Intention	Int_you	The extent of a respondent's intention to conduct disaster risk reduction behaviour by him/herself
	Int_com	The extent of a respondent's intention to conduct disaster risk reduction behaviour through mutual help in the community
Knowledge	Dis_ed_bef	Disaster education before typhoon Haiyan
	Dis_ed_aft	Disaster education after typhoon Haiyan
	Storm surge	Knew the word "storm surge" before Haiyan
Community	Community	Community evacuation drill
	Community	Construction of disaster management facilities in the community

Survey implementation activities were conducted during the period of October 1 to 12 in 2018. The tasks of the survey enumerators were to (1) visit households in each barangay; (2) interview the household head or his/her representative; and, (3) write down the responses and other notes. One person per household were sampled from barangays located near the coast. Households were randomly chosen by the enumerators with the help of barangay or community leaders who knew which households belonged to which barangay. Approximately 100 sample observations were collected from each barangay. After cleaning the data, the valid observations totalled 282 with the following breakdown: 92 in Anibong, Tacloban; 99 in San Joaquin, Palo; and, 91 in Bislig, Tanauan.

4 ANALYSIS AND FINDINGS

Based on the conceptual framework described in Section 3, a structural equation model (SEM) is applied to empirically test the behavioural intention model. After several iterations, we obtained results shown in Fig. 3. The Chi-square statistic is 41.758 and CMIN/DF is 2.198. The overall model fit is a GFI value of 0.965, AGFG value of 0.933, and RMSEA value of 0.65. These represent goodness of fit in the specified structural equation model.

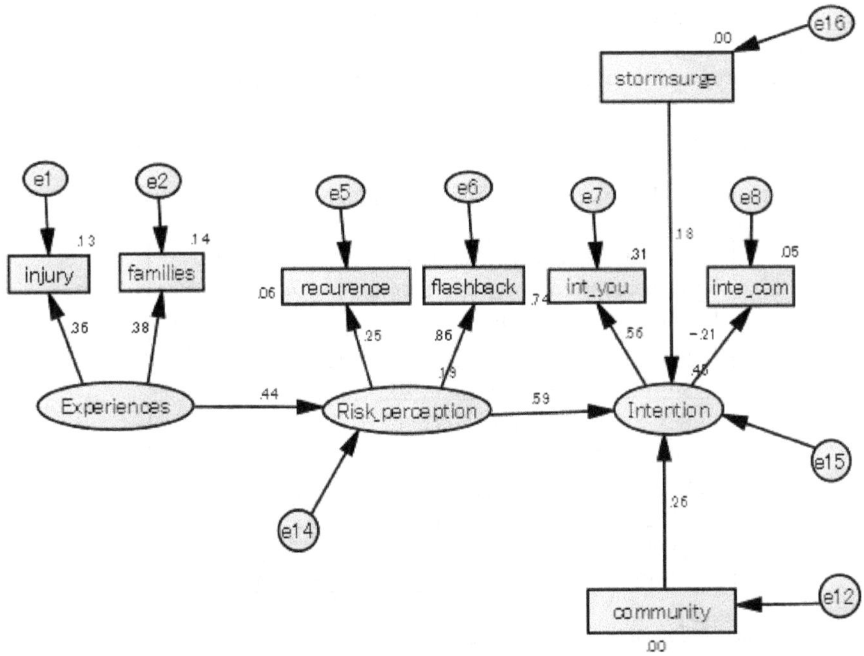

Figure 3: Structural equation modelling (SEM) analytical results.

4.1 Influences of intention to conduct disaster risk reduction behaviour

The results show that the variable for "experiences" affects "risk perception" significantly which in turn affects the individual's "intention to conduct disaster risk behaviour" significantly. The measured variables of "injury" and "loss of families" (for the latent variable of "disaster experiences") influence "risk perception" with relative significance. Measurable variables of the latent variable "demographic attributes", such as "age", "sex" and "education" did not affect "risk perception" in this model, and the goodness of fit of the model was not satisfactory, thus, latent variable "demographic attributes" were eliminated from the final model.

Simulation of the measurable variables of "risk perception" ("recurrence" and "flashback") yielded highly significant coefficients which imply compatibility of the model and significant influence on "intention". Especially, "flashback" accounts for "risk perception", and it indicates that people who responded that they do not want to be reminded about Haiyan but still have flashbacks or nightmares about it are more likely to have the intention to conduct disaster risk reduction behaviour. It means that people who take risks more seriously and feel some anxiety tend to have the intention to conduct disaster risk reduction behaviour. Although the level of significance of the coefficient of "recurrence" accounting for "risk perception" is low, it means that people who think strong typhoon like Haiyan will occur again in the near future tend to have intention to conduct disaster risk reduction behaviour strongly. The flipside of the coin implies that people who perceive low risks of a strong typhoon like Haiyan occurring again soon, tend to have no intention to conduct disaster risk reduction behaviour.

"Intention" explained by measurable variables "int_you" and "int_com" yields compatibility of the model and statistically significant coefficients. Coefficients accounting for "intention" of "Int_you" are relatively large and that of "int_com" is negative. It indicates that people who are capable of self-help or initiating disaster management activities tend to have intention for risk reduction behaviour while people who expect help from the community are less likely to have the intention to engage in disaster risk reduction behaviour.

Table 4: Significance of path coefficients.

Measurable and latent variables	*P*-values
Risk_perception <--- Experiences	0.438 ($p<.05$)
Intention <--- community	0.263 ($p<.01$)
Intention <--- risk_perception	0.594 ($p<.01$)
Intention <--- stormsurge	0.183 ($p<.1$)
Injury <--- experiences	0.356 ($p<.05$)
Families <--- experiences	0.377 ($p<.1$)
Recurrence <--- risk_perception	0.252 ($p<.05$)
Flashbacks <--- risk_perception	0.859 ($p<.01$)
Int_you <--- intention	0.558 ($p<.05$)
Int_com <--- intention	-0.213 ($p<.05$)

4.2 Effects of knowledge and community efforts

Based on the empirical results, "knowledge" and "community disaster risk reduction" have relatively small marginal effects on the individual's "intention to conduct disaster risk behaviour". Analysis of the model using the latent variable "knowledge" with measurable manifestations such as disaster-related "education before Haiyan" and "education after Haiyan" did not yield statistically significant coefficients. However, the results for the observed variable of "(pre-Haiyan) knowledge about storm surge" were highly significant which imply compatibility with the behavioural intention model. The above explains that "disaster experiences" as well as "knowing about storm surges (or other natural hazards)" strongly affect "risk perception".

5 CONCLUSION

We formulated a behavioural intention model built on the hypothesis that having previous disaster experience affects risk perception which in turn affects the intention to engage in disaster risk behaviour. We empirically test this behavioural intention model using data collected from Tacloban, Palo and Tanuan in Leyte, Philippines. We find that previous disaster experiences positively increase awareness or enhance risk perception that lead to adaptive behaviour for disaster risk reduction suitable for building-back better process. Moreover, although influences of knowledge and community efforts for disaster reduction were not observed significant at this time, it is necessary to continue efforts to provide disaster knowledge and involve people in community-based disaster risk reduction activities as it takes time to see effects of those efforts in the long-term process of building-back better and resilient communities.

ACKNOWLEDGEMENTS

We are grateful to the staff and residents of the barangays for their cooperation in the questionnaire survey. The results of this study will be shared with the barangays as a resource for building resilient communities in Leyte. We also express our appreciation to Japan's Ministry of Education and Hyogo Prefecture for providing research funds for this study.

REFERENCES

[1] EM-DAT: The Emergency Events Database. Universite Catholique de Louvain (UCL), CRED, D. Guha-Sapir. www.emdat.be, Brussels.

[2] Fishbein, M. & Ajzen, I., *Belief, Attitude, Intention and Behavior: An Introduction to Theory and Research.* Addison-Wesley: Reading, MA, 1975.

[3] Ajzen, I. & Fishbein, M., *Understanding Attitudes and Predicting Social Behavior.* Prentice-Hall, Inc: Englewood Cliffs, 1980

[4] Tatsuki, S. et. al., The impact of risk perception, disaster scheme, resources, intention, attitude, and norms upon risk aversive behavior among Marikina City residents: Structural equation modelling with latent variables. *Proceedings of Asia Conference on Earthquake Engineering*, vol. 1, pp. 267–272, 2004.

[5] Lejano, R. et. al., Communicating risk: Learning from Typhoon Haiyan. *Nature*, **518**(7537), p. 35, 2015.

[6] Tuhkanen, H. et al., A typology framework for trade-offs in development and disaster risk reduction: A case study of typhoon Haiyan recovery in Tacloban, Philippines. *Sustainability*, **10**(6), 2018.

[7] Bustillos Ardaya, A., Eversa, M. & Ribbe, L., What influences disaster risk perception? Intervention measures, flood and landslide risk perception of the population living in flood risk areas in Rio de Janeiro state, Brazil. *International Journal of Disaster Risk Reduction*, pp. 227–237, 2017.

[8] Lechowska, E., What determines flood risk perception? A review of factors of flood risk perception and relations between its basic elements. *Natural Hazards*, **94**(3), pp. 1341–1366, 2018.

[9] Paton, D., Disaster preparedness: A social cognitive perspective. *Disaster Prevention and Management*, **12**(3), 2003.

[10] Paton D. & Tedim, F., Enhancing forest fires preparedness in Portugal: Integrating community engagement and risk management. *Planet at Risk*, **1**(1), 2013.

[11] Philippine Local Government Code of 1991, Official Gazette. www.officialgazette.gov.ph/downloads/1991/10oct/19911010-RA-7160-CCA.pdf. Accessed on: 8 Jul. 2019.

THE FIRE OF NOTRE DAME: ECONOMIC LESSONS LEARNED

WADAD KATHY TANNOUS
School of Business, Western Sydney University, Australia

ABSTRACT

On the 14th April 2019, a major fire damaged Notre-Dame Cathedral in France. The damage was estimated to the value of billions of dollars in terms of lost art and built material. This study aims to assess the impact of this event and its predictability and potential preventability. The study uses primary data from surveys of response agencies, response personnel, structural engineers, fire engineers, insurance assessors, and heritage specialists. The study examines the economic cost of the fire in the immediacy of the incident, the short term and the long term. In addition, the environmental impact of the fire incident is examined. This includes the internal environment of the church, the chemicals that may be used in the restoration, the chemicals that may be released into the general environment and what they mean for response agency personnel and the impact on their health. The economic impact of the fire of Notre Dame is significant and will be long lasting on the residents in the immediate surroundings and wider vicinity of the church; the response workers; and on the country. Our findings provide lessons for assessing the costs to implementing preventive measures and improving fire preparation for older style buildings. In particular, measuring the economic costs of iconic buildings, such as Notre-Dame Cathedral, whose damage or destruction are horrific for the short and long term.
Keywords: disaster, fire safety, environmental impact, economic costs.

1 INTRODUCTION

On 15th April 2019 at 6:18 pm a fire began in the roof of the French gothic Notre-Dame Cathedral in Paris France [1] with the first alert was sound at 6:20 pm local time [2]. The landmark's famous spire and vaulted interior roof (known as "the forest") provided ample fuel for the flames as they were built with wood, primarily 13th century oak trees [3]. Over five hundred firefighters responded and it took nine hours to control the fire and fifteen hours until the fire was extinguished [3], [4].

Notre-Dame cathedral is a Parisian icon that had inspired artists, poets, novelists and Francophiles over many generations [5]. It is more than just a place of worship but also an architectural marvel for others [6]. It has further reach as being the mascot of a Disney movie, and a backdrop for many other recent and past movies, and as Victor Hugo novel *The Hunchback of Notre Dame*, 1931 [7], [8]. The fire incident has been described as a devastation for the building but also for the city. Notre-Dame Cathedral is the single most visited cultural site in Paris with 12 million visitors in 2017 double the number that visit the Eiffel Tower, with 6.2 million visitors in the same year [9]. The building is over 850 years old and its famous spire of the cathedral was undergoing €6 million restoration project [10]. Notre Dame had an extensive fire warning system that took six years to put together and involved thousands of pages of diagrams, maps, spreadsheets and contracts [11]. The system was based on prevention and detection with two guards on site monitoring the roof structure, day and night and having it checked regularly [12]. The fire alarms in Notre-Dame did not notify the fire department but alerted the guard of the fire. A number of subsequent events resulted in significant delay in the alerting the response agencies including the guard checking on the wrong church and the need for the personal check of the attic to confirm that the fire was there that involved the climb of steep set of stairs [11], [12]. The fire in Notre

WIT Transactions on The Built Environment, Vol 190, © 2019 WIT Press
www.witpress.com, ISSN 1743-3509 (on-line)
doi:10.2495/DMAN190051

Dame has been described as a symptom neglect of the building [13]. Paris public prosecutor's office said that their preliminary findings suggested the fire had been started accidentally.

The fire safety experts underestimated the risk from fire but also the costs if and when the incident did occur [12]. In addition, they were most conservative in their approach to preserving the historic wooden structure in unadulterated form that they did not install protective measures of sprinklers or fire walls. Even back to base alarms were not installed due to concerns of false alarms.

The costs of the fire are still being determined and for some of the destroyed contents, they are priceless. However, the economic costs of this incident extend beyond the building and extend to the impact of this event on tourism to Paris and France itself. In addition, unplanned costs and effects have also started to surface from this incident of lead contamination. Notre-Dame's spire and roof housed upwards of 400 tonnes of lead which melted in the fire, releasing toxic dust and particles across Île de la Cité and the surrounding neighbourhoods [14], [15].

Section 2 will discuss the damage that Notre-Dame cathedral sustained from the fire incident and touch on the resources used to contain the incident. Section 3 will describe the environmental costs and potential ongoing health costs from the lead contamination. Section 4 will detail the restoration process and challenges. Section 5 will provide a simulation model of the potential lost income, most conservatively, over the planned five-year restoration period. The final section will describe the lessons learned from this event.

2 DAMAGE TO NOTRE-DAME CATHEDRAL

2.1 Damage done

While the Notre-Dame cathedral received extensive damage in the fire, it is difficult to make a true estimate of the exact cost of the damage. As Walt [16] explained, "two-thirds of the roof collapsed in the fire, in the process also destroying some of the centuries-old statues of saints that were perched on the spire… part of the nave and the choir are also gone" [16]. The ceiling vaults were made of 5,000-year-old oak trees had seen some of the most severe damage, adding that much of the damage to the cathedral and its content was "difficult to calculate" as they are considered "priceless" [16]. One clear loss was the famous spire of the cathedral. When the fire broke out, Notre-Dame's spire was undergoing a €6 million restoration project [10]. As a result of this, many valuable items, including sixteen copper statues of saints, had fortunately been removed from the premises mere days before the fire erupted [17]. French Culture Minister Franck Riester stated that many of France's "most precious treasures" were spared from destruction, including the crown of thorns, allegedly worn by Jesus, and the tunic of St. Louis [17], [18]. The famous stained glass Rose Windows were spared from catastrophe, as well as the organ. The large artwork titled the "May de Notre-Dame", along with other artworks, were moved to the Louvre museum, where they would "be dehumidified, protected, conserved and restored" [19]. While major parts of the church, as well as relics and artworks inside, were destroyed or damaged by fire, smoke and water, it is still considered to be too early to estimate the cost of the damage [20]. The cathedral's two bell towers and outer walls stood firm, while their insides and the upper structure were eviscerated by the blaze [2].

3 ENVIRONMENTAL COSTS

Notre-Dame's spire and roof housed upwards of 400 tonnes of lead that coated Notre-Dame Cathedral's spire and roof framing was released into the air and surrounding environment across Île de la Cité and the surrounding neighbourhoods when the cathedral burned [14], [15], [21]. The vaulted ceiling is just below the roof and had been detailed to have stopped the lead from falling out of the roof space. It was trapped close to the blaze that burned at over 800°C that some of the lead would have vaporized and oxidized to feed more heat into the reaction and accelerating the vaporization and oxidization [21], [22]. The city officials issues no warning to residents of any potential dangers related to lead contamination; in fact, it was not until April 27, nearly two weeks after the fire, that the first warning of elevated lead levels in the area surrounding Notre-Dame was issued [14].

On 27th April, the Parisian police issued a warning of high levels of neurotoxic lead dust in the immediate area around the church. The areas around the cathedral, such as the gardens, have been closed with advice that residents in the area use wet wipes to remove dust from surface and furniture. Some of the fine particles including lead oxides may have deposited on surrounding soils or were transported by wind. Another part of the lead is assumed to have dispersed in the Seine river given the location of the cathedral on a river island called "Île de la Cité" and the large amount of water that was used by the firefighters on the blaze [22]. The concern raised is the impact of lead vaporization and lead poisoning. The first results provided by the French authorities of lead (Pb) soil concentration on the order of 10 g kg^{-1} that demonstrates the intensity of lead contamination and likely other related metals such as antimony or arsenic [22]. The areas showing high levels of lead contamination were the plaza and gardens surrounding Notre-Dame as well as inside the cathedral itself, all of which were already closed to the public [23].

A number of prevention and protection of the population have been undertaken to minimize the health consequences from lead pollution. In the 18th July 2019 Health Notice by the Agence Régionale de Santé, samples were be taken from all establishments that have young children near the cathedral or a road network where a high value of lead (>5000 $\mu g/m^2$) was found in the dust [24] and rates of >1000 $\mu g/m^2$ for outdoor spaces of schools and other types of facilities [25]. Samples were taken of indoor spaces and playgrounds and when values were abnormal, work measures and cleaning were undertaken with subsequent analyses to ensure that the measures had been effective [24]. Three elementary schools and one kindergarten were found to have rates above 1000 $\mu g/m^2$ requiring excavation of the playground, access to be removed and coverage of the patio by flexible slabs to be made. In addition, the City of Paris widen the geographical scope of testing and measurements [25]. The costs remediating the playground at one school Saint-Benoît was 200,000 € with additional costs of treating the polluted bitumen as these hazardous material [25].

The risk from lead poisoning is predominately with young children, especially those under the age of 7, and pregnant women and the children they carry [25]. Health authorities aim to protect cathedral restoration workers and to continuously conduct longer-term testing of the exposed areas [21]. The forecourt of Notre-Dame and the adjacent streets have been identified to require specific treatment as they measured very high concentration of lead [25]. In late July, clean-up work at the site was stopped with workers sent home from the site due to concerns that the anti-contamination measures may be insufficient [26].

In June, a child living on Île de la Cité was found to have high levels of lead in his blood. This prompted authorities to suggest blood tests for pregnant women and families with kids under seven years old living on Île de la Cité [27]. Officials, however, maintained that lead contamination was not a problem in the areas around Notre-Dame; on July 5, Paris's regional health office stated that "all the interior samplings taken in the residences of families living near the cathedral are beneath regulation levels" [14]. It was not until weeks later that the same agency declared, "lead pollution is very significant on Île de la Cité and around the Cathedral", but maintained that "no health impact that can be attributed to the pollution caused by the fire has been thus far observed" [14]. At the same time, an environmental group called Robin de Bois filed a lawsuit against French authorities, accusing them of minimising the danger and failing to provide adequate warnings to local residents. The head of the organisation stated that lead contamination could easily spread within a mile of the cathedral, affecting Paris's 6th arrondissement, including nearby schools and the Place Saint-Michel, as well as the Left Bank, an area on the southside of the Seine. Robin de Bois observed cafes and bouquinistes on the Left Bank still operating as usual and pedestrians walking right up to the barricaded plaza around Notre-Dame to take photos [14], [28]. In early August, decontamination efforts began for schools and nurseries within several hundred metres of the cathedral, and Notre-Dame itself was sealed off on August 13 to commence clean-up operations [15], [29]. This was the second attempt at decontaminating the cathedral after efforts in July were halted due to concerns around lead poisoning. Concurrently, 162 local children were tested for lead contamination – 16 were found to have levels that need monitoring and one child was found to have a worryingly high level, but officials said it was unclear if this was linked to Notre Dame or his home [15].

France's healthcare system is largely financed by government health insurance: in 2015, France spent 11.5% of its GDP on healthcare, the third highest in all of Europe [30]. The risk of lead poisoning as a result of the Notre-Dame fire could bear the government with an increased financial burden, on top of the already astounding costs of rebuilding the cathedral. As lead is a cumulative toxin, risk of poisoning increases with length of exposure, and seemingly "safe" levels with no apparent symptoms can still lead to irreversible neurological and behavioural damage [31]. The attempts to decontaminate Notre-Dame and the surrounding areas remain strong, but we will not know the effects of the potential contamination for years to come.

4 COSTS AND TIME OF OTHER RESTORATIONS

Upon news of the fire, pledges poured in immediately for the costs of reconstruction and reached over €750 million in just the first 10 days [32]. This amount is equivalent to nearly three years of France's entire national restoration budget [33]. Several months on, questions remain as to the cost and viability of reconstruction as well as the likely time frame. The original structure took over 200 years to build and was in need of significant repairs and restorations prior to the devastating impacts of the recent fire [34].

Accurately estimating the likely cost and time frame of repairs to the cathedral is difficult for a number of reasons, one being concerns about the availability of resources to recreate damaged areas. In particular, the original wooden ceiling was made from approximately 5,000 primeval oak trees which simply no longer exist in such large quantities. Another reason is the limited number of tradespeople with the skills and techniques utilised to achieve certain original features of the building to the standard they were [35]. Furthermore, the building is not considered safe or structurally sound enough for workers to enter, inspect and determine the true extent of the damage. Franck Riester, France's Culture Minister, said Notre-Dame remained unstable and vulnerable – in particular its ceiling, which can potentially still collapse [36]. This initial step of inspection, cleanup and stabilising the remaining structure has already experienced delays due to concerns about lead contamination from the melted roof.

Work has only recently recommenced with strict new lead-protection measures in place to protect workers onsite, including "throwaway full-body clothing, obligatory showers and a decontamination zone to ensure that no one tracks pollution outside the site" [37]. These important measures will likely remain throughout the duration of the project but will nonetheless make for a more costly, complicated and lengthy process.

4.1 Time frame: Looking to precedents and determining approach

Despite President Macron's desire to have Notre Dame rebuilt in 5 years, ostensibly in time for the 2024 Paris Olympics, architects and reconstruction experts were quick to cast doubts on the viability of this time frame. Frédéric Létoffé, president of a group of companies specialising in the restoration of historic buildings and monuments, warned that a comprehensive restoration of Notre-Dame would likely take longer, between 10 and 15 years [10]. Eric Fischer, who oversaw the restoration of France's 1,000-year-old Strasbourg Cathedral, indicated it might take decades [38]. Medieval historian Mickaël Wilmart cited precedents of smaller buildings from the same era that had taken longer to restore:

> The Nantes Cathedral suffered a similar roof fire in January of 1972. It was closed for three years while the roof was rebuilt. But it took another ten years of further work before it was completely restored... and the parliament in [the French region of] Brittany [which burned in 1994] took five years, and it wasn't as big as Notre-Dame [35].

Marine de la Guerrande, an architect with the Ile de France Order of Architects, warned that it was far too early to determine a timeline. She cited a 17th-century building, nowhere near the scale of Notre-Dame but similarly devastated by fire that took five years to rebuild, needing "two years just for initial conservation measures, to monitor and dry the structure" [35]. This is due to the risk of thermal shock caused by cold water proceeding the fire's powerful heat, which can cause fractures and corrosion to the stone. If this were the case at Notre-Dame, the entire vault may need to be destroyed and rebuilt, which would obviously add a large amount of work, time and cost to the project [35]. However, some experts are advocating that with enormous support the project could be finished in the ambitious time frame. One of the key determiners will be the approach taken to reconstructing the building, which is yet to be resolved. If there are attempts to recreate and restore Notre-Dame using original materials and techniques, there will be associated challenges and a significant investment of time and expertise required. However, the French government is open to innovation in design, technique and materials – at least for the spire, a 19th-century addition [3]. They are running an open, worldwide competition for architects to submit a design either for rebuilding the old spire or for a new, modern spire [10]. Many experts have indicated that openness to the innovative use of technology in design, materials and construction will be vital to meeting the five-year time frame put forward [34].

4.2 Costs: Still no official estimate and even educated guesses differ

No official cost estimate has been put forth by the French government. However, since the fire, several external organisations have made estimates regarding the cost of reconstruction. One estimate came from Untec, the national union representing construction economists, who indicated costs of reconstruction would likely be between €300 and €600 million. Robert Read, head of insurance agency Hiscox, stated costs could reach over €1bn, but cautioned making estimates this early on without a comprehensive understanding of the potential consequences [32]. While field experts can make estimates, the reality is that these are not based on an actual assessment of the site for damages. The cost alone of securing the building to make it safe for restoration workers to enter is estimated to reach €20 million [39]. Even those working on the official restoration team that have been able to enter the cathedral remain unable to accurately assess the costs of restoring Notre-Dame due to many of the same reasons discussed above. Both cost and time frame are inextricably linked and ultimately unknowable until Notre-Dame is safe for inspection and assessment and until decisions are made about the approach to reconstruction from the perspective of design, techniques, materials and quality. What is clear is that there are many important decisions to be made regarding the future of Notre-Dame and only then can we understand the true cost and time it will take to see this vision realised.

Decisions to be made are significant and include which of the 19th-century additions, such as the spire that was destroyed in the fire, will it be replicated or replaced [4]. Because of the church's significance, history, and religious worth, renovators will need to consult with scholars, architects and church officials [2].

5 SIMULATION MODEL OF FUTURE LOST INCOME

The number of tourists visiting France from the year 2013 to 2018 was collected from DGE and Banque de France, EVE survey of visitors from abroad. The number of tourists visiting the Notre-Dame cathedral was 12 million in 2017 which was about 13.82% of the total tourists coming to France. We have calculated the number of tourists visiting the Cathedral for the years 2013–2018, assuming that the percentage does not vary significantly across time. We have forecasted the estimated number of visits to this tourist attraction in three steps. First, we calculate the annual percentage changes in the number of tourists for the Cathedral from the available data. Secondly, we estimate the average annual growth rate. In the last step, we forecast the number of tourists visiting the Notre-Dame cathedral by summing up the previous year visitors and change in visitors for a given year. The forecast provides the estimated number of visitors if the fire event did not occur. We can make different assumptions in the reduction of the number of tourists in different years and provide estimates of lost revenue in different sectors.

5.1 Lost revenue from souvenirs

For the years 2019–2025, we have estimated revenue lost from souvenir sale assuming the reduction in number of tourists at the Cathedral from 20% to 70%. In case of 2019, the calculation is done after the incident. The average spending per tourist on souvenir at this attraction assumed to vary from EUR 10 to EUR 40. We have also included different scenarios where the percentage of people buying these souvenirs varies from 20% to 70%, while visiting the Notre-Dame cathedral. We divided our estimates into three scenarios: best case, base case and worse case. If the reduction in number of tourists is 20%, we define it as best case, whereas 50% and 70% reductions are defined as base case and worse case respectively.

Table 1 shows revenue lost from souvenir sales which would have otherwise taken place in the absence of the fire incident.

5.2 Lost revenue from entry fees

We have estimated the fees lost by multiplying the number of tourists with relevant fees of entry to the Tower or the Crypt or the Treasury of the Cathedral. We have assumed the same scenarios for the calculation of revenue forgone. We use the average fees of entry to the Tower and the Crypt are EUR 9 (average for EU and non-EU) and EUR 7 along with the entry fee to the Treasury is EUR 3 in the calculation. We have also included different scenarios where the percentage of people visiting these places within the Cathedral varies from 20% to 70%. Table 2 shows revenue lost from entry fees which would have otherwise earned in the absence if the event of fire did not happen.

Table 1: Revenue lost from souvenir sales.

Year	% of tourists buying souvenirs	Total revenue lost (in million Euro)								
		Best case (20% reduction in tourists)			Base case (50% reduction in tourists)			Worse case (70% reduction in tourists)		
		Average spending: EUR 10	Average spending: EUR 20	Average spending: EUR 40	Average spending: EUR 10	Average spending: EUR 20	Average spending: EUR 40	Average spending: EUR 10	Average spending: EUR 20	Average spending: EUR 40
2019*	20%	3.6	7.2	14.3	8.9	17.9	35.8	12.5	25.0	50.1
	50%	8.9	17.9	35.8	22.4	44.7	89.4	31.3	62.6	125.2
	70%	12.5	25.0	50.1	31.3	62.6	125.2	43.8	87.6	175.2
2020	20%	5.1	10.1	20.3	12.7	25.4	50.7	17.8	35.5	71.0
	50%	12.7	25.4	50.7	31.7	63.4	126.8	44.4	88.8	177.5
	70%	17.8	35.5	71.0	44.4	88.8	177.5	62.1	124.3	248.5
2021	20%	5.1	10.3	20.6	12.9	25.7	51.4	18.0	36.0	72.0
	50%	12.9	25.7	51.4	32.1	64.3	128.5	45.0	90.0	179.9
	70%	18.0	36.0	72.0	45.0	90.0	179.9	63.0	125.9	251.9
2022	20%	5.2	10.4	20.8	13.0	26.1	52.1	18.2	36.5	72.9
	50%	13.0	26.1	52.1	32.6	65.1	130.3	45.6	91.2	182.4
	70%	18.2	36.5	72.9	45.6	91.2	182.4	63.8	127.6	255.3
2023	20%	5.3	10.6	21.1	13.2	26.4	52.8	18.5	37.0	73.9
	50%	13.2	26.4	52.8	33.0	66.0	132.0	46.2	92.4	184.8
	70%	18.5	37.0	73.9	46.2	92.4	184.8	64.7	129.4	258.8
2024	20%	5.4	10.7	21.4	13.4	26.8	53.5	18.7	37.5	74.9
	50%	13.4	26.8	53.5	33.5	66.9	133.8	46.8	93.7	187.3
	70%	18.7	37.5	74.9	46.8	93.7	187.3	65.6	131.1	262.3
2025	20%	5.4	10.9	21.7	13.6	27.1	54.3	19.0	38.0	76.0
	50%	13.6	27.1	54.3	33.9	67.8	135.6	47.5	94.9	189.9
	70%	19.0	38.0	76.0	47.5	94.9	189.9	66.5	132.9	265.8
Total	20%	35.1	70.1	140.2	87.6	175.3	350.5	122.7	245.4	490.8
	50%	87.6	175.3	350.5	219.1	438.2	876.4	306.7	613.5	1226.9
	70%	122.7	245.4	490.8	306.7	613.5	1226.9	429.4	858.8	1717.7

*From 16 April 2019.

Table 2: Revenue lost from entry fees.

Year	% of tourists entering Treasury/Tower/Crypt	Total revenue lost (in million Euro)								
		Best case (20% reduction in tourists)			Base case (50% reduction in tourists)			Worse case (70% reduction in tourists)		
		Treasury	Crypt	Tower	Treasury	Crypt	Tower	Treasury	Crypt	Tower
2019*	20%	1.1	2.5	3.2	2.7	6.3	8.1	3.8	8.8	11.3
	50%	2.7	6.3	8.1	6.7	15.6	20.1	9.4	21.9	28.2
	70%	3.8	8.8	11.3	9.4	21.9	28.2	13.1	30.7	39.4
2020	20%	1.5	3.6	4.6	3.8	8.9	11.4	5.3	12.4	16.0
	50%	3.8	8.9	11.4	9.5	22.2	28.5	13.3	31.1	39.9
	70%	5.3	12.4	16.0	13.3	31.1	39.9	18.6	43.5	55.9
2021	20%	1.5	3.6	4.6	3.9	9.0	11.6	5.4	12.6	16.2
	50%	3.9	9.0	11.6	9.6	22.5	28.9	13.5	31.5	40.5
	70%	5.4	12.6	16.2	13.5	31.5	40.5	18.9	44.1	56.7
2022	20%	1.6	3.7	4.7	3.9	9.1	11.7	5.5	12.8	16.4
	50%	3.9	9.1	11.7	9.8	22.8	29.3	13.7	31.9	41.0
	70%	5.5	12.8	16.4	13.7	31.9	41.0	19.2	44.7	57.4
2023	20%	1.6	3.7	4.8	4.0	9.2	11.9	5.5	12.9	16.6
	50%	4.0	9.2	11.9	9.9	23.1	29.7	13.9	32.3	41.6
	70%	5.5	12.9	16.6	13.9	32.3	41.6	19.4	45.3	58.2
2024	20%	1.6	3.8	4.8	4.0	9.4	12.0	5.6	13.1	16.9
	50%	4.0	9.4	12.0	10.0	23.4	30.1	14.1	32.8	42.2
	70%	5.6	13.1	16.9	14.1	32.8	42.2	19.7	45.9	59.0
2025	20%	1.6	3.8	4.9	4.1	9.5	12.2	5.7	13.3	17.1
	50%	4.1	9.5	12.2	10.2	23.7	30.5	14.2	33.2	42.7
	70%	5.7	13.3	17.1	14.2	33.2	42.7	19.9	46.5	59.8
Total	20%	10.5	24.5	31.5	26.3	61.3	78.9	36.8	85.9	110.4
	50%	26.3	61.3	78.9	65.7	153.4	197.2	92.0	214.7	276.1
	70%	36.8	85.9	110.4	92.0	214.7	276.1	128.8	300.6	386.5

*From 16 April 2019.

Table 3: Revenue lost from accommodation fees.

Year	% of tourists staying less nights in accommodation	Total revenue lost (in million Euro)											
		Reduction of 0.25 night						Reduction of 0.50 night					
		Best case (20% reduction in tourists)		Base case (50% reduction in tourists)		Worse case (70% reduction in tourists)		Best case (20% reduction in tourists)		Base case (50% reduction in tourists)		Worse case (70% reduction in tourists)	
		EUR 100	EUR 170	EUR 100	EUR 170	EUR 100	EUR 170	EUR 100	EUR 170	EUR 100	EUR 170	EUR 100	EUR 170
2019*	20%	4.5	7.6	11.2	19.0	15.6	26.6	8.9	15.2	22.4	38.0	31.3	53.2
	50%	11.2	19.0	27.9	47.5	39.1	66.5	22.4	38.0	55.9	95.0	78.2	133.0
	70%	15.6	26.6	39.1	66.5	54.8	93.1	31.3	53.2	78.2	133.0	109.5	186.2
2020	20%	6.3	10.8	15.9	26.9	22.2	37.7	12.7	21.6	31.7	53.9	44.4	75.4
	50%	15.9	26.9	39.6	67.4	55.5	94.3	31.7	53.9	79.2	134.7	110.9	188.6
	70%	22.2	37.7	55.5	94.3	77.7	132.0	44.4	75.4	110.9	188.6	155.3	264.0
2021	20%	6.4	10.9	16.1	27.3	22.5	38.2	12.9	21.8	32.1	54.6	45.0	76.5
	50%	16.1	27.3	40.2	68.3	56.2	95.6	32.1	54.6	80.3	136.5	112.4	191.1
	70%	22.5	38.2	56.2	95.6	78.7	133.8	45.0	76.5	112.4	191.1	157.4	267.6
2022	20%	6.5	11.1	16.3	27.7	22.8	38.8	13.0	22.1	32.6	55.4	45.6	77.5
	50%	16.3	27.7	40.7	69.2	57.0	96.9	32.6	55.4	81.4	138.4	114.0	193.7
	70%	22.8	38.8	57.0	96.9	79.8	135.6	45.6	77.5	114.0	193.7	159.6	271.2
2023	20%	6.6	11.2	16.5	28.1	23.1	39.3	13.2	22.4	33.0	56.1	46.2	78.6
	50%	16.5	28.1	41.3	70.1	57.8	98.2	33.0	56.1	82.5	140.3	115.5	196.4
	70%	23.1	39.3	57.8	98.2	80.9	137.5	46.2	78.6	115.5	196.4	161.7	274.9
2024	20%	6.7	11.4	16.7	28.4	23.4	39.8	13.4	22.8	33.5	56.9	46.8	79.6
	50%	16.7	28.4	41.8	71.1	58.5	99.5	33.5	56.9	83.6	142.2	117.1	199.0
	70%	23.4	39.8	58.5	99.5	82.0	139.3	46.8	79.6	117.1	199.0	163.9	278.7
2025	20%	6.8	11.5	17.0	28.8	23.7	40.4	13.6	23.1	33.9	57.6	47.5	80.7
	50%	17.0	28.8	42.4	72.1	59.3	100.9	33.9	57.6	84.8	144.1	118.7	201.7
	70%	23.7	40.4	59.3	100.9	83.1	141.2	47.5	80.7	118.7	201.7	166.1	282.4
Total	20%	43.8	74.5	109.5	186.2	153.4	260.7	87.6	149.0	219.1	372.5	306.7	521.4
	50%	109.6	186.2	273.9	465.6	383.4	651.8	219.1	372.5	547.7	931.2	766.8	1303.6
	70%	153.4	260.7	383.4	651.8	536.8	912.5	306.7	521.4	766.8	1303.6	1073.5	1825.1

*From 16 April 2019.

5.3 Revenue lost from accommodation fees

We have calculated and forecasted the forgone income due to the fire incident of the Notre-Dame cathedral with three scenarios. In this case we assume two different average prices of accommodation: EUR 100 and EUR 170. Table 3 shows the estimated forgone revenue for the years 2019–2025.

6 LESSONS LEARNED FROM NOTRE-DAME FIRE

The reaction of onlookers and the extensive news coverage worldwide is a demonstration of the significance of Notre Dame as a structure. It is also noted as a symbol of Christianity and the people's ability to feel a personal and emotional connection through the building to God [6]. The appropriate maintenance of older structures is often done without appropriate reference to scientific evidence such as the addition of a fire sprinkler system. This is often avoided due to erroneous concerns that doing so might alter the historical authenticity of a building, or water would damage the building and its historical collections, or associated electrical wiring would present a fire hazard [12], [13]. The reasons for not putting in place the fire prevention measures is due to cost or aesthetics. However, the cost of not minimising risk is priceless, as once it is gone, the original is gone forever. Any rebuilding is just a rebuild and not original. In addition, for older buildings like Notre Dame, the costs of fire need to be viewed from multiple dimensions inclusive of the environmental and health impact. The economic costs of the fire have been discussed mildly in this paper as the full damage is yet to be understood and with every day new information is being released. One of the groups that needs to be monitored closely is the first responders and people who work or live in the vicinity with regards to their health and ongoing effects of exposures to different toxicities.

ACKNOWLEDGEMENT

This research acknowledges support provided by Moin Uddin Ahmed and Kathleen Quilty.

REFERENCES

[1] Chung, F., How did the Notre Dame Cathedral blaze start? 16 April 2019. www.news.com.au/travel/travel-updates/how-did-the-notre-dame-cathedral-blaze-start/news-story/0047a8551efcbe8574ff958c5c641904. Accessed on: 20 Aug. 2019.

[2] El-Bawab, N., Newburger, E. & Steinberg, M., Notre Dame will be rebuilt within the next five years, French President Emmanuel Macron says. CNBC World News, 16 April 2019. www.cnbc.com/2019/04/15/paris-notre-dame-cathedral-on-fire-reuters.html. Accessed on: 24 Aug. 2019.

[3] Vandoorne, S., Bell, M. & Fox, K., Devastating Notre Dame blaze was "likely accidental". CNN, 16 April 2019. https://edition.cnn.com/2019/04/16/europe/notre-dame-cathedral-fire-intl/index.html. Accessed on: 30 Aug. 2019.

[4] El-Bawab, N., Restoration of the Notre Dame Cathedral could take years and cost upward of $1 billion, experts say. CNBC, 17 April 2019. www.cnbc.com/2019/04/17/notre-dame-fire-experts-weigh-in-on-timeline-and-cost-of-restoration.html. Accessed on: 1 Sep. 2019.

[5] Morshed, A.Z., The wrong kind of fire. *The Daily Star*, 18 April 2019. www.thedailystar.net/opinion/the-grudging-urbanist/news/the-wrong-kind-fire-1730437. Accessed on: 30 Aug. 2019.

[6] Latham, M.D., Gothic cathedrals: A shift in Christians' relationship with God. *Young Historians Conference 2019*, Portland State University, Oregon, 2019.

[7] Gross, M., Uncovering the roots of religion. *Current Biology*, **29**(11), pp. R426–R429, 2019.

[8] Sanchez, O., Notre Dame Cathedral: 14 classic movie scenes at the Paris landmark. The Wrap, 15 April 2019. www.thewrap.com/notre-dame-cathedral-10-films-shot-set-paris-landmark/. Accessed on: 30 Aug. 2019.

[9] Statista, Number of visitors to cultural sites in Paris in 2017, 2019. www.statista.com/statistics/991935/cultural-sites-attendance-paris-france/. Accessed on: 2 Sep. 2019.

[10] Prisco, J., France announces competition to rebuild Notre Dame's spire. CNN, 17 April 2019.https://edition.cnn.com/style/article/notre-dame-spire-competition-intl/index.html. Accessed on: 30 Aug. 2019.

[11] Peltier, E., Glanz, J., Grondahl, M., Cai, W., Nossiter, A. & Alderman, L., Notre-Dame came far closer to collapsing than people knew. This is how it was saved. *New York Times*, 18 July 2019. www.nytimes.com/interactive/2019/07/16/world/europe/notre-dame.html. Accessed on: 30 Aug. 2019.

[12] Bennhold, K. & Glanz, J., Notre-Dames safety planners underestimated the risk, with devestating results. *New York Times*, 19 April 2019. www.nytimes.com/2019/04/19/world/europe/notre-dame-fire-safety.html. Accessed on: 1 Sep. 2019.

[13] Wells, J.C., Science for built heritage. *Science*, **364**(6439), p. 413, 2019.

[14] Nossiter, A., Notre-Dame fire released toxic lead that authorities dismissed, lawsuit says. *New York Times*, 31 July 2019. www.nytimes.com/2019/07/31/world/europe/notre-dame-fire-lead-lawsuit.html. Accessed on: 30 Aug. 2019.

[15] Willsher, K., Notre Dame cathedral sealed off for huge lead decontamination operation. *The Guardian*, 13 August 2019. www.theguardian.com/world/2019/aug/13/notre-dame-fire-lead-contamination-clean-up-begins-around-cathedral. Accessed on: 25 Aug. 2019.

[16] Walt, V., We tried to save Notre Dame too late, says champion of cathedral restoration. *Time*, 16 April 2019. https://time.com/5571554/paris-fire-notre-dame-shock-damage/. Accessed on: 22 Aug. 2019.

[17] Li, D.K., What was lost and what survived devastating Notre Dame fire. NBC News, 17 April 2019. www.nbcnews.com/news/europe/what-was-lost-what-survived-devastating-notre-dame-fire-n995026. Accessed on: 20 Aug. 2019.

[18] Gajanan, M., The Notre Dame fire put priceless art and artifacts at risk. Here's what survived – and what didn't. *Time*, 16 April 2019. https://time.com/5571542/notre-dame-fire-art-artifacts-lost/. Accessed on: 30 Aug. 2019.

[19] Ries, B. et al., Firefighters saved many precious artworks from the Notre Dame blaze. CNN, 16 April 2019. https://edition.cnn.com/world/live-news/notre-dame-fire/h_37d7f4960c561e868ce2c03adc111d0d. Accessed on: 30 Aug. 2019.

[20] Lough, R. & Pineau, E., French President Macron hopes to rebuild Notre-Dame in five years. Reuters, 16 April 2019. www.reuters.com/article/us-france-notredame-probe/french-president-macron-hopes-to-rebuild-notre-dame-in-five-years-idUSKCN1RS0AV. Accessed on: 30 Aug. 2019.

[21] Howes, L., Lead contamination risk near Notre-Dame cathedral. *American Chemical Society*, Report No.: 0009-2347, 30 April 2019.

[22] Le Roux, G., De Vleeschouwer, F., Weiss, D., Masson, O., Pinelli, E. & Shotyk, W., Learning from the past: Fires, architecture, and environmental lead emissions. *Environmental Science & Technology*, **53**(15), pp. 8482–8484, 2019.

[23] Chrisafis, A., Notre Dame fire: Police say air not toxic despite high lead levels on the ground. *The Guardian*, 10 May 2019. www.theguardian.com/world/2019/may/09/paris-police-say-no-danger-of-toxic-inhalation-from-air-near-notre-dame. Accessed on: 30 Aug. 2019.
[24] Agence Regionale de Sante, Fire Notre-Dame: Health opinion of 29/08 and situation update, France, 2019.
[25] Ville de Paris, Lead: Update on the situation after the Notre-Dame fire Paris, 2019. www.paris.fr/pages/incendie-de-notre-dame-l-essentiel-concernant-la-pollution-au-plomb-7028.
[26] Chrisafis, A., Notre Dame fire: Activists launch lawsuit over "toxic fallout". *The Guardian*, 30 July 2019. www.theguardian.com/world/2019/jul/30/notre-dame-fire-activists-launch-lawsuit-over-toxic-fallout-paris. Accessed on: 29 Aug. 2019.
[27] Williams, S., Young, pregnant urged to take blood tests for lead after Notre Dame fire. CTVNEWS, 4 June 2019. www.ctvnews.ca/health/young-pregnant-urged-to-take-blood-tests-for-lead-after-notre-dame-fire-1.4451376?cache=yes%3FclipId%3D86116%3Fot%3DAjaxLayout%3Fot%3DAjaxLayout. Accessed on: 1 Sep. 2019.
[28] Cigainero, J., Notre Dame repair crews are back to work, but Paris' lead concerns remain. NPR, 20 August 2019. www.npr.org/2019/08/20/752565861/notre-dame-repair-crews-are-back-to-work-but-paris-lead-concerns-remain. Accessed on: 23 Aug. 2019.
[29] Associated Press in Paris, Notre Dame fire: Lead decontamination of schools begins. *The Guardian*, 8 August 2019. www.theguardian.com/world/2019/aug/08/notre-dame-fire-lead-decontamination-of-schools-begins. Accessed on: 30 Aug. 2019.
[30] Ballas, D., Dorling, D. & Hennig, B., *The Human Atlas of Europe*, Policy Press: Bristol, 2017.
[31] World Health Organization, *Exposure to Lead: A Major Public Health Concern*, World Health Organization: Switzerland, 2010.
[32] Cuddy, A. & Boelpaep, B., Notre-Dame fire: Has too much money been given to rebuild it? BBC News, 25 April 2019. www.bbc.com/news/world-europe-48039770. Accessed on: 2 Sep. 2019.
[33] Casert, R., The Notre-Dame fire was a warning bell, but will Europe listen? The Globe and Mail, 22 April 2019. www.theglobeandmail.com/arts/art-and-architecture/article-the-notre-dame-fire-was-a-warning-bell-but-will-europe-listen/. Accessed on: 29 Aug. 2019.
[34] Fleming, S., France wants to rebuild Notre Dame in just 5 years. Here's how new technology can help. World Economic Forum, 30 April 2019. www.weforum.org/agenda/2019/04/france-wants-to-rebuild-notre-dame-in-just-five-years-here-s-how-new-technology-can-help/. Accessed on: 24 Aug. 2019.
[35] Trouillard, S. & Mufson, C., Restoring Notre-Dame: Tough decisions ahead. France 24, 17 April 2019. www.france24.com/en/20190417-notre-dame-cathedral-fire-restoration-realistic-macron-rebuild-five-years. Accessed on: 30 Aug. 2019.
[36] AP, Notre-Dame celebrates first Mass since devastating April fire. *Sydney Morning Herald*, 16 June 2019.
[37] Charlton, A., Lead scrubbed from Paris streets as Notre Dame work resumes. The Columbian, 19 August 2019. www.columbian.com/news/2019/aug/19/lead-scrubbed-from-paris-streets-as-notre-dame-work-resumes/. Accessed on: 2 Sep. 2019.
[38] Marin, L., "We Will Rebuild": Macron vows to restore Notre-Dame within five years. France 24, 17 April 2019. www.france24.com/en/20190417-macron-vows-rebuild-notre-dame-five-years. Accessed on: 30 Aug. 2019.

[39] McCarthy, N., How much will it cost to repair Notre Dame?. Statista, 25 April 2019. www.statista.com/chart/17801/estimated-repair-costs-for-notre-dame/. Accessed on: 30 Aug. 2019.

IMPORTANCE OF SELF-HELP AND MUTUAL ASSISTANCE AMONG MIGRANTS DURING NATURAL DISASTERS

MARIA MAKABENTA IKEDA[1] & ARLENE GARCES-OZANNE[2]
[1]Kyoto Sangyo University, Japan
[2]Otago University, New Zealand

ABSTRACT

In this study, we examine the factors that influence how migrants cope after a natural disaster. We surveyed two different samples of migrants: Filipinos living in Japan after the 2011 Great East Japan earthquake and tsunami and Filipinos living in New Zealand during the 2010/11 Christchurch earthquakes. We examine their risk perception and capability to manage risk on two levels: self-help and mutual assistance and we hypothesize that if migrants are proactive in information gathering and community involvement, they are more likely to be resilient, to self-help and to assist others. Survey responses were analysed using a multinomial logit model yielding results that show how socioeconomic factors affect migrant capability for self-help and mutual assistance and dependence on public or government assistance. Our results suggest that the migrants with the following characteristics are likely to be resilient: (1) long-staying, educated, and permanently employed; (2) engaged in communities, (3) share/discuss disaster risk-reduction (DRR) information; (4) those who have a lower perception of risks and less conscious of other's needs are less likely to be resilient. On the other hand, testing for vulnerability, we find that the average probability of experiencing some serious damage is higher, for migrants: (1) without social or community involvement, (2) who are only somewhat conscious of the risks and needs of others, and (3) have no or few sources of information.

Keywords: social cognitive theory, self-help, self-efficacy, mutual assistance, bayanihan as collective action, 2011 Great East Japan earthquake and tsunami, 2010/2011 Christchurch earthquake, Filipino migrants, coping, multinomial logit.

1 INTRODUCTION

Japan and New Zealand have two similarities. First, both countries are vulnerable to natural hazards due to their geographical location in the Pacific Rim of Fire. Second, in recent years, both countries have seen a steady growth in the number of foreign nationals with permanent-residency status. As a response to the labour shortage in Japan, the government has begun a quiet revolution of opening its labour market to foreign workers. As of the end of 2018, the number of foreign residents who are legally staying in Japan had reached a historical record high of 2.73 million, roughly 2.1% of total population and an increase of approximately 20% in the past three years [1]. The Ministry of Justice reports that this represents an increase of 6.6% at the end of 2018 from a year earlier, while number of those who overstayed their visas increased to 74,167 up by 11.5% as of 1 January 2019 [2], [3]. On the other hand, New Zealand's estimated resident population as of end of December 2018 was 4,882,500. Available statistics on the number of overseas-born people living in New Zealand (based on the census of 2013) was 1,001,787, a sizeable portion of the country's total population [4], [5].

Japan's national government's willingness to tap foreign labour pool has not been matched by ample provision of services for foreigners in several cities. In a poll taken by Nikkei Research in November and December 2018 among 334 localities, approximately 60% lack support offices to help foreign residents adjust to life in Japan [6] due to "limited administrative resources in terms of personnel and costs".

WIT Transactions on The Built Environment, Vol 190, © 2019 WIT Press
www.witpress.com, ISSN 1743-3509 (on-line)
doi:10.2495/DMAN190061

As the frequency of extreme weather events increase annually, many have voiced concern about reviewing risk management practices particularly in localities with growing number of migrants. According to the United Nations, the term *migrant* means "*any person who lives temporarily or permanently in a country where he or she was not born, and has acquired some significant social ties to this country*" [7]. In a broad sense, "migrant" includes migrant workers, international students as well as immigrants who are regularly and permanently present in a country [8]. Migrants hurdle various cultural barriers by learning how to cope, adjust and behave according to the rules and norms of society. The social vulnerability of migrants calls for more inclusive disaster risk awareness programs designed to enhance capacity building at the community level which are important to enable self-help as well as mutually cooperative activities in crisis situations.

The literature on disaster resilience in Japan and New Zealand has been extensively examined from a social capital perspective. Similar to the current study, Ikeda and Ozanne [9] conducted a pilot survey of Filipino migrants in Tohoku and Kanto areas as well as in Christchurch and noted the importance of social networks and communication skills as prerequisites to having a proactive attitude towards disaster risk management particularly in an environment with considerable cultural and language barriers. Uekusa and Matthewman's [10] qualitative study highlights this social vulnerability by conducting in-depth interviews with immigrants and refugees in Canterbury and Tohoku confirm some of the findings in Ikeda and Ozanne [9] about the importance of social capital in resilience; those who actively interacted with others were able to procure supplies not only for their own families but also for others in need.

Based on a survey sample from Tohoku after the earthquake, Sawada and Kuroishi [11] find that damage caused by a disaster tend to have present bias on behaviour which in turn coincides with a high level of trusting people within the same community. This present bias is closely related to social capital as formal and informal bonding within each community as a form of risk-coping behaviour to deal with adverse disaster effects. Aldrich [12] on the other hand points out that social capital proved to be a more significant factor for recovery than physical damage or economic conditions in the aftermath of the 1995 Kobe earthquake. Aldrich observes that cohesive communities are competent at leveraging resources and their bonding which provide needed support in dire situations works like a form of *de facto* insurance. Because of these social capital benefits, individuals are more likely to be empowered and thus less likely to leave a devastated community. In a study about disaster reconstruction in Japan, Aota [13] reviews the government's concept of the so-called "new public commons" as the foundation of Japan's disaster risk-reduction (DRR) strategy with the following three main components: a) self-help, b) mutual assistance and c) support from the government or public–private partnerships. Social responsibility and mutual assistance are the tenets of Japan's resilience in an era of uncertainty and disruption. Mutual assistance dynamics run on social capital that emanates from trust, norms of reciprocity and networks. Harada [14] summarizes well how resilience under the new public commons in Japan is implemented: each person autonomously makes decisions about personal safety which involves preparing oneself on a regular basis in order to be able to cope in a potentially worst disaster scenario where he or she will be on their own with no one else to depend on. For mutual assistance, "formation and maintenance of tight networks based on regular information sharing and collaborative relationships" [14] is crucial. The government provides last-resort support and reassurance for the public.

In this paper, we clarify important factors affecting how migrants particularly those who are living in vulnerable environments (other than their places of birth) exhibit DRR behaviour. We formulate a model based on social cognitive theory and provide empirical evidence using a sample of Filipinos in Japan and New Zealand circa the 2011 natural disasters. We analyse the vulnerability of migrants and their capability to engage in self-help and mutual assistance initiatives to cope with disaster risks, help others and build resilience in their own communities. We ask which migrant characteristics are related to higher vulnerability to disaster risks and whether migrants self-help and/or help others in a disaster.

2 CONCEPTUAL FRAMEWORK: SOCIAL COGNITIVE MODEL FOR MIGRANT DISASTER RISK REDUCTION (DRR) BEHAVIOUR

This section provides a conceptual analysis of the different factors and processes through which migrant capability to self-help and assist others affect DRR behaviour. A social cognitive model is conceptualized to analyse the factors affecting how migrants conduct self-help and engage in mutual assistance strategies to disaster resilience.

2.1 Vulnerability and resilience

Combaz [15] defines "disaster resilience as the ability of individuals, communities to adapt to and recover from hazards, shocks or stresses without compromising long-term prospects for development." Disaster resilience and vulnerability are intrinsically related in a complex and multidimensional manner. While reducing risk behaviour can potentially enhance resilience, it is misleading to conflate less vulnerability with increased resilience. In our conceptual framework based on social cognitive theory, we depict vulnerability and resilience to be affected by what Bandura calls "triadic reciprocality" [16] of personal experiences, behaviour and the environment. However, vulnerability is represented not as a mirror image or binary opposite of resilience (Fig. 1). The literature cites various forms of resilience (natural or physical, adaptive, restored, etc.), so migrants can be resilient in some but not other aspects due to differences in personal characteristics, competencies, knowledge, experiences, practices or how they interact with and learn from their environment.

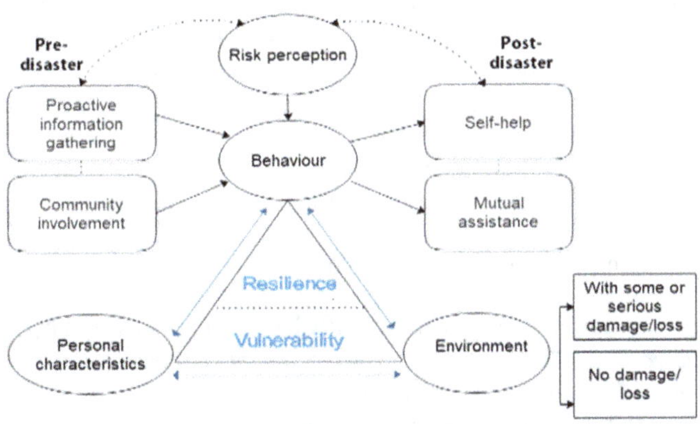

Figure 1: Migrant disaster resilience and social cognitive theory.

2.2 Factors affecting self-help, mutual assistance and disaster risk reduction

To understand the factors of self-help and mutual assistance, we studied the concepts of self-efficacy and collective efficacy in social cognitive theory. Bandura explains that the key lies in the "belief in one's own or group's capability to organize and execute the courses of action to manage often stressful situations and that such beliefs influence how people think, feel, motivate themselves and act". These beliefs influence choice sets and capability to execute a behaviour successfully. Bandura proposes the concept of triadic reciprocity and defines human behaviour as a dynamic, and reciprocal interaction of a) personal factors, b) behaviour, and c) environment. Individuals operate cognitively on their social experiences and these cognitions then influence behaviour [16].

Paton applies social cognition concepts to disaster preparedness such that an individual's risk perception and hazard anxiety is affected by the level of social consciousness or how much people are consciously thinking and discussing about disaster risks in undisrupted periods of quiescence which motivate individuals towards protective or mitigation action [17]. Paton calls this motivation phase as pre-cursor variables linking intentions and belief in one's capability to prevent adverse outcomes through preparation. In our conceptual framework shown in Fig. 1, we adapt Paton's view about *pre-disaster* variables and indicate factors such as proactive information gathering, community involvement and risk perception, and personal characteristics which affect beliefs on his or her ability to mitigate hazards through self-help and/or collective initiatives.

According to a recent study by Babcicky and Seebauer [18], collective efficacy or a group's shared belief in its joint capabilities to achieve an objective, influences risk perception, anxiety, and self-efficacy towards protective action. These studies [17], [18] indicate a complex interrelatedness between the beliefs that buttress self-efficacy and collective efficacy.

In this study, we consider personal characteristics, risk perception, information sources, community involvement and behavioural attitudes before and after a disaster: (1) personal characteristics: age, residency/visa status, gender, marital status, number of years staying in the country (Japan or New Zealand), number of years staying in the immediate disaster area; (2) community involvement: in any community group (Filipino, local, neighbourhood or professional associations, etc.); (3) behaviour: pre-disaster (proactive self-initiated DRR information gathering, drills and community involvement) and post-disaster (share/discuss DRR and recovery information, help others, volunteer in drills and/or recovery activities, receive information from others; utilise government sources of information and accept assistance from others); (4) risk perception: whether one is always/sometimes/never conscious of disaster risks and the needs of others; (5) information: sources of DRR information (family, friends, neighbours, TV, radio, news, social media, government; (6) environment: severity of disaster outcome experience (no/some/serious damage or loss).

2.3 Hypothesis building and model formulation

We hypothesise that migrant engagement in DRR behaviour is affected by factors including *personal characteristics, social capital (prosocial or community involvement, shared information, community coping) as well as the capability to self-help and help others*. Here, we hypothesize proactive or action-oriented self-help akin to our prior description of social cognition that incorporates risk perception and how individuals are conscious of other people's needs. The role of self-help plays a key role in risk reduction and quality of coping in crisis situations.

Collective action is defined as when two or more people coordinate their actions in space and time. Cultural factors may play a role as Filipinos harness community involvement and practice a custom called *bayanihan*. Engagement in their communities not only among Filipinos but also with the local communities is found to enhance their social competence and capability to recover as well as to help others and engage in community recovery [9].

Thus, we expect that community involvement or some form of social capital affects the intention to conduct disaster risk reduction behaviour.

Based on the social cognitive model of migrant disaster resilience in Fig. 1, we formulate the following hypotheses: (1) migrants learn from each other and from their environment; (2) personal characteristics, behaviour, risk perception and environmental factors influence vulnerability and disaster resilience; (3) individuals who are more proactive in DRR information gathering and who are more socially connected are more likely to either engage in self-help or mutually assistance; (4) capabilities to self-help or mutually assist each other affect resilience; (5) self-help and mutual assistance substitute for reliance on government support.

3 RESEARCH METHODOLOGY

Based on the literature review and components of social cognition described above, we hypothesized that certain migrant characteristics promote behavioural attitudes that enhance migrant resilience either through self-initiated or mutually cooperative DRR activities.

3.1 Collection of data

Field work and face-to-face interviews in Christchurch, New Zealand, and Sendai, Kessenuma, Ishinomaki and Higashi Matsushima, Japan were conducted in 2015 in order to have an initial understanding of the earthquake experiences of Filipino migrants in these areas. From these interviews, we developed a pilot online survey questionnaire (in English and Filipino) with 40 questions, which we pre-tested in Christchurch in January 2016. However, due to the low response rate and feedback that the questionnaire was too long, we reduced the questions to 18 for the succeeding surveys in Christchurch, Tohoku and Kanto, to enable respondents to complete the survey within 10 minutes. We ran the surveys from January 2016 to March 2017 in New Zealand and Japan.

The survey used a respondent-driven sampling (RDS) method which is a variation of snowball sampling. This particular sampling method is appropriate because it contends that those who are best able to determine members of target populations are their own peers, and therefore allows the researchers (through their initial contacts) to locate people of a specific population (Filipinos affected by the earthquakes). This sampling method, combined with the online survey questionnaire, yield a simple and efficient data collection method.

3.2 Characteristics of respondents

We find that the social connectedness of the Filipino migrants surveyed is relatively strong. About 76% of those surveyed in Japan are involved in some kind of social or community group, and 85% in New Zealand. Further, on average, approximately 70% of those surveyed in Japan and New Zealand participate, discuss and share information about disaster preparedness, 90% indicate that they are conscious of the risks and needs of people during and after disasters, 75% provide material help (money, food, clothing, shelter), and 62% volunteer in their community's earthquake preparedness and recovery activities.

We also find that although the respondents in Japan and New Zealand are generally proactive when it comes to accessing information either through their own initiatives or through family and friends, on average, the New Zealand respondents (on average 79%) were relatively more proactive than the respondents in Japan (on average 59%). It is also interesting to note that 72% of the New Zealand respondents also sought information from government agencies, compared to only 21% of the Japanese respondents.

3.3 Description of the variables and logistic regressions

We briefly summarize and describe the variables of the empirical model in Table 1. We ran logistic regressions to *determine whether certain socio-demographic characteristics (education, employment, length of residency in disaster area, social or community group involvement) have any effect on the probability of an individual being resilient during disasters* (Model 1). We also tested *whether certain activities, for example, participation in disaster drills, sharing or discussing disaster-related information, and/or volunteering in disaster preparedness and recovery activities have any effect on the probability of an individual being vulnerable during disasters* (Model 2). Our proxy indicator of resilience is based on whether or not an individual received any assistance or support after the disaster, and vulnerability is based on how severely an individual was affected by the disaster.

Table 1: Description of the variables.

Latent variables	Measurable variables	Description
Personal characteristics	Age	Age
	Residency	Residency/visa status
	Gender	Sexual orientation
	Marital	Marital status
	Dis. years	Number of years living in the disaster area
	Country years	Number of years living in Japan or New Zealand
	Educ.	Educational attainment
	Employ	Employment/job status
Behavioural	Social (pre-disaster)	Community/social involvement
	Drills (pre-disaster)	Participation in DRR drills before 2011 disasters
	Self-help	Self-initiated gathering of DRR related information
	Mutual	Received information from family or friends
	Government	Utilised government-provided information
	Share (post-disaster)	Share or discuss DRR and recovery information
	Donate (post-disaster)	Donate money, food, supplies, clothing, shelter/room
	Volunteer (post-disaster)	Voluntarily participate in DRR and/or recovery activities
Risk perception	Conscious	Conscious of risks and needs of other people
Information	Info	Number of sources of DRR-related information
Environment	No damage/loss	Experienced no post-disaster damage/loss
	Some damage/loss	Experienced some post-disaster damage/loss
	Serious damage/loss	Experienced serious/severe post-disaster damage/loss

Model 1 determines what factors in general affect individuals' resilience to natural disasters, where *Yi* takes the value of 1 if the individual did not receive any assistance or donation, and 0 otherwise. There are two ways to interpret the resilience of individuals with respect to whether or not she received any help. First, an individual who did not receive any help is resilient because she did not require any help during or after the disaster and is able to attend to her own needs. On the other hand, an individual who received help can also be resilient because this individual knows how to get the help she needs and to harness the aid she received under scarce and dire conditions. For these reasons, we do not have any a priori hypothesis regarding the sign of the coefficients of the explanatory variables for resilience.

We run independent binary logistic regression models in which one outcome is chosen as the "base" outcome and the other outcome is separately regressed against this base outcome. For example, we chose the outcome: did not receive any assistance or donation as the base, and estimated eqn (1) using maximum likelihood:

$$ln\frac{\Pr(Y_i=1)}{PR(Y_i=0)} = \beta \cdot X_i. \qquad (1)$$

The regressors (X_i) include personal socio-demographic characteristics of the respondent and also variables that measure individual's behavioural attitudes related to accessing disaster-related information and social networking. We hypothesise that *individuals who are more proactive with respect to information gathering and who are more socially active are characteristics of resilient individuals.* Specifically:

$$X_i = \begin{pmatrix} Country_i, Age_i, Residency_i, Gender_i, Marital_i, DisYears_i, CountryYears_i, \\ Educ_i, Employ_i, Social_i, Info_i, Selfhelp_i, Mutual_i, Government_i, Drills_i, \\ Conscious_i, Share_i, Donate_i, Volunteer_i \end{pmatrix}. \qquad (2)$$

Model 2 determines the factors that affect individuals' vulnerability to natural disasters. We used multinomial logistic (MNL) models to explore these. Vulnerability is measured in terms of the individuals' self-reported assessment of how severely they were affected by the crisis, that is, whether or not they experienced damage or injury to themselves and/or their household because of the disaster. For K possible outcomes: K_1 = no damage/injury; K_2 = some damage/injury; and K_3 = serious damage/injury, we ran K_{-1} independent binary logistic regression models in which one outcome is chosen as the "base" outcome and the other K_{-1} outcomes are separately regressed against this base outcome. For example, we chose outcome K_1 (i.e., the individual experienced no damage/injury) as the base, and estimated the following eqns simultaneously using maximum likelihood:

$$ln\frac{\Pr(Y_i=K2)}{\Pr(Y_i=K1)} = \beta_1 \cdot X_i. \qquad (3)$$

$$ln\frac{\Pr(Y_i=K3)}{\Pr(Y_i=K1)} = \beta_2 \cdot X_i. \qquad (4)$$

Note that for each possible outcome there is an identical set of regressors (X_i). The regressors include and factors that capture the extent of individuals' involvement in their respective communities and how they access information about disasters. Specifically:

$$X_i = \begin{pmatrix} Social_i, Info_i, Selfhelp_i, Mutual_i, Government_i, Drills_i, \\ Conscious_i, Share_i, Donate, Volunteer_i \end{pmatrix}. \qquad (5)$$

4 ANALYSIS AND FINDINGS

Table 2 presents average marginal effects of all (significant) explanatory variables on the probability that an individual received some form of help because of the disaster. Marginal effects show the change in probability when one explanatory variable increases by one unit, while keeping all other variables constant. For continuous variables this represents the instantaneous change since the "unit" may be very small. For categorical variables, the marginal effects show the predicted possibilities for a specific category relative to a base or reference category, and for binary variables, the change is from 0 to 1.

Table 2: Logistic regression: Base Outcome: Received assistance/donation.

Log likelihood = -45.352555		LR chi2(38) = 80.90; Prob > chi2 =0.0001	
Number of observations = 124		Pseudo R2 = 0. 4714	
Question/variable	Response	Average marginal effect	Standard error
Country	Japan	0.8097***	0.1450
Residency	Citizen/permanent resident in Japan or NZ		
	Trainee/student visa/permit	0.3677***	0.0796
	Spouse/partner/dependent of citizen/resident	0.2828***	0.0751
Marital status	Married		
	Single	0.1748*	0.0907
	Divorced/separated	0.2321**	0.1149
Years in disaster area	10 years or more		
	4–9 years	-0.3200***	0.0757
	Less than 4 years	-0.4839***	0.0671
Years in Japan/NZ	10 years or more		
	4–9 years	0.3196***	0.0712
Education/qualification	University graduate		
	High school	0.1998**	0.0979
	Vocational or technical training	0.2117*	0.1122
	University postgraduate	-0.2027***	0.1771
Current work	Employed full time		
	Self-employed	0.2458*	0.1408
Sources of information	Many different sources		
	Few sources	-0.1882*	0.0967
	None	-0.3471**	0.1560
Participate in DRR Drills	Always/many times		
	Never	-0.2831**	0.1161
Conscious of risks and others' needs	Always/Often		
	Sometimes	-0.2961***	0.0614
	Never	0.3587***	0.0681
Share or discuss DRR information	Always/many times		
	Sometimes	0.1633*	0.0937
	Never	0.3025***	0.1114
Donate	Always/many times		
	Sometimes	0.3207***	0.0889
Volunteer in community DRR	Always/many times		
	Rarely	-0.2484**	0.1148

Note: ***, ** and * indicate statistical significance at the 1%, 5% and 10% level, respectively.

An intuitive way of interpreting these average marginal effects that essentially compares the “typical” individual (the reference group) with another individual who differs on one category. The reference group in Model 1 represents a typical individual: who has lived in the disaster area for 10 years or more, a university graduate, employed full-time, is able to access vital disaster information by himself/herself and participates in social, community activities.

Based on our results, the following socio-economic characteristics are statistically significant for individuals who did not receive any assistance or donation: residency, number of years living in the disaster area and in the country, education and work status. We find that Japanese residents are more likely than New Zealanders to have received assistance or donation. Compared to citizens/permanent residents, students, and partners/dependents of citizens/permanent residents are also more likely to have received assistance/donations. We also find that new settlers in the affected regions are less likely to have received any assistance. For new settlers, not receiving any assistance can be an indication of higher vulnerability because they do not know where to go for help that they need in these localities.

We also find that those with post-graduate qualifications are less likely to have received any assistance. We can also think of a postgraduate qualification as a proxy for financial well-being, and so those with postgraduate qualifications would have more financial security to cope with disasters and require less assistance. Relative to those with university qualifications, those with only a high school qualification or vocational/technical training are 20 and 21 percentage points respectively, more likely to have received assistance. Compared to those with a full-time job, those who are self-employed are 24 percentage points more likely to have received assistance.

Of the social-networking variables, we find that those who are less socially aware, e.g. those who are not conscious of other people’s needs and those who do not share or discuss information with others are more likely to receive assistance.

Finally, Table 3 presents average marginal effects of all (significant) explanatory variables on the probability on observing different outcomes related to how an individual has been affected by the disaster (no/some/serious damage or injury).

Our multinomial logistic regressions confirm that various mutual help and social networking variables influence the level of engagement in disaster preparedness and thus lead to reduced vulnerability outcomes (whether she experienced damages and the degree of severity such as (no/some/serious) losses). The base (significant) predictors are: involvement in Filipino/Japanese/New Zealand, other community gatherings; sought/received information from various sources (family, friends, colleagues, news, etc); received information from government sources; active participation in disaster drills; active consciousness of people’s risks and needs; active sharing of information about disasters; frequency of donations made; and active volunteering in disaster preparedness and recovery activities. The measure of self-perceived level of proactive behaviour is operationalized based on questions such as: “How often do you participate in earthquake/tsunami/fire etc drills?”; “How often do you volunteer in community’s earthquake preparedness/recovery activities?”; “Are you conscious of own risks as well as needs of others during and after natural disaster episodes?” to which respondents assess themselves based on levels of frequency (always/many times, sometimes, rarely, never) or degree/intensity (Yes, always/sometimes; No, rarely/never) conscious of risks. We use this measure of self-perceived proactivity as an indicator for self-help as it deals with the subjective assessment that a person makes about one’s perceived capability to make things happen in crisis situations and serves as an independent predictor of resilience.

Table 3: Multinomial logistic regression.

Log likelihood = -82.091531				LR chi2(38) = 105.26; Prob > chi2 =0.0000			
Number of obs = 148				Pseudo R2 = 0.3907			
Question/variable	Response	No damage		Some damage		Serious damage	
		Average marginal effect	Standard error	Average marginal effect	Standard error	Average marginal effect	Standard error
Social or community involvement	Filipino/Japanese/NZ/ Other communities						
	Not involved	-0.212**	0.1027			0.239*	0.124
Source of information	Many sources						
	Few sources	-0.196**	0.0874	0.218**	0.093		
	Received no information	-0.428***	0.1118	0.394**	0.163		
Information from government	Yes						
	No	0.230***	0.0688	-0.202***	0.074		
Participate in DRR drills	Always/many times						
	Sometimes	-0.256***	0.084	0.255***	0.0885		
Conscious of risks and others' needs	Always/many times						
	Sometimes					-0.055*	0.029
	Rarely	-0.029**	0.145			0.325**	0.133
Share or discuss DRR information	Always/many times						
	Rarely			-0.321***	0.093	0.425***	0.076
	Never					-0.073***	0.025
Donate	Always/many times						
	Sometimes					-0.1345**	0.0636
	Rarely					-0.205***	0.045
	Never			0.2362*	0.1217	-0.142***	0.049
Volunteer in community DRR	Always/many times						
	Sometimes	0.344***	0.095	-0.373***	0.095		
	Rarely	0.522***	0.114	-0.510***	0.111		
	Never	0.308***	0.118	-0.223*	0.120	-0.085***	0.305

Note: ***, ** and * indicate statistical significance at the 1%, 5% and 10% level, respectively.

Consistent with our hypotheses, we find that the average probability of experiencing no damage is lower, and the average probability of experiencing some serious damage is higher, for individuals who have no social or community involvement, those who are only conscious of the risks and needs of others sometimes. For those who have no or few sources of information, the average probability of experiencing some damage is higher, while the average probability of experiencing no damage is lower. We think that the more sources of information a migrant has access to, the more she is able to validate acquired information that can be utilized to reduce risks.

For effects of mutual assistance, we find evidence that the average probability of experiencing no damage is higher, and for experiencing some and serious damage is lower for those people who always engage in sharing/discussing information about disaster preparedness and recovery; for those who donate in cash or kind to disaster victims; and for those who volunteer in preparedness and recovery activities. Our survey results concur with our interviews that some of the migrants were able to cope with the disaster effects and in the process experience a sense of psychological and social growth.

Our field interviews reveal anecdotal evidence that indicate Filipino migrant communities are self-helping groups. It was the first time they experienced a massive natural disaster and yet when asked why they actively helped others during the relief and recovery period, many replied, "to divert focus away from my own pain or loss". Many respondents felt the need to be useful in their communities "like many others around them who were just thankful to be alive" and realized a self-affirming change in themselves as a member of the Filipino community by actively helping others after the disaster and by earning recognition not only in their own communities but also in media for their civic-minded efforts.

Finally, for those who did not get information from government sources, the average probability of experiencing no or some damage is also higher. This may have two important implications. First, weak public information dissemination on disaster risks have not reached overseas-born residents due to either government implementation weakness or migrant lack of communication skills particularly among respondents in Japan who have low Japanese language proficiency. Second, social cohesiveness and collective efficacy prove our hypothesis that social connectiveness or community involvement of migrants is vital as migrants learn and empower each other to either self-help or help others.

5 CONCLUSION

We studied how migrants in Japan and New Zealand coped during episodes of massive natural disasters in 2010–2011. Using questionnaire survey data collected from Filipino migrants in these countries, we empirically test a model of migrant disaster resilience and vulnerability based on social cognitive theory. Using multinomial logit regression, we find evidence for mutual assistance as a strong determinant of reduced vulnerability among Filipino migrants living in Japan and New Zealand. Our findings suggest that vulnerability to some or serious damage is higher for migrants who are not community involved and only somewhat conscious of disaster risks. We find stronger evidence for community involvement and mutual assistance than for self-help in Filipino migrant DRR behaviour.

In addition, this study provides evidence that public information dissemination on disaster risks have not reached nor appealed to most of the foreign-born residents that responded to our survey. Our findings also show that social cohesiveness enhance mutual cooperation and can effectively reduce migrant vulnerability to natural disasters to the extent that it may substitute for lack of or weak government support. Community involvement of migrants lessens their direct dependence on government support. These findings on the importance of self-help and mutual assistance are considerably relevant in vulnerable places where population of migrants or overseas-born individuals is steadily growing in the face of limited or lack of public resources for migrant support services.

For policy recommendations, to reach those who do not have strong bonds with other migrants nor local communities, government authorities need to implement inclusive information dissemination in mainstream and social media to increase awareness on disaster risks and consequences of ill-preparedness. Finally, tapping non-government organizations and other civil service organizations that help improve or deepen linkages between migrants and their neighbours or locals, need to be further harnessed at the micro or community-level.

Due to time and data constraints, the analysis of our paper is limited in scope and we encourage others empirical analyse the interrelatedness of self-help and mutual help motivations of locals and foreign-born residents to examine how they adapt to and learn from each other in a vulnerable disaster setting.

ACKNOWLEDGEMENTS

We thank all the Filipinos who accepted our requests for interviews and/or participated in our online survey. We are grateful to the Hyogo Prefecture for providing support in an earlier phase of this study as well as to Japan's Ministry of Education for financial support.

REFERENCES

[1] Osumi, M., Number of foreign residents in Japan rose 6.6% in 2018, while number of overstayers grew almost twice as much, government data shows. *The Japan Times.* www.japantimes.co.jp/news/2019/03/22/national/number-foreign-residents-japan-rose-6-6-2018-number-overstayers-grew-almost-twice-much-government-data-shows. Accessed on: 27 Jun. 2019.

[2] Ministry of Justice, Japan, About the number of foreign residents in Japan as of Yearend December 2018. (In Japanese.) www.moj.go.jp/nyuukokukanri/kouhou/nyuukokukanri04_00081.html. Accessed on: 20 Aug. 2019.

[3] Statistics Bureau of Japan, Ministry of Internal Affairs and Communications, Population estimates by age (five-year groups) and sex. (In Japanese.) www.stat.go.jp/data/jinsui/2.html#monthly. Accessed on: 20 Aug. 2019.

[4] StatsNZ, Summary figures for the New Zealand resident population, December 2018. www.stats.govt.nz/topics/population. Accessed on: 25 Aug. 2019.

[5] StatsNZ Archive, 2013 Census QuickStats about culture and identity. https://archive.stats.govt.nz/Census/2013-census/profile-and-summary-reports/quickstats-culture-identity/birthplace.aspx. Accessed on 25 Aug. 2019.

[6] Yamamoto, K., Japanese cities lack support for foreign residents, poll shows. *Nikkei Asian Review*. https://asia.nikkei.com/Spotlight/Japan-immigration/Japanese-cities-lack-support-for-foreign-residents-poll-shows. Accessed on: 25 Aug. 2019.

[7] UNESCO, Glossary of migration related terms: Migrant/migration. www.unesco.org/new/en/social-and-human-sciences/themes/international-migration/glossary/migrant/. Accessed on: 17 Sep. 2019.

[8] International Organization for Migration (IOM), Key migration terms. www.iom.int/key-migration-terms#Migrant. Accessed on: 17 Sep. 2019.

[9] Ikeda, M. & Ozanne, A., Human Security, social competence and natural disasters in Japan and New Zealand: A case study of Filipino migrants. *Japan Social Innovation Journal*, **6**(1), pp. 42–60, 2016.

[10] Uekusa, S. & Matthewman, S., Vulnerable and resilient? Immigrants and refugees in the 2010–2011 Canterbury and Tohoku disasters. *International Journal of Disaster Risk Reduction*, **22**, pp. 355–361, 2017.

[11] Sawada, Y. & Kuroishi, Y., How to strengthen social capital in disaster affected communities? The case of the great east Japan earthquake. *Disaster Risks, Social Preferences, and Policy Effects: Field Experiments in Selected ASEAN and East Asian Countries*, eds Y. Sawada & S. Oum, ERIA Research Project Report FY2013, No. 34, Jakarta: ERIA, pp. 163–199, 2015.

[12] Aldrich, D.P., *Building Resilience: Social Capital in Post-Disaster Recovery*, University of Chicago Press, 2012.
[13] Aota, R., Consideration of "new public commons" characteristics for disaster reconstruction. *Japan Social Innovation Journal*, **2**(1), pp. 1–17, 2012.
[14] Harada, H., Social capital in disaster: From the great east Japan earthquake. *The Senshu Social Capital Review*, **3**, pp. 5–21, 2012.
[15] Combaz, E., *Disaster Resilience: Topic Guide*, GSDRC, University of Birmingham: Birmingham, 2014.
[16] Bandura, A., Self-efficacy: Toward a unifying theory of behavioral change. *Psychological Review*, **84**(2), p. 191, 1977.
[17] Paton, D., Disaster Preparedness: a social cognitive perspective. *Disaster Prevention and Management*, **12**, p. 3, 2003.
[18] Babcicky, P. & Seebauer, S., Collective efficacy and natural hazards: differing roles of social cohesion and task-specific efficacy in shaping risk and coping beliefs. *Journal of Risk Research*, 2019. DOI: 10.1080/13669877.2019.1628096.

DIRTY THE WATERS: MOTHERS' EXPERIENCE OF A CHEMICAL DISASTER IN WEST VIRGINIA, USA

EMILY E. PARSONS & EMILY DIAMOND
The Wright Institute, USA

ABSTRACT

The World Health Organization estimates that 12.6 million deaths a year are attributable to unhealthy environments, while modern industry uses more than 100,000 different chemicals in their operations, most of them understudied. On 9 January 2014, a major chemical spill in Chemical Valley, West Virginia, polluted the water of 300,000 residents across nine counties of this Appalachian region of the United States. At the time of the disaster, and even now, there is very limited knowledge about the chemical in terms of health effects. Approximately 10,000 gallons of 4-Methylcyclohexanemethanol (MCHM), which is used in coal processing, began leaking from a 48,000-gallon tanker in the early morning hours. Residents were not notified of a "Do not use" order until later that evening, after which people had no potable water, and no water for sanitation. This study explores, through structured interviews, the experience of mothers, some pregnant, some with ill children, others with multiple children, in their attempts to manage during the crisis. The study focuses on their levels of trust in systems that many felt failed them throughout the course of the disaster. Communication (official and non-official), the accessibility of clean water, community resilience and coping, caring for their children, immediate and long-term health risks, and the psychological and economic impacts of this disaster will be discussed. This study focused on 35 mothers. It's the first study to explore this particular demographics' experience and their continued adjustment in the following years. The structured interview used for this project holds promise for better understanding the experience of mothers in other chemical disasters, in which parents confront limited information, the need to make difficult choices, limited resources, and the lasting echoes of those decisions. It's hoped that it can be used in other contexts to deepen our understanding of disaster management.

Keywords: chemical spill, toxic environments, 4-Methylcyclohexanemthanol, Chemical Valley, West Virginia water crisis, Elk River, MCHM, polyglycol ethers, water contamination, freedom industry, epigenetic effects, family environmental health.

1 INTRODUCTION

On 9 January 2014, 48,000 gallons of 4-Methylcyclohexanemethanol (MCHM) leaked out of Freedom Industries' Tank #396 into the Elk River, contaminating an area populated by over 300,000 people spanning nine counties, and affecting the drinking water of one-sixth of West Virginia's population. MCHM is a chemical slightly soluble in water, used to clean coal, by separating the coal from rocks and debris [1]. Annually, more than hundred million tons of coal are mined from underground seams, surface mines and mountain top removal, and then processed in the state [2]. MCHM is one the chemicals used in this process, and smells somewhat like licorice. Ten-thousand gallons of MCHM seeped into the municipal water system, along with polyglycol ethers (PPH), a solvent also used to further clean coal, which is faintly yellow in colour. Together they contaminated the state's largest water treatment plant situated a mile upriver. This water treatment plant served 15% of West Virginia's population [3], [4]. The smell and the slight yellow colour were the primary warnings to the population that the water had been contaminated. Late that evening, President Obama declared a state of emergency, which would last for 50 days.

At the time, people knew very little about this chemical, which is used to "bathe" and clean coal before it's burned for use [5]. A search of the US National Library of Medicine, National Institutes of Health Library, PubMed, holds no health studies of the chemical prior

WIT Transactions on The Built Environment, Vol 190, © 2019 WIT Press
www.witpress.com, ISSN 1743-3509 (on-line)
doi:10.2495/DMAN190071

to this event. Even today, there is not much that is known about MCHM, including whether it could cause birth defects, cancer, or epigenetic changes, or how it might work synergistically with other chemicals, or its potential to cause ecosystem damage.

The site of this disaster was in southern West Virginia, in and around the state's capital, and one of the most economically depressed areas of the United States. For nearly a century, this area had been known as Chemical Valley, as it contained the largest number of chemical plants in the United States. Coal and salt mining factories were well established in West Virginia as far back as the 1700s. However, Chemical Valley has its roots in World War I, when weapons were being produced for the war effort, and this continued on through the Vietnam era. In fact, during the Vietnam War, Agent Orange and other defoliants were produced in Chemical Valley.

It's likely that the magnitude of this leak could have been avoided. Weeks earlier, a few local residents reported a pungent smell they identified as "smelling like licorice" to the West Virginia Department of Environmental Protection. No preventative action was taken. On the day of the major spill, a number of complaints were filed, beginning at 7:30 am and continuing throughout the day. Many of the complaints were reported on social media, and some news agencies picked up the story. Still, no action was taken. The official "Do not use" water order was finally issued at 5:36 pm, with the exception of flushing the toilet [6]. That evening, the governor, Earl Ray Tomblin, went on the local news to caution that the water was not safe for "drinking, cooking, washing or bathing" [7]. Information about the spill was inadequately disseminated. Many didn't know about the spill until they watched the evening news, and some people hadn't seen the news or have access to this information.

The governor's order forced the closure of approximately 2,000 water-dependent facilities, 200 schools and many businesses [7]. The estimated cost to the local economy was $19 million per day [8]. Federal Emergency Management Agency (FEMA) and the National Guard were sent to deliver water to the area, particularly to hospitals and nursing homes. However, this was a limited effort that did not benefit all the people affected by the spill. In addition to the struggle to find clean water to drink and for household use, many community markets and convenience stores inflated their prices; others had empty shelves.

In the following days, the public was urged to watch for "symptoms of exposure, including rashes, nausea, vomiting, and wheezing". In the immediate aftermath, the West Virginia Poison Center received over 1,900 calls, and over the ensuing three days after the spill, more than 200 people went to local hospital emergency rooms complaining of rashes, nausea, and other symptoms [5], [9].

On the fourth day, the governor held a press conference in which he announced that the risk to public health was decreasing, which was widely disbelieved. In fact, as the governor lifted the ban on the drinking water, emergency room visits rose for "skin rashes, eye irritation, nausea, vomiting, anxiety, and migraines" [5]. In their study the following year, Schade et al. [7], found that the days following the spill marked the largest acute illness outbreak caused by water contamination in United States history.

2 LITERATURE REVIEW

Across the Great Smoky Mountains from West Virginia, lies the US Marine Corps Base, Camp Lejeune. Much like Chemical Valley, it has a long history of using and manufacturing weapons. The base housed families, and from 1968 through 1985, three potent chemicals are known to have contaminated the water supply, trichloroethylene, tetrachloroethylene, and benzene. Families noticed health problems. Looking back at the health of mothers and children, two kinds of problems emerged among children, pre-term birth and being born at term, but having low birth weight; both of which can cause long lasting developmental problems [10]. The base in now what is called a Superfund site, an area identified as a risk to human health by the Environmental Protection Agency and eligible for the federal funding necessary for toxic clean-up. Anyone at Camp Lejeune who drank the water for 30 days or more, and has one or more of several kinds of cancer is entitled to free medical care for their treatment [11].

Travelling further South from Camp Lejeune is the Mississippi Delta region where Texas, Louisiana, Alabama and Florida form the Gulf of Mexico. On 20 April 2010, a British Petroleum oil well in the Gulf began to leak, and this became the biggest marine oil spill in history. The spill discharged about 5 million barrels of oil before the leak was capped 87 days later. It is one of the largest environmental disasters in the country's history, impacting the health of marine life, and the lives, which were nourished by fishing, both at the table and through the jobs it created. An environmental activist and mother, Marylee Orr stated, "It began for me with concern for the men on the rig, who would be alive and who wouldn't. And then it came from bayou wives who called to tell me their husbands were vomiting, had chest pains and nausea, headaches, and generally, were very sick". Her son Michael Orr said of the accumulation of disasters and the poverty of the region, "There's no real sense to me of bouncing back. It's clinging on" [12].

Perhaps important to how these events are now handled is a mother named Lois Gibbs. Love Canal was a 70-acre (28 ha) suburban development near Niagara Falls, New York. The area had a long history of being a dumping ground for chemical waste. Beginning in the 1940s, Hooker Chemical Company used the land to dump 21,800 tons of chemical waste from the manufacturing of a variety of products, such as synthetic resins, dyes, perfumes, rubber, solvents and dioxin. In 1953, now owned by Occidental Chemical Corporation, the site was sold to the local school district. In the 1970s, Lois Gibbs was raising a young son with seizures and other inexplicable health issues. For years, people had wondered about a black fluid, seeping up through the ground, and in the canal. Community members complained about odors they couldn't identify that were on the school ground and elsewhere in the neighbourhood. It was Lois Gibbs' persistent attempts to alert elected officials that eventually led to biological sampling in 1978, which in turn led to the evacuation of hundreds of families. Borne out of her concerted efforts to be heard, President Jimmy Carter used emergency funds for a toxic disaster for the first time in the nation's history. The federal program, called Superfund, is now in place to identify and remediate places like Love Canal and Camp Lejeune [13]. The mothers of Woburn, Massachusetts and Hinkley, California spoke out to guide research towards toxins in their water, and the mothers in Wilmington, California are currently doing the same about their air quality. Despite these mothers' powerful voices, it remains a neglected area of public health and health research to more comprehensively, and strategically collect their concerns.

3 AIMS OF THE STUDY

Mothers and their children are often in the crucible of vulnerability. This is particularly true of disasters. Mothers may be pregnant and caring for children; some are caring for children and their own parents. In cases of divorce, mothers in the US are often the sole or primary care providers of children. This study focused on two things: one was to learn about the short and longer-term consequences of this disaster, as well as concerns of mothers through semi-structured interviews who had gone through the West Virginia Water Crisis. These interviews were conducted in order to gain a more granular view and understanding of their experience of how they navigated risk, the actions they took during and after the disaster, and the adequacy of information they had. The interview also addressed how mothers made decisions about staying or leaving the area, and other thoughts about the area and their futures in it.

The second goal was to begin the development of a semi-structured interview protocol that could be used in this disaster and potentially others. This would aid in the furthering of our combined knowledge of how different toxic disasters vary by chemical, by region, by the economic resilience of the community, and by the different ways in which the disaster is communicated, information imparted, risks mitigated, and follow-up put in place. This arose because toxic disasters are likely to increase in the coming years, as they become connected to severe weather events such as fires, hurricanes, and flooding, which are projected to increase in both frequency and intensity in the future.

4 METHODS

This project relied on qualitative methodology to explore mothers' experiences of the 2014 Freedom Industries spill in Chemical Valley, West Virginia. The creation of the initial semi-structured interview protocol was a joint endeavor, and allowed both for the strategic collection of information, but also room to ask follow-up questions as needed. The idea was to begin the development of a semi-structured interview protocol that could be used in other disasters, thus allowing for cross-comparisons between different kinds of events by chemical, by age, gender, and location. Furthermore, the general history of these narratives is that they are often told to reporters. It is equally important and, perhaps, more so that they are also captured by researchers in healthcare. The semi-structured interview and protocol received IRB approval. The list of interview questions is provided in the Appendix.

Participants were recruited through social media and local newspaper ads to inform area residents of the study. To be included in the study, participants had to be a mother of a child 18 or younger, and living within the geographical zone affected during the toxic spill. The first 35 to meet this criterion were interviewed. The process of interviewing was a powerful emotional experience for those who participated; many reported being flooded with feelings they had during the time of the crisis. Unfortunately, some were unable to participate. One potential participant was in hospice care for cancer, and while she met the criteria, sadly failing health made it too difficult to participate. Another participant who endured a miscarriage during the spill found the idea of discussing her experience too emotionally challenging.

Throughout the interview, participants were asked to freely add to their answers and were offered the opportunity to contact the researcher if anything came to mind after the interview had taken place. This partnership created an opportunity to uncover ideas, thoughts, and questions that we, as researchers may not have considered. It also produced narratives that involved both the participant and researcher. It was thought that research need not only be the extraction of information, but itself part of a larger process of feeling greater control. All participants were told that what was learned from the project would be shared with them.

The interviewer for this project was born and raised in West Virginia. Rural communities have been known to be skeptical of outside researchers, particularly those that identify themselves as associated with mental health, which is often stigmatized in this region. It is likely that the interviewer's shared heritage with the mothers aided in creating a safe and comfortable space in which to share their stories.

All interviews were transcribed, and resulting transcripts were read, analyzed, and then coded with Quirkos software. The tapes, the transcriptions and the software allowed for the close analysis of text including content as well as the emotional overlay of the interviews. The themes generated were the effort of both authors. Much of the speech was in the vernacular of West Virginia, which does not come across as profoundly as in the mothers' voices themselves.

5 PARTICIPANT DEMOGRAPHICS

Thirty-five mothers participated in this project. The mothers' ages ranged from 24–43. Of the participants, 45% were married, while 55% were either not married, separated, or divorced. 60% of participants had one or two children, and 40% had three or more children. Children ranged widely in age, with the majority (40%) falling between 3 and 6 years of age. The mothers came from a diverse range of socio-economic backgrounds. 26% of the participants were stay at home mothers, while the other 74% came from varied occupations that included lawyers, social workers, educators, artists, government employees, and bankers. Educational backgrounds varied: 23% of participants had a high school diploma, 20% had a 4-year college degree, and 20% possessed a master's degree and beyond, while another 20% reported having some college education. This group of participants likely have more years of formal education than is typical of West Virginia; the percentage graduating from college according to 2010 data, was 29.5% of people [14]. The vast majority (86%) of participants reported having relatives living in the area. Most of those interviewed were white, which reflects the state's population at 93.34% Caucasian [15].

6 RESULTS

Nearly all the mothers spoke of deep ties to the area and strong feelings of being rooted in the land and culture of West Virginia. One mother remarked, "My generation, there's lots of family – I have 102 first cousins … most of them still reside in Charleston". This connection to the area, and network of family ties was intricately linked to the emotional experience of those who went through the West Virginia Water Crisis. The following gives an overview of the mothers' thoughts and emotions, with special attention to those that might help in providing better health care, specifically mental health care.

All mothers were deeply impacted during and after the disaster. Most were afraid for their children at the time of the spill, and worried about their children's future health. Nearly all felt keenly disappointed with what they perceived was a delay in being notified, all the while describing the difficulty in accessing clean water for them and their families. Many conveyed a sense that there was little to no justice, particularly given that the company who was responsible has since gone bankrupt. Mothers were also burdened with the expectation of no help for emergent problems, particularly those that were health related. Several envisaged the environmental health of their children's generation as being worse and more challenging to mitigate in the future.

All participants were asked about their experience of the day they learned of the toxic spill. One mother described the smell of the water, "It smells like licorice, so that sort of made you think of food, and not something that could hurt you". Another mother said, "I remember … I drove through town thinking something stinks, you know, like different than the normal chemical smell you have going through South Charleston". Describing the water coming out of her tap, one mother stated, "It was kind of just like a yellowish color, and then basically it just had like this very Listerine smell". She describes that non-essential workers were excused from work, and that black garbage bags were put over all the fountains, and they remained there for a year. One mother described doing the same in her home, to keep her daughter from touching the water, and perhaps to try and contain the fumes of the solvent as it evaporated. A pregnant woman dashed to the stores looking for bottled water, only to find empty shelves. She said of the water, "I think being pregnant for me was the scariest part, and how much had I taken in?" Another said she felt, "sheer desperate fear".

Some spoke of empty shelves, others recalled price gouging. One mother described it this way, "water became gold". A few left the state, but most stayed in the area. Mothers of sick children found themselves needing clean water, but unable to leave home to stand in the long lines to get clean water.

Not surprisingly, medical issues arose for many, in different ways across the generations. For a single mother whose baby was born at 652 grams, and who needed intensive home care, the scarcity of clean water for formula, and for sterilizing her baby's medical equipment, combined with her poverty, caused what she described as "a big depression". Not having a partner, she wasn't free to go out in search of clean water. One mother who has a son with asthma said that she had learned from others that, "when I flushed, I should not have the kids in the house". For one mother, there was the emergence of an unknown illness and high fever which needed hospitalization, and she needed to be evacuated to a hospital out of the area, as the local hospital couldn't spare the water to make the ice to keep her cool. The water caused rashes for some, and they were told to avoid contact. One mother said, "We all showered in it because we didn't have a choice, and we just weren't going to work dirty". Another participant said that her mother needed clean water for her CPAP breathing machine. Water was part of a lifeline for the sick and the well, as one woman put it, "Water is life".

While numerically not a large number of women, a few were pregnant at the time, and for them, the event was particularly difficult. One woman went into labor during the crisis, "We had a stillborn with our second (baby), and you know, who's to know if those things (chemicals) affected me. I mean, I don't think I even connected that until right now. She was already 12 inches long". One mother relayed that her son was born prematurely, requiring neo-natal intensive care, "He was born at 37 weeks and came out having breathing issues". Another mother noted, "My daughter was diagnosed in utero with a congenital heart defect. The correlation with that (chemical spill) has never been proven". Each of these women spoke about the distress in part stemming from not knowing. For one mother, pregnant at the time of the toxic spill, her child has since been diagnosed with autism. While she understood that there were several possible causes, she does come back to the toxic spill as a probable cause.

Worries about future health problems were also very common, "I was very, very scared for my baby. He had low immune system (functioning), anyway. I didn't know what he had been exposed to … will we find out ten years down the road we were exposed to a cancer-causing agent? And we knew from the get-go, nobody had our backs". One mother said, "I've known a lot of people that have passed. I don't know if it has anything to do with it, but have passed from cancer … What's the future going to hold … for my family?" Not only is there worry, but many also some spoke about a lack of responsibility, "I worry it's going to be one of those things where everybody develops like cancer, or like a brain tumor … some kind of mystery health issue, and it's going to be very prevalent here – and then they're going to be like, oh it's not our fault, but then it is, you know?"

Compounding this future worry is the observation of one of the mothers, "We've seen a lot of doctors leave. We have to travel pretty far to get healthcare services that are specialized … We just can't keep doctors here".

When the official water ban was lifted, one mother who was divorced talked about not wanting her child to use the tap water, but her ex-husband challenged her, not wanting their son going through life afraid. Four years later, a majority of participants still do not drink water from the tap. One woman said, "Currently, I cannot tell you that I trust the water source. We do bathe with the water, but I don't drink tap water. I don't prepare my food with tap water. I have zero faith that that situation was properly taken care of".

When asked about leaving the area, some mothers reported that life would not be that much different outside of the state. One such mother grew up in Flint, Michigan, in which a problem of lead contamination in the municipal water supply was uncovered in 2014, the same year the present crisis occurred. She had moved to Charleston, West Virginia before the chemical spill occurred. As both Flint and Charleston have very similar median incomes, it's likely that economics played some role in the search for affordable housing. She noted: "I have it in my mind that it could just happen anywhere. If people in other states aren't having it happen to them right now, it could actually be happening to them, and they don't even realize it. Growing up in Flint, we never knew anything was wrong with our water, but come to find out there was something wrong the entire time. So it's almost as if you know, you're not really safe anywhere". For the majority of mothers, it was family ties that kept them from moving away. A mother described her family obligations: "I think I would stay here until something would happen with my parents. I feel an obligation to stay and take care of them. They are elderly. After that, I'm not sure that my ties to the mountain state will remain". Another mother said, "We're so rooted in this area, and this is where my family is. You know, my dad is older and sick, and he won't go anywhere. So, we're just kind of tied to the area". For a divorced mother, she couldn't imagine being able to take the children out of the state without a court battle.

Some did leave the area, and for those left behind, such as this mother, she recalls losing her network of friends, "the people that would have just came in my house and sat down…my entire girlfriend network left. They left because they could … Within literally a year of the Water Crisis, I lost my community".

For some, this event has taken an economic toll. "I think financially we really put ourselves in a bind because of all the extra expenses. You don't think about bottled water, paper plates, paper towels. We bought adult washcloths, I mean, adult baby-wipes, things that you did not realize cost so much because you don't buy them that frequently". The Supplemental Assistance Program, or SNAP, helps low-income families buy food. One mother receiving the food allowance estimated that she used about "thirty to sixty dollars a month on water". While the toxic water spill eventually led to a lawsuit in which the plaintiffs won, with checks averaging several hundred dollars going out in September of 2018, it often didn't make up for the expenses that were incurred during the disaster, or the change in buying habits which ensued in the following years. A mother of three noted: "Show me some studies 15, 20, 30 years down the road and then elaborate that $400 was sufficient for what happened to our state. But I suppose time will tell".

Mothers talked about what they wanted other mothers to know, much of it having to do with being prepared. A mother with a sick child said she would caution mothers to have extras of all the necessities. Another mother said, "Rely on your gut, do everything you can from a mother's standpoint to protect your child for the future. No one else has your back. It's on you". This sentiment was echoed by another, "I hope it gets better. Don't rely on your government officials to take care of the situation for you". As far as chemicals and what is safe, one mother said there was no testing on what would constitute a safe level of a chemical on premature babies or infants so "to make sure that you're getting the most accurate and up-to-date information". This sentiment summarized the feeling of needing to stay strong, "Just keep pushing through and it will get better eventually … do what you got to do to survive".

Mothers were asked about what their child's generation would be contending with environmentally. Here almost all mothers felt the situation would worsen. Speaking about the environment, one mother said, "I would assume that my kids will have it much harder". While mothers throughout the interviews expressed love and concern for their children, at one point a mother said, "I am honestly scared for my children, and some days, I feel bad that we made the choice to have children". One of the causes of the despair was, "the regulations are loosening instead of tightening". As a consequence, a mother noted, "I believe that medical issues and illnesses are going to just continually worsen". Of her children's generation, one mother stated, "I hope they take better care of the resources, and of each other".

7 DISCUSSION

Prominent to many disasters which impact whole communities, including this one, is despair and anxiety about future health problems, and the fate of the land and all that it allows for the community, emotionally and economically. Health practitioners focus on single patients at a time, but what happens when the community is the patient? The mothers in this project voiced a wide range of concerns stemming from the spill. No one can know what health impacts there might be in the long run, or the fate of the Elk River, which flows through the cultural identity of the community, going back to when its sole inhabitants were Native Americans and elk roamed the banks.

In response to the crisis of the Deep Horizon oil spill, national research funding went to the Gulf Coast Health Alliance, a consortium that was in part university researchers, and also the community itself [16]. Community-based Participatory Research (CBPR), in which researchers partner with the community, to not only define the questions being asked, but to make sure that the perspectives of ordinary citizens are part of the data, is itself a way of treating a community. It addresses the mistrust and the feelings of being side-lined, while assuring that people's perspectives are incorporated into the findings. This research can also make sure that data is collected regarding the long-lasting health concerns that people worry about. Encouraging this form of citizen science is to acknowledge that the community has a role. Disasters take their toll on communities in part because for a moment in time, sometimes days, sometimes years, no one has a role that they once had, and one of the most prominent roles they do have, is that of victim.

Every mother who participated in this project interviewed with someone raised in West Virginia. Each person had the opportunity to revisit their interview and add things they felt were important to add. Each of them will get a synopsis of the project so that they understand that their stories were heard and are part of the story of their community. Healthcare's basic model is linked to the bio–psycho–social understanding of the individual. Additionally, to a large extent, the training of those in health care is disease or condition specific. With structured interviewing to help us learn more about major disasters, we hope that we can provide integrated care, which is *event specific*. It is hoped that these narratives help those in healthcare better understand this event and its long shadow.

From the research standpoint, we felt the need to develop a more systematized way of gathering information, so that we could further the knowledge of how they compare across events, places, and people.

There are several findings from this project relevant to future disaster management. On the largest level, the United States does not subscribe to the Precautionary Principle, the principle used throughout the EU and other places stating that a chemical or pharmaceutical must be proven to be safe, *before* it's introduced into public use. As it stands, currently in the US, people must demonstrate that they have been harmed for a chemical to be taken out of use. US industry uses more than 100,000 different chemicals, so the traditional scientific methodologies of public health find it increasingly difficult to establish whether any one chemical has harmed an ecosystem or negatively impacted human health [17]. This is because chemicals are released into an environmental context of other untested chemicals, or with other untested chemicals, and the synergistic effects produced when combined are unknown. Further, the focus of the spill was on two chemical compounds, MCHM and PPH, yet commercial products often have other ingredients, which go unexamined because they aren't considered active ingredients, and those too may have important health effects.

The Hazard Communication Standard, which was revised in 2012, requires chemical manufacturers, or the distributor, to provide a 16-point Safety Data Sheet, formally known as the Material Safety Data Sheet. The current Safety Data Sheets are part of an international unified hazard communication system so that people using chemicals, and also first responders, can quickly understand the hazard potential and necessary first aid. Looking up the Safety Data Sheet for 4-Methylcyclohexanemethanol, this chemical is reported, "For Laboratory Use Only". First aid includes things that were not possible for those in the impacted area, such as "washing off with soap and water". Further, the first version of the Safety Data Sheet was issued on 26 March 2014, nearly four months after the spill [18].

Many mothers are worried about the long-term health effects to their children. Not only should we look at harm in the conventional ways of potentially causing cancers, but also focus on potential reproductive harm, epigenetic effects, and synergistic effects of chemicals as they combine with others during environmental releases. Of the small sample of 35 mothers, three reported reproductive problems.

This region lacked an appropriate disaster communication system that could have reached cell phones and landlines, or sounded warning alarms. Acting as its own notification system, part of the way that people knew something was wrong with the water was its smell and colour. There are of course numerous gasses and chemicals which are odorless, and if that was the case, it's conceivable that there would have been much more human exposure. It caused people to have burning in their eyes, respiratory issues, as well as nausea, so while little was known about the chemicals, the "Do not use" notification may have not only been slow in dissemination, but misleading. This was not only a toxic water disaster, but it was also an issue of toxic vapor, where exposure was occurring as it evaporated in toilets, where there is almost always standing water, and in the rivers and tributaries which were contaminated.

There has been a move in the US for several decades towards greater transparency. In 2004, the US National Library of Medicine and the Environmental Protection Agency created Toxmap. For those in disaster management, risk management, public health and medical research, this site has been invaluable. Selected industries, which are using an amount of a chemical thought to be potentially harmful to human or environmental health, are required to track their usages. The industries are mapped, and site-specific chemical use and waste is catalogued in a searchable format, which is accessible to the public. Toxic waste sites were also geospatially mapped. As it currently stands, the website reads, "TOXMAP website will be retired in the fall of 2019" [19]. Different municipalities and academic institutions may try and save the data, but importantly, it may not be kept up to date. In an era projected to have more natural disasters and, in turn, infrastructural damage, the loss of this knowledge is of great concern.

While it may go without saying, economics played a major role in this disaster, as it does in most. It could be considered a disaster within a disaster. These are often the most difficult to remediate in the long run. According to the 2018 Behavioral Risk Factor Surveillance System (BRFSS), 19% of West Virginians live in poverty. More than a quarter, 26.3%, consider their health fair to poor. West Virginia ranks the 3rd highest among the states in cancer prevalence [20]. Their current adult asthma prevalence as of 2017 is the 2nd highest in the nation, with 12.7% of adults having asthma. Importantly for children, the infant mortality rate is 23% higher than for the US as a whole. Regarding mental health, the suicide rate is 27% higher than the national rate, according to the Appalachian Regional Commission's Health Disparities report [21]. It's likely reasonable to say that Chemical Valley had for years been caught between the need for chemical industry jobs, and perhaps the private desire for a healthier environment, so that lack of knowledge helped to ease the bind that many found themselves in. So in a disaster, it was harder to relay full information, plan evacuations, and work on appropriate disaster signalling in preparation for a toxic release.

While certainly there are limitations to this research, in that a granular view of a subset of people may not generalize to the whole population, it's hoped that it still provides an important range of challenges and obstacles, both in the short and long-term that mothers experienced.

In summary, better safety knowledge, more timely and accurate communication, and the preservation of systems of transparency are essential. As disasters are likely to increase in frequency and intensity, those in medical and mental health need to have educational training in meeting the needs of people, both during the crisis and in its long aftermath. Issues of water quality are numerous, and the long shadow that single events cast can last years, as this one illustrates. We look forward to using our protocol to examine other disasters in future years, to see the details of human experience that may help those in the frontlines of healthcare do the best they can.

ACKNOWLEDGEMENT

We would like to acknowledge Dr Patricia Wood for her substantial contribution to the ideas articulated in this text and for helping us guide this project forward.

APPENDIX: INTERVIEW QUESTIONS

1. How long have you lived in the area?
   a. What are your historical/emotional ties to the area?
   b. Before the spill happened – what would you say were your main concerns for your family and community?
2. What was it like to go through the chemical spill?
   a. Remembering back to those days, what was your initial response to the spill?
   b. Did your response change as time passed?
   c. What were your main worries?
   d. What were your worries for your family/children?
   e. What are your current worries? How have they changed?
   f. Have you gone through something similar in the past?
3. Can you speak a little about the aftermath of the spill, the days and weeks following?
   a. How did you cope?
   b. What if anything helped you to cope better?
   c. What if anything made it harder to cope?
   d. What resources, supports – if any – do you wish you had had to cope better?
4. Do you feel, having gone through the event, more prepared for other potential environmental disasters? Less prepared?
   a. How did, or do you prepare?

5. Do you see the rivers eventually getting cleaned up?
   a. If yes: How would that happen? What would it take for that to happen?
   b. If no: What will keep that from happening?
6. Do you see your child's generation also having to worry about the environmental things you do? Do you feel like their concerns might be the same as yours? How might they be different?
7. What do you think or feel are some of the biggest consequences of water pollution for you and your family?
8. Sometimes when people go through an environmental disaster, they think about moving. In your answering, there can be emotional factors, economic factors, or practical reasons; all of them are okay to talk about.
   a. a. Did you think about moving?
   b. What were some of the reasons you decided to stay?
   c. What were some of the reasons you had considered moving?
9. In terms of this spill, do you feel there was accountability? Who is or was responsible?
10. Having gone through this, if you had a platform to talk to mothers across the country who are now facing disasters in their communities – what, if anything, might you want to say to them?
11. What are your hopes and dreams for your children?
12. Is there anything else you would like to say about this experience that you haven't mentioned?

REFERENCES

[1] Horzmann, K.A., de Perre, C., Lee, L.S., Whelton, A.J. & Freeman, J.L., Comparative analytical and toxicological assessment of methylcyclohexanemethanol (MCHM mixtures associated with the Elk River chemical spill. *Chemosphere*, **188**, pp. 599–607, 2017.

[2] West Virginia Office of Miners' Health and Safety, Coal: West Virginia Coal Mining Facts. www.wvminesafety.org/wvcoalfacts.htm. Accessed on: 7 Jun. 2019.

[3] Cooper, W.J., Responding to crisis: The West Virginia chemical spill. *Environmental Science and Technology,* **48**(6), 2014.

[4] Ward, D., West Virginia clean up. *Aquosus Potentia*, pp. 2–10, 2014.

[5] Osnos, E., Chemical Valley. *The New Yorker*. www.newyorker.com/magazine/2014/04/07/chemical-valley. Accessed on: 12 Aug. 2017.

[6] Whelton, A. et al., Residential tap water contamination following the Freedom Industries chemical spill: Perceptions, water quality, and health impacts. Division of Environmental and Ecological Engineering. https://pubs.acs.org/doi/suppl/10.1021/es5040969/suppl_file/4es5040969_si_001.pdf. Accessed on: 31 May 2019.

[7] Schade, C.P., Wright, N., Gupta, R., Latif, D.A. & Jha, A., Self-reported household impacts of large-scale chemical contamination of the public water supply, Charleston, West Virginia, USA. *PLoS One*, pp. 1–14, 2015.

[8] Ginty, M., The waterborne toxic event: Why the West Virginia spill was not a freak occurrence. *In These Times*, 2014.

[9] TOXNET: Toxicology Data Network, 4-Methyclcyclohexanemethanol. https://toxnet.nlm.nih.gov/cgi-bin/sis/search/a?dbs+hsdb:@term+@DOCNO+8182. Accessed on: 4 Jun. 2019.

[10] Ruckart, P., Bove, F. & Maslia, M., Evaluation of contaminated drinking water and preterm birth, small for gestational age, and birth weight at Marine Corps Base Camp Lejeune, North Carolina: A cross-sectional study. *Environmental Health*, **13**(99), 2014.

[11] US Department of Veterans Affairs, Camp Lejeune: Past water contamination. www.publichealth.va.gov/exposures/camp-lejeune/. Accessed on: 1 Jul. 2019.

[12] Sullivan, J. & Rosenberg, B., I remember the mental chaos while they tried to seal the well and clean up the oil spill – How much fear and uncertainty everyone felt: An interview with Marylee and Michael Orr, Louisiana Environmental Action Network. *New Solutions: A Journal of Environmental and Occupational Health Policy*, **28**(3), pp. 467–486, 2018.

[13] Gibbs, L.M., Excerpt from Love Canal: My story. Housewife's data. *American Journal of Public Health*, **101**(9), pp. 79–82, 2011.

[14] US Department of Education, New state by state college attainment numbers show progress towards 2020 goal. www.ed.gov/news/press-releases/new-state-state-college-attainment-numbers-show-progress-toward-2020-goal. Accessed on: 5 Jun. 2019.

[15] West Virginia Population 2019. www.worldpopulationreview/com/states/west-virginia-population. Accessed on: 5 Jun. 2019.

[16] Sullivan, J. et. al., Building and maintaining a citizen science network with fishermen and fishing communities post deepwater horizon oil disaster using a CBPR approach. *New Solutions*, **28**(3), pp. 416–447, 2018.

[17] Henretig, F., Kirk, M. & McKay, C., Hazardous chemical emergencies and poisonings. *The New England Journal of Medicine*, pp. 1638–1655, 2019.

[18] Eastman Chemical Company, Safety data sheet: Crude MCHM. www.msdsonline.com/sds-search/. Accessed on: 6 Jun. 2019.

[19] EPA's Toxic Release Inventory (TRI) and Superfund Programs. https://toxmap.nlm.nih.gov/toxmap/. Accessed on: 31 May 2019.

[20] West Virginia Department of Health and Human Resources, 2018 behavioral risk factor surveillance system. https://dhhr.wv.gov. Accessed on: 2 Jun. 2019.

[21] Appalachian Regional Commission. www.arc.gov. Accessed on: 5 Jun. 2019.

FROM SHELTER TO COMMUNITY RECOVERY: A RESEARCH PROJECT ON AN SAE AREA

CLAUDIA DELLA VALLE & VINCENZO ROMANIA
Department of Philosophy, Sociology, Education and Applied Psychology, University of Padua, Italy

ABSTRACT

Disastrous events raise issues about the territories and the affected population's future. Providing adequate housing for displaced people is both a challenge and a crucial point for any post-disaster policy. In this paper we will focus on the effects of long-term permanent housing solutions on displaced people. Anticipated data consist of the research we have conducted previously on the emergency housing solutions destined for displaced people from the Central Italy earthquake of 2016 who could not leave the territory. In our paper, we will briefly introduce the methodology and first results of our ongoing research, which extends the one we conducted in the earthquake area. Through ethnographic methodological tools and some interviews with actors involved in the emergency process, our main objective is to explore how the models of social interaction are reproduced and transformed in SAE areas. Small and medium-sized villages consist of single-family and earthquake-resistant houses, which will offer housing to the displaced population until the end of the reconstruction. We look forward to understanding how the brand new forms of settlement and social aggregation will affect the reconfiguration of social bonds. The new housing solutions push people to experience more frequent face-to-face interaction and with the challenge of community recovery. Then, the research intends to investigate whether, and how, the community recovery can lead to the formation of social capital and how it can be configured as a significant element capable of affecting the adaptive abilities, therefore resilient, of individuals, families and local community.

Keywords: qualitative disaster research, social capital, community, recovery, temporary housing, ethnography, Central Italy earthquake.

1 INTRODUCTION

Although in recent years interest in the topic of disasters has grown considerably and specific study paradigms have developed, the issue of what is meant by disaster and what physical, ecological or social events should be referred to, has long been difficult to clarify [1]. In the field of social sciences, scholars now agree that disasters should be considered as a social phenomenon, observable over time and through space; it disrupts the daily activities of social entities, which implement unplanned adaptive actions. Attention is no longer dedicated to the event or to the impact, but to the ways in which disasters interact with vulnerabilities, as weaknesses inscribed in the social structure [2], [3]; they derive from well-established social, political and economic processes that condition the manner and the intensity with which people are exposed to the disaster, and react to it [4]. The disaster, therefore, does not passively involve individuals but is socially constructed and actively implemented, through practices and processes of social interaction that take place at an individual, family, community and institutional level [1].

The post-disaster phase involves a variety of actors, both institutional and other types, who are called upon to respond to the challenge of recovery. In it, the importance of interactions and social ties is now widely recognized, but it must be supported by adequate post-emergency choices, in particular, concerning the housing dimension. The focus of this research is on the relationship between community, place and recovery process, in the hope that it can contribute to critical reflection on the importance of putting the community at the centre of the post-disaster phase.

2 THEORETICAL FRAMEWORK

Beyond the breaking of normal social systems, the destruction of places and, sometimes, of human lives, disasters often involve the loss of houses. As a place of refuge and protection, the house must be a central point in the action of governments that, following a disaster, are required to provide a rapid and effective response to this need. Major international agencies dealing with emergency management, such as the United Nations High Commissioner for Refugees (UNHCR), the United Nations Human Settlements Program (UN-HABITAT) or the International Federation of Red Cross and the Red Crescent Societies (IFRC) consider the right to post-disaster accommodation related to the more general right of individuals to adequate housing, as enshrined in Article 25 of the Universal Declaration of Human Rights or in Article 11 of the International Convention on Economic, Social and Cultural Rights (ICESCR) [5]. Despite its recognized centrality, the topic of housing has become an integral part of disaster research only very recently.

Quarantelli [6], [7] identifies four typologies of post-disaster accommodation. The first one is emergency sheltering, i.e. those places where displaced people find shelter for a short time, usually for a few hours after the disaster. These are often spontaneous solutions, arising from immediate needs, and can include schools, gyms, churches, airports or any other building available for the first reception of the population. The second category, temporary shelter, indicates the spaces that offer temporary hospitality to the displaced people, once the first period of the emergency has passed. These solutions, which certainly require more planning than previous ones, are not limited to offering an emergency shelter but allow a whole series of individual daily needs to be satisfied: usually thought of as mass interventions, they provide shelter to the affected population, guarantee the distribution of water and food and the circulation of information. The resumption of daily activities and family responsibilities marks the difference between sheltering and housing. All those accommodations that allow a first, albeit temporary, restoration of domestic routines refer to temporary housing. The inhabitants are aware that this type of housing goes beyond the emergency and can extend for weeks and months, if not years. These solutions are characterized by a certain ambivalence: on the one hand they represent a significant improvement of the housing conditions for some individuals, on the other they could contribute to slowing down or inhibiting the search for a definitive home. Finally, permanent housing is defined as the condition of those who return to live permanently in their homes, following restoration work, or in new homes. The four typologies proposed do not always develop in a linear way, but they are configured as a social process that is not static; moreover, the differences between them are very often not so well-defined [6]–[8].

The restoration of housing is fundamental for the recovery process, at the individual, family, company or community level; the recovery of permanent housing allows individuals to restore and carry out normal domestic and daily activities. Delays in housing assignments very often lead to slowdowns in many of the other recovery dimensions [8]. For these reasons, the primary objective of the institutions should be to give the population the possibility of regaining ownership of their family habits and domestic routines following the disaster. This restitution of the "normal" everyday life can only happen through correct and careful planning of the new housing, or an adequate restoration of the old one, with the full knowledge that they can have a positive impact on displaced populations [9]. On the other hand, incorrect or careless planning can generate negative effects: in some cases, for example, long-term housing problems, determined by particular urban-architectural choices, may be related to the increase of pathologies triggered by disorientation processes, loss of the sense of place or they can create mechanisms that reproduce pre-existing structural vulnerabilities [10].

The destruction of material and human capital is given a lot of attention by multiple studies on disasters, widely supported by media coverage: the destroyed houses, the collapsed buildings, the rubble or the search and rescue phases of the population are shown. Less attention is often dedicated to social capital, because it is less tangible and more difficult to represent in the media. However, among all forms of capital, it is less damaged and less affected by the disaster; on the contrary, during the various phases of the emergency it is renewed and rapidly strengthened [11].

Theories of social capital refer to a multiplicity of definitions, given its complex and multidimensional nature. Although this article will not reconstruct the wider debate on the subject, it is beneficial to distinguish between a structural, relational or micro approach and a collective, community or macro approach [12]. The former sees social capital as an individual resource and focuses on the individual relations and social network; from the processes of social interaction it is possible to obtain gains and advantages [13] and achieve objectives [14], [15]. From a macro perspective, in contrast, social capital is as a public and collective resource, which facilitates the well-being of a community. Robert Putnam, one of the most authoritative exponents of this approach, writes that social capital refers to "features of social organizations, such as networks, norms, and trust, that facilitate coordination and cooperation for mutual benefit" [16, p. 35]. The author distinguishes between bonding social capital, which characterizes strong exclusive ties and strengthens solidarity and belonging in the group, and bridging social capital, which is more inclusive, is identified with the weakest ties, and which generates wider identities and reciprocity, including outside the group [17]. Some recent works in disaster research identify a third type of social capital, the linking one, which describes the relationships of trust between citizens and institutions. They also show that social capital positively affects all phases of the disaster: mitigation and adaptation, preparation and evacuation, response and impact, recovery [12], [18]–[20]. In this last phase, in particular, social capital plays a central role, both for individuals and families as well as for the communities, especially when state interventions are slow or non-existent.

According to Aldrich [18] and Aldrich and Meyer [19], the role of social capital is highlighted by three main mechanisms, through which networks can influence, and accelerate, the recovery process. Firstly, social ties can act as "informal insurance", offering subjects help and economic, logistical, psychological and emotional support. Secondly, the social capital is also linked to a more effective collective action, which allows greater participation in the dialogue with the authority, increasing the chances of satisfying the requests and needs. Finally, it hinders the strategy of exit, which consists of the abandonment of the affected communities by individuals, through an increase in the social cost. Thus, it is more likely that the population, through the strategy of voice, works collectively to overcome the crisis. From an interdisciplinary perspective, Spokane et al. [21] suggest that social capital should also be taken into account in the design of temporary houses, so as to facilitate short and long-term recovery process, especially for more vulnerable groups. The authors encourage the adoption of a synergistic or eco-systemic vision in the reconstruction of the community, possible only when the emergency physical structures are designed with attention placed on social and cultural networks.

However, some studies point to the ambivalent dimension of social capital in the disaster recovery process. Buckland and Rahman [22], for example, affirm that although it favours cooperation, fuelled by mutual trust, social capital can lead to a greater conflict in the decision-making process, due to the horizontal social structure that it promotes. Despite this, social capital is now considered as a key resource for communities, on a par with education, work, safety and health [12]. It also has a central role in a new perspective, called Community-Based Disaster Management: promoting a bottom-up approach to implementing emergency policies, while not undermining the institutions, local communities are supported in the analysis process and in raising their awareness of their own risk conditions, vulnerability and capacity, in order to respond promptly and flexibly to the disaster [23], [24].

The sociological literature suggests some dimensions on which to analyse social capital, for example, interpersonal trust, social cohesion, quality and density of ties and networks, associations and citizen participation. In order to investigate social capital in relation to the disaster and the recovery process, Minamoto [25] identifies three categories of indicators: the social norms, the behaviours and the attitudes of people during reconstruction; the characteristics of the organizations in the community and, finally, the changes in networks during the reconstruction. However, social capital, when not referring to a specific "object", should from time to time be interpreted in relation to the actors, the context and the aims that the research intends to pursue. Thus, it is a "situational and dynamic concept" [26, p. 395].

3 CASE STUDY: THE CENTRAL ITALY EARTHQUAKE

The case that we will analyse in this research is particularly suitable for exploring the dynamics of social capital that we have just discussed. We will study, in particular, the temporary houses assigned to the population following the seismic events that struck central Italy between August 2016 and January 2017. It was a complex situation, unprecedented in Italian history because of the territorial and the temporal extent of the disaster. A very large area, involving four distinct regions, was affected for a relatively long time. The earthquake affected some internal areas of the central Apennines: those areas are significantly far from the large and medium urban centres, as well as from the main poles of essential services, which have important environmental and cultural resources and constitute a profoundly diversified territory, the result of the dynamics of natural systems and of age-old processes of anthropization [27]. Like the Italian mountains, the internal areas of the central Apennines are subject to progressive depopulation and an aging population [28].

This territorial peculiarity is accompanied by an equally particular form of emergency management that is unprecedented in Italian history. Following the earthquake of 24th August 2016, which claimed 299 lives and resulted in around 12,500 damaged buildings, the institutions set up 43 tent camps and, at the same time, prepared for the reception of the population in habitable structures in the territory. From the beginning, however, Fabrizio Curcio, then head of the Civil Protection Department, underlined the intention to quickly dismantle the tent camps and identified some alternative housing solutions, contained in the Ordinance of the Head of the Civil Protection Department, 19th September 2016 n. 394: the granting of the autonomous accommodation contribution (CAS), the hospitality in public and hotel structures and the use of empty or second homes.

The seismic events of 26th and 30th October 2016 and of 18th January 2017, together with the worsening meteorological conditions, considerably complicated the scenario: there were another 34 fatalities; the so-called seismic crater expanded, including 140 municipalities; the number of damaged buildings increased, as well as the number of displaced persons, now reaching about 50,000. In addition to the housing assistance measures already provided for as a result of the first earthquake, the institutions added the Collective Housing Modules (MAC): temporary modular containers, consisting of accommodation modules with a maximum of three beds each, connected to shared toilets and collective spaces, such as refectories and living rooms. The MACs were installed in nine municipalities between Umbria and Marche, with a total of 23 residential settlements and 1,746 beds; moreover, they differed in size, hosting around 21 to 400 people. The MACs were to be considered as local temporary solutions, for those citizens with specific and urgent needs related, for example, to their work activity. In a previous study, Della Valle [29] further explored this solution, showing its limits and criticalities in terms of habitability. In addition to highlighting the fact that the most vulnerable population converged in the MACs, the research showed that the concept of comfort seemed to be absent, particularly in terms of its psychological–environmental meaning, which considers it as that "condition, belonging to – and sought after in – everyday life, from which the uncertainty and the unexpected are expelled" [30, p. 104]. The housing dimension, more than any other area of everyday life, should represent this variation of comfort, just because the house "is above all the place of the known, of the familiar, as opposed to the external world" [30, p. 104]. Thus, it is possible to highlight that the MAC areas, on the contrary, were characterized by dynamics that are not only foreign to the sphere of comfort but that even amplified the uncertainty, the unpredictability and the precariousness of the population that lived there. The experiences of hardship and suffering experienced by the population, the feeling of being forgotten by the institutions, the uncertainty about the future, the impossibility of regaining their domestic habits and their autonomy, among other things, cause us to reflect on whether MACs can actually be considered housing; indeed, they have certain characteristics that are more related to shelter.

The housing solutions briefly outlined so far represent the institutional responses offered to the population in the phase of the first post-earthquake emergency, which should include the removal of the rubble, the reopening of the disaster zones and the conclusion of the light reconstruction, thereby allowing those who have suffered non-structural damage to return to their homes. In order to guarantee long-term accommodation, however, for citizens with destroyed or severely damaged homes, or those located in the disaster zone, there are Emergency Housing Solutions (SAE), which were the subject of a European tender proposal by the Department of Protection Civil in April 2014 and awarded in August 2015. The tender involved the supply, transport and assembly of prefabricated anti-seismic housing units, which will host the population until the end of the reconstruction. Each housing unit was installed in settlements of variable sizes, whose aggregate layout was left to the discretion of the contracted company, as well as the choice of the types of module foundations and urbanization works. Although the tender provided for the possibility of two-storey solutions, the companies decided to install single-family and single-storey housing units; this, together with the absence of prescriptions guaranteeing the effective temporary nature of the modules, suggests a lack of attention on behalf of the institutions regarding the territorial impact of these structures, which were built according to the standards of permanent constructions, often compromising the local territory [31].

Although the Civil Protection Department stated that the realization of the SAE would take about seven months, only 1,054 out of 3,702 orders were delivered in October 2017, corresponding to 28.5% of the total [32]. After about two years from the first earthquake, the data published on 17th August 2018 show that 3,639 SAEs out of 3,857 ordered, 94.3%, have been completed [33].

4 RESEARCH QUESTION AND METHODS

Within such a scenario characterized by uncertainty and prolonged waiting, it is interesting to investigate how the inhabitants of temporary houses reproduce and modify their models of social interaction and how they perceive the living space that has been assigned to them, taking into account of the heterogeneity between the current settlements and the original context in which people lived. The physical environment is made up of objects, as the product of social interaction, that individuals and groups know and recognize, through an attribution of meaning. In order to understand how the actors develop their actions, therefore, it is essential on the one hand to identify the objects that make up the environment in which they live and act, and on the other hand to explore how this is perceived by the individuals, through a continuous formation and interpersonal transmission of meanings [34].

The assumption of this perspective, which recognizes the environment not as a passive substrate of human interaction but as an element with an active function, capable of conditioning action and producing territorial singularities [35], lays the foundations for a socio-territorial community study, focusing on the ways in which new housing configurations influence social ties and the possibility that they promote, or inhibit, the formation of social capital. Since the second half of the 20th century, the long sociological tradition of community studies has offered multiple, important contributions, among which *Middletown* by Lynd and Lynd [36]; *Marienthal: The Sociography of an Unemployed Community*, by Jahoda et al. [37]; *Street Corner Society* by Whyte [38]; *The Moral Basis of a Backward Society* by Banfield [39] or *The Levittowners*, written by Gans [40]. Although 20th century community studies have lost importance in today's scientific landscape, due to the lack of a precise definition of the research object and of a strong theoretical apparatus to refer to, it is possible to recognize a renewed vitality of this trend of studies. This is only possible if it is accepted, as an essential prerequisite, that the community does not constitute a fact, a homogeneous social group lived to a specific space, but rather an "object of a social construction by cooperating, competing or even conflicting actors" [35, p. 73], "a stake, or the outcome of a process that involves the project activity of a multiplicity of actors" [35, p. 79].

The approach that we want to support, in addition to recognizing the centrality of the community in the emergency and post-emergency phase, as suggested by Community-Based Disaster Management approach [23], [24], takes up a typical concept of the Chicago School, according to which social organization is configured not as a fact, but as a process. In a famous work, first published in 1918, Thomas and Znaniecki [41] develop the theory of social organization, within ecological theory, which underlines this procedural character. Conceiving society as being in perpetual change, the authors indicate three moments that belong to the continuous cycle of social life: social organization, social disorganization and social reorganization [42].

The characteristics of the research question, consistent with classical community studies, require a qualitative methodological approach, able to better understand the interactions and subjective interpretations of individuals and groups living in SAE areas. In particular, it was decided to refer to a SAE settlement whose housing units have been assigned to some citizens residing in a municipality of the Marche hinterland, which has few inhabitants but has an area of 78 km^2 in the province of Macerata. This choice is due to the fact that the socio-demographic, territorial and economic characteristics of the municipality, while reflecting the general tendencies of the internal areas of central Italy, present peculiar aspects, compared not only to national averages, but also to those of the other municipalities in the seismic crater. Of particular interest is the fragmentation of the municipal area, which has particular characteristics in terms of types of inhabited locality. They can be divided into three different categories: the inhabited centre, characterized by the presence of contiguous or nearby houses with interposed public services, constituting the condition for an autonomous form of social life; the inhabited nucleus, that is, an aggregate of houses, with at least five families, even if they neighbour each other, however, they do not constitute a place of social aggregation due to a lack of public services; the scattered houses, which are scattered across the municipal territory over such a distance that they cannot form an inhabited nucleus [43]. Before the disaster, the largest proportion of the population residing in the municipality (44.1%) lived in scattered houses, which represents 39.9% of total residential properties. This data is particularly significant if compared with the housing situation in the areas of the seismic crater. In fact, of all the population affected by the earthquakes, only 12.7% lived in scattered houses, which represent 16.8% of the residential buildings used. The difference is even more marked if compared to the national average data: the scattered houses represent 12% of the residential buildings inhabited, in which only 6% of Italians live [44].

In order to understand the dynamics preceding the disastrous event, the research will use second level data relating to the housing and territorial situation preceding the disaster, together with biographical interviews with some inhabitants of the SAE area. The ethnographic method, on the other hand, which combines observation, participation and dialogue, will allow us to explore in greater depth the context where social interaction usually takes shape, that is, in the SAE area [45]. Ethnographic notes and interviews represent the empirical material through which we will attempt to answer the research question, within the framework of the theory of argumentation. The qualitative methodological framework is also consistent with that widely used in Disaster Research, as an independent field of academic studies that was formalized in the 1960s with the foundation at the Ohio State University of the Disaster Research Center, the first research centre dealing with the study of disasters from a sociological perspective. The pioneering study by Prince in 1920 [46], the research conducted by the scholars of the National Opinion Research Center and of the Disaster Research Center, as well as those of the most recent research centres, share a marked sensitivity to qualitative methods. Indeed, they are better able to grasp the complexity of individuals and communities, which change rapidly and unexpectedly following a disaster. Qualitative Disaster Research, although often highlighting problems and inadequacies, such as an uneven use of data collection techniques or a lack of longitudinal research, can give voice to individuals and develop processes of individual and community empowerment [47].

5 FROM SHELTERING TO HOUSING: AN ETHNOGRAPHY IN THE SAE AREA

The results presented derive from the first phase of field exploration, consisting of three distinct ethnographic days. This indispensable phase of the research aims to achieve two complementary and interconnected objectives: on the one hand, the understanding of a sphere of social life that is foreign to the researcher; on the other, the possibility of developing and refining research in such a way that data and interpretations arise and remain rooted in the empirical context of study [34].

The SAE settlement was built in a flat agricultural area owned by the municipality, not far from the provincial road, near which there are some commercial activities. The SAEs were delivered to the mayor, then to the population, in December 2017, 16 months after the first earthquake and more than a year after the October 2016 shocks, which had a devastating effect on this territory, forcing most of the population to permanently abandon their homes. After the earthquakes of 26th and 30th October 2016, the mayor arranged for the first reception of the citizens, including many of the inhabitants of the SAE area, in the municipal hostel, the only public structure remaining accessible in the municipal territory. The temporary shelter identified by the mayor in place of the tent camps consisted of dormitories, each of which housed about 10 people, shared bathrooms and a common refreshment area. Volunteers from some local associations distributed the three daily meals for free.

From the stories of inhabitants it emerged that this first emergency phase represented a very difficult moment: in addition to the fear and desperation due to the events suffered, critical issues emerged regarding the overcrowding of the dormitories and the difficult balance between the schedules of the hostel and the daily and working life of individuals. In a short time, therefore, many of them chose alternative housing solutions. Some preferred those provided by the institutions, such as the CAS, public contributions with which to rent a house, or hospitality in hotels present on the territory or along the Adriatic coast.

Alternatively, others have implemented informal housing solutions, being able to count on the support of family or friendship networks. The mayor, who at first identified two areas in which to place Collective Housing Modules (MAC), decided not to install them. Pending the assignment of the SAE, in this municipality, as in many other affected places, the housing solutions adopted by the population were different, mainly depending on the varying possibilities and resources, therefore on the different forms of capital (economic, social and cultural) [14], of each individual or family. For some, the assignment of the SAE represented the possibility of returning to their territory of origin; for others, the opportunity to regain their own, albeit precarious, domestic autonomy. Overall, it is possible to affirm that the assignment of SAEs has constituted, for the earthquake-affected population, the transition from shelter to housing, as conceptualized by Quarantelli [6], [7].

The housing settlement in question consists of 19 SAEs, in which about 60 individuals live, the majority of whom were known only superficially or not known at all before the assignment. The housing units are distributed on two small parallel streets, each three metres wide, which span out from the car park adjacent to the area. In each street, the SAEs are arranged opposite each other, at a distance of six metres. The aggregation layout chosen by the construction company is defined as "terraced": it provides for the contiguous distribution of the housing units, leaving two free fronts (Fig. 1). They present a standard structure, imposed by the technical specifications of the European tender issued by the Civil Protection Department, but differ in size, according to the number of household members: typology A, of 40 m^2, is composed of a kitchen/living room, a bathroom and a bedroom and is intended for families of one or two members; typology B, of 60 m^2, has a second room, used to accommodate families of three or four individuals; finally, typology C is 80 m^2, it has three bedrooms and is intended for families of five or six people. In front of each SAE there is a covered outdoor area, a veranda, to ensure shelter from the sun and rain, designed as an extension of the living area and where tables and chairs are placed.

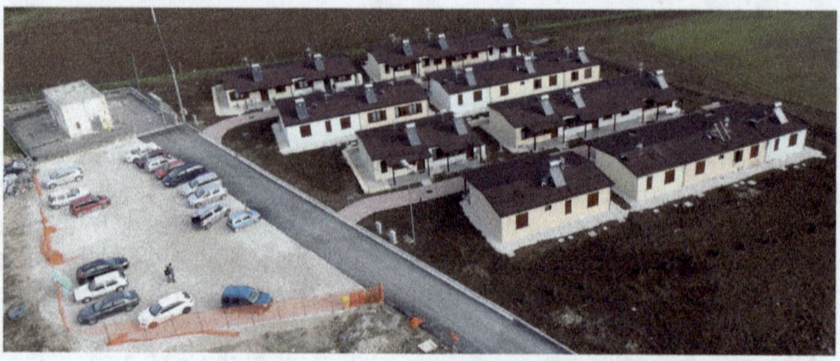

Figure 1: Photo of the SAE area. (*Source: Website Marche Region.*)

From a first exploration of the field it emerged that the demographic structure of the SAE settlement reproduces, at least in part, that of the municipality before the disaster. According to Istat data from July 2016, the population was 3,479 inhabitants, of which 9.5% foreigners. The demographic structure of the municipality showed a certain weakness, linked both to the incidence on the territory of people over 65 (29.6%) and to the limited presence of young people (10.5%), which results in a rather high old age index: 281.7 against 210.6 of the seismic crater municipalities and 161.4 of the Italian average. Furthermore, the low generational turnover is accompanied by a higher structural dependence, as the ratio between the non-active and working age population, equal to 66.8 compared to 59.6 of the seismic crater municipalities and 55.5 of Italy [44].

Similarly, in the SAE area there is a prevalence of elderly inhabitants, living alone or in pairs, and a limited number of households with children. Foreign families, on the other hand, are overrepresented, because they live in about one SAE out of three. The interesting question is that they, almost in their totality, were assigned SAEs located in one of the two streets of the housing settlement. The result is a strong ecological division of the area, which influences the forms and ways through which the inhabitants interact with each other. In fact, the inhabitants of each street are more likely to interact with their neighbours and minimise social contact with the other individuals in the settlement. If compared to a much larger scale, like the reality of a big metropolis, this is what probably some sociologists of the Chicago School, including Park [48], would have called natural areas, characterized by a certain degree of socio-cultural homogeneity that promotes interpersonal knowledge and, often, the creation of ties of solidarity. However, as Castrignanò [49] points out, in areas of study that are territorially and numerically smaller, as in the case of the SAE area, it is more appropriate to refer to urban interstices (buildings, condominiums, street crossings or small streets) or to "non-public collective spaces", meaning, for example, courtyards and walkways inside buildings but outside homes, "able to act as incubators to establishment of relationships, with a high 'recognition coefficient' that allows rooting in a known and familiar environment" [50, p. 203].

In the SAE area, each street often turns into a place of meeting and socializing; the veranda of each house, under which individuals, especially the older ones, sit and spend a good part of the day, becoming the privileged observation point over what is happening, but also the prevailing communicative space, given the spatial proximity between the housing units. This aspect, if related to the pre-disaster housing situation, is very interesting. Individuals have, in fact, passed from an extremely disaggregated mountain-housing context, characterized by a considerable presence of scattered houses, to an aggregated context, similar to that which can be found in the city. Informal interviews with some inhabitants show an increase in the perception of security related to this new housing configuration. Individuals can now count on the help and support of others if something happens, such as a new earthquake. Some have pointed out that it is sufficient to raise their tone of voice to be heard by neighbours, unlike the situation in their previous homes. Others have said that they willingly sacrificed some features of mountain life, being in contact with nature, in exchange for the advantage of the spatial and social proximity they now have. Experiencing the dramatic event of the earthquake, and the subsequent emergency phase, has certainly upset them but, at the same time, it has brought them closer. Within each street, in fact, individuals can count on the help and goodwill of neighbours. There is no lack of reciprocal exchanges of small daily favours, such as shopping or borrowing something; sometimes there is even the creation of fiduciary and solidarity ties demonstrated, for example, by the possibility that some inhabitants entrust their children to neighbours for a short period of time.

6 CONCLUSIONS

In conclusion, the exploration phase of the SAE area has revealed some important elements, to be further explored during the research. Among these, there is certainly the perception, by the inhabitants, of both the individual living space and the non-public collective spaces [50]; the modalities of assigning SAEs by the institutions, in an attempt to understand the reasons underlying the ecological division of the settlement; the creation and reproduction of social capital, bridging, bonding or linking, within the two streets that compose the SAE area, in order to reflect on the role of the community in the recovery process. Finally, reading the disaster with the conceptual triad proposed by Thomas and Znaniecki [41], the exploratory phase has brought out an interesting suggestion, which will certainly be explored further later. Just as the disaster would mark the passage from a phase of social organization to one of social disorganization, the assignment of SAEs, or the transition from shelter to housing, would allow a first social reorganization, which, in the post-recovery phase, would stabilize into a new social organization. This, in line with what has been argued in the theoretical part, could have repercussions on exit routes and strategies, especially for the most vulnerable individuals. While not considering these as linear and orderly moments, but being characterized by fluidity and dynamism, the result is a circular reading of the disaster, which actively involves communities and territories, during a continuous process, from the pre-disaster phase to post-recovery one.

REFERENCES

[1] Ligi, G., *Antropologia dei disastri,* Laterza: Roma, 2009.
[2] Perry, R.W., Defining disaster: An evolving concept. *Handbook of Disaster Research*, eds H. Rodríguez, W. Donner & J.E. Trainor, Springer: Cham, pp. 3–22, 2018.
[3] Quarantelli, E.L., A social science research agenda for disasters of the 21st century: Theoretical, methodological and empirical issues and their professional implementation. *What is a Disaster: New Answers to Old Questions*, eds R.W. Perry & E.L. Quarantelli, Xlibris Publishers: Philadelphia, pp. 325–396, 2005.
[4] Wisner, B., Blaikie, P., Cannon, T. & Davis, I., *At Risk: Natural Hazards, People's Vulnerability, and Disaster*, Routledge: London, 2004.
[5] Bennicelli Pasqualis, M., *Case Temporanee. Strategie Innovative per L'emergenza Abitativa Post Terremoto*, Franco Angeli: Milan, 2014.
[6] Quarantelli, E.L., General and particular observations on sheltering and housing in American disasters. *Disasters*, **6**(4), pp. 277–281, 1982.
[7] Quarantelli, E.L., Patterns of sheltering and housing in US disasters. *Disaster Prevention and Management: An International Journal,* **4**(3), pp. 43–53, 1995.
[8] Peacock, W.G., Dash, N., Zhang, Y. & Van Zandt, S., Post-disaster sheltering, temporary housing and permanent housing recovery. *Handbook of Disaster Research*, eds H. Rodríguez, W. Donner & J.E. Trainor, Springer: Cham, pp. 569–594, 2018.
[9] Corsellis, T. & Vitale A., *Transitional Settlement, Displaced Populations*, Oxfam: Oxford, 2005.
[10] Ciccozzi, A., I pericoli della ricostruzione: antropologia dell'abitare e rischio sociosanitario nel dopo-terremoto aquilano. *Epidemiologia & Prevenzione*, **40**(2), pp. 93–97, 2016.
[11] Dynes, R.R., *Community Social Capital as the Primary Basis for Resilience*. Disaster Research Center, University of Delaware, Preliminary paper 344, 2005.
[12] Meyer, M.A., Social capital in disaster research. *Handbook of Disaster Research*, eds H. Rodríguez, W. Donner & J.E. Trainor, Springer: Cham, pp. 265–286, 2018.
[13] Lin, N., *Social Capital: A Theory of Social Structure and Action*, Cambridge University Press: New York, 2001.
[14] Bourdieu, P., The forms of capital. *Handbook of Theory and Research for the Sociology of Education,* ed. J.G Richardson, Greenwood: New York, pp. 241–258, 1986.
[15] Coleman, J.S., *Foundations of Social Theory*, Belknap Press: Cambridge and London, 1990.

[16] Putnam, R.D., The prosperous community: Social capital and public life. *The American Prospect*, **4**(13). 1993. http://prospect.org/article/prosperous-community-social-capital-and-public-life. Accessed on: 5 May 2019.
[17] Putnam, R.D., Thinking about social change in America. *Bowling Alone. The Collapse and Revival of American Community,* ed. R.D. Putnam, Simon & Schuster: New York, pp. 12–27, 2000.
[18] Aldrich, D.P., Social capital in post disaster recovery: Towards a resilient and compassionate East Asian community. *Economic and Welfare Impacts of Disasters in East Asia and Policy Responses*, eds Y. Sawada & S. Oum, ERIA: Jakarta, pp. 157–178, 2012.
[19] Aldrich, D.P. & Meyer, M.A., Social capital and community resilience. *American Behavioral Scientist*, **59**(2), pp. 254–269, 2015.
[20] Hawkins, R.L. & Maurer, K., Bonding, bridging and linking: How social capital operated in New Orleans following Hurricane Katrina. *British Journal of Social Work*, **40**, pp. 1777–1793, 2010.
[21] Spokane, A.R., Mori, Y. & Martinez, F., Housing arrays following disasters: Social vulnerability considerations in designing transitional communities. *Environment and Behavior*, **45**(7), pp. 887–911, 2013.
[22] Buckland, J. & Rahman, M., Community-based disaster management during the 1997 Red River Flood in Canada. *Disasters*, **23**(2), pp. 174–191, 1999.
[23] Allen, K.M., Community-based disaster preparedness and climate adaptation: Local capacity-building in the Philippines. *Disasters*, **30**(1), pp. 81–101, 2006.
[24] Pandey, B. & Okazaki, K., Community based disaster management: Empowering communities to cope with disaster risks. United Nations Centre for Regional Development, Japan, 2012. http://citeseerx.ist.psu.edu/viewdoc/download?doi=10.1.1.467.1932&rep=rep1&type=pdf. Accessed on: 5 May 2019.
[25] Minamoto, Y., Social capital and livelihood recovery: Post-tsunami Sri Lanka as a case. *Disaster Prevention and Management*, **19**(5), pp. 548–564, 2010.
[26] Piselli, F., Capitale sociale: Un concetto situazionale e dinamico. *Stato e mercato*, **3**, pp. 395–417, 1999.
[27] Barca, F., Casavola, P. & Lucatelli, S., Strategia nazionale per le Aree interne: Definizione, obiettivi, strumenti e governance. *Materiali Uval*, **31**, 2014.
[28] Fondazione Montagne Italia, *Rapporto Montagne Italia 2016.* www.dropbox.com/s/f76iz9bmebgx32c/RAPPORTO%20MONTAGNE%20ITALIA_STAMPA.pdf?dl=0. Accessed on: 5 May 2019.
[29] Della Valle, C., Con-vivere con il terremoto. Il sisma dell'Appennino Centrale e le soluzione-container nelle Regioni Umbria e Marche, Masters thesis, University of Bologna, 2018.
[30] Marrone, V., La costruzione sociale dell'efficienza energetica. Un approccio sistemico a CasaClima. *Sociologia Urbana e Rurale*, **114**, pp. 95–112, 2017.
[31] Emidio di Treviri, *Sul fronte del sisma. Un'inchiesta militante sul post-terremoto dell'Appennino centrale (2016–2017)*, DeriveApprodi: Roma, 2018.
[32] Terremoto Centro Italia, i numeri dell'emergenza a un anno dalle scosse del 26 e 30 ottobre. Dipartimento della Protezione Civile – Presidenza del Consiglio dei Ministri. www.protezionecivile.gov.it/media-comunicazione/comunicati-stampa/dettaglio/-/asset_publisher/default/content/terremoto-centro-italia-i-numeri-dell-emergenza-a-un-anno-dalle-scosse-del-26-e-del-30-ottobre. Accessed on: 5 May 2019.

[33] Dipartimento della Protezione Civile – Presidenza del Consiglio dei Ministri, I numeri del sisma in Centro Italia. www.protezionecivile.gov.it/resources/cms/documents/Aggiornamento_dati_Terremoto_Centro_Italia.pdf. Accessed on: 5 Mar. 2019.

[34] Blumer, H., *Symbolic Interactionism. Perspective and Method,* University of California Press: Englewood Cliffs, 1969.

[35] Mela, A., Per una nuova generazione di studi di comunità. *Sociologia Urbana e Rurale*, **110**, pp. 71–85, 2016.

[36] Lynd, R.S. & Lynd, H.M., *Middletown: A Study in American Culture*, Harcourt, Brace and World: New York, 1965.

[37] Jahoda, M., Lazarsfeld, P.F. & Zeisel, H., *Marienthal: The Sociography of an Unemployed Community*, Tavistock: London, 1972.

[38] Whyte, W.F., *Street Corner Society: The Social Structure of an Italian Slum*, University of Chicago Press: Chicago, 1943.

[39] Banfield, E.C., *The Moral Basis of a Backward Society*, The Free Press: Illinois, 1958.

[40] Gans, H.J., *The Levittowners: Ways of Life and Politics in a New Suburban Community*, Pantheon Books: New York, 1967.

[41] Thomas, W.I. & Znaniecki, F., *The Polish Peasant in Europe and America*, Alfred A. Knopf: New York, 1927.

[42] Romania, V., La Scuola di Chicago e la sua eredità. *Lezioni Italiane. L'eredità Della Scuola di Chicago*, ed. V. Romania, Orthotes: Napoli and Salerno, pp. 41–71, 2018.

[43] Glossario Istat, http://dawinci.istat.it/daWinci/jsp/MD/misc.jsp?p=7._Accessed on: 16 May 2019.

[44] Caratteristiche dei territori colpiti dal sisma del 24 agosto, 26 ottobre e 30 ottobre 2016 e 18 gennaio 2017, Istat. www.istat.it/it/archivio/199364. Accessed on: 5 May 2019.

[45] Cardano, M., *La Ricerca Qualitativa*, Il Mulino: Bologna, 2011.

[46] Prince, S.H., *Catastrophe and Social Change. Based upon a Sociologic Study of the Halifax Disaster*, Columbia University Press: New York, 1920.

[47] Phillips, B., Qualitative methods and disaster research. *International Journal of Mass Emergencies and Disaster*, **15**(1), pp. 179–195, 1997.

[48] Park, R.E., *Human Communities: The City and Human Ecology,* The Free Press: Glencoe, IL, 1952.

[49] Castrignanò, M., Il concetto di comunità: quale spendibilità per la sociologia urbana? *Sociologia Urbana e Rurale*, **88**, pp. 73–88, 2009.

[50] Micheli, G.A., "Vis resistiva": Come indurre a ridefinire lo spazio-azione dell'anziano, *Le sfide dell'esclusione: metodi, luoghi, soggetti*, ed. E. Mingione, Il Mulino: Bologna, pp. 197–217, 1999.

SCIENCE DURING CRISIS: THE ROLE OF SCIENCE IN DISASTER RESPONSE

GARY E. MACHLIS
Clemson University, USA

ABSTRACT

The number, scale, intensity, impact, and cost of environmental and technological disasters is increasing, from Category 5 hurricanes/typhoons to earthquakes in dense and growing urban spaces. Since 2014, the international community has experienced 1,639 man-made and natural disaster events that collectively have caused over 75,000 fatalities and US$917 billion in damages and recovery costs. Protecting human health, reducing risk, and improving outcomes requires science-informed decision-making. Hence, science during crises is of critical importance, and improved collaboration between scientists and disaster-response practitioners is essential. In this paper, based on the recent US Academy of Arts and Sciences report *Science During Crisis*, a set of best practices, research needs, and policy priorities are presented, along with case examples. Best practices range from the creation of interdisciplinary research teams, expanded joint training of emergency response and scientific communities, to central, curated clearinghouses for available data and insights deliverable in ways that response practitioners can use. Research needs to include improved baseline information, scenario-building to better understand cascading consequences, and more effective communication of science to managers, decision-makers, and the public during a disaster event. Policy priorities range from improving accessibility through to published scientific information and developing a code of conduct for scientists engaged in response. Case examples include the Gulf of Mexico Deepwater Horizon oil spill (2010), the Haitian earthquake (2010), the Fukushima Daiichi nuclear accident in Japan (2011), Typhoon Haiyan in the Philippines (2013), the South American and Caribbean zika virus emergency (2016), and Hurricane Maria in Puerto Rico (2017). A call to action is presented to improve the management, operation, and application of science during crises, in ways that increase the use, applicability, and value of science to disaster-response personnel.

Keywords: science, crisis, best practices, research needs, policy priorities.

1 INTRODUCTION

The number, scale, intensity, impact, and cost of environmental and technological disasters is increasing, from Category 5 hurricanes/typhoons to earthquakes in dense and growing urban spaces. The types of large-scale disasters range from the Gulf of Mexico Deepwater Horizon oil spill (2010), the Haitian earthquake (2010), the Fukushima Daiichi nuclear accident in Japan (2011), Typhoon Haiyan in the Philippines (2013), the South American and Caribbean zika virus emergency (2016), to Hurricane Maria in Puerto Rico (2017) and more. Since 2014, the international community has experienced 1,639 man-made and natural disaster events that collectively have caused over 75,000 fatalities and US$917 billion in damages and recovery costs [1]. These weather and climate disasters – along with natural hazards such as earthquakes, public health crises arising from disease outbreaks, and human-caused disasters such as contaminant spills and industrial accidents – threaten human lives and pose challenges to relief efforts, restoring ecosystems, and rebuilding communities.

Science – including biological, physical, social, behavioral, cultural, engineering, and medical disciplines – plays an important role in responding to such crises. Physicians and geochemists collaborated in assessing the short- and long-term health impacts of dust from the September 11, 2001 attacks on the World Trade Center [2]. In 2010, scientists and engineers with expertise in oceanography, geology, engineering, physics, public health, and ecology helped contain the Deepwater Horizon oil spill and assess the extent of its damage to the Gulf Coast. Immediately following the 2010 Haitian earthquake, the European

doi:10.2495/DMAN190091

Commission's Joint Research Council analyzed satellite imagery to produce a rapid damage assessment to inform prioritization of emergency response actions [3]. When Hurricane Sandy made US landfall in 2012, scientists and engineers were summoned to evaluate structural damage, assess health and environmental risks, and provide direction for response and recovery efforts. During the emergency response to the 2013 Typhoon Haiyan in the Philippines, the UN Office for Coordination of Humanitarian Affairs coordinated crowd-sourced mapping along with satellite and other data to develop emergency response maps. In 2016, when the Zika virus threatened the well-being of Caribbean, South American, and US citizens, experts from a variety of scientific fields worked together to assess human-health and environmental impacts and develop interventions ranging from genetically modified mosquitoes to chemical spraying [4]. In each case, science during crisis was essential to an effective response.

A rich literature on preparing for crises exists, but strategic deployment of scientific expertise and application of scientific information *during* crisis events is understudied. There is a critical need to develop best practices to collect relevant data; work together with affected communities; establish interdisciplinary teams; coordinate scientists, engineers, crisis managers, and decision-makers when disaster strikes; and ensure their collaboration through the crisis, response, and recovery.

2 WHAT COMPRISES SCIENCE DURING CRISIS

Crisis events are most often acute disruptions (such as a 5.9 Richter magnitude earthquake) and place-specific (such as the L'Aquila earthquake in the Abruzzo region of Italy), with consequences for both natural and human systems. Science during crisis includes conducting scientific research and analyzing data, as well as organizing, staffing, communicating, and archiving scientific and technical resources during the crisis event – which for many events like earthquakes can last far beyond when the main shock and intense aftershocks end [5].

Science during crisis requires the engagement of scientists and engineers across a broad range of disciplines, as well as emergency managers, resource managers, policy-makers, and the public. Because crises impact people and infrastructure and/or environmental assets of societal value, science during crisis is necessarily human-centric. Science during crises helps guide decision-making, from search and rescue operations and environmental remediation plans to health monitoring and evacuation planning. Further, scientific work in emergency response directly impacts the lives and livelihoods of survivors in a crisis-affected area.

Science during crisis has distinctive characteristics. For scientists serving in a crisis response, the protocols and time-scales of conducting research during the crisis differ from the usual practice of science. Typically, scientific research is deliberate and iterative, with peer-reviewed publications the hallmark of success. In contrast, science in support of emergency management is rapid, decisive, and typically delivers results necessarily based on more limited and uncertain information. Success is gauged by lives saved, injuries reduced, ecosystem and infrastructure services restored, speed of recovery, and development of mitigation tools for future disasters. These differing strategies and goals can impair coordination and information-sharing during response [6]. They can also jeopardize careful consideration of challenges, risks, and ethical protections inherent in scientific undertakings. Little formal training in emergency response, ethical issues, or legal obligations is available for scientists to inform their work during crises. Similarly, there are few examples available of technical training in the sciences or the application of science for emergency managers.

3 THE IMPORTANCE OF SCIENCE DURING CRISIS

While weather and climate crises, natural hazards, public health crises, and technological disasters are inevitable, so are their cascading consequences across social, economic, and environmental systems. The challenges are exacerbated by significant human population growth, socioeconomic disparities, environmental factors including climate change, and diminishing natural resources. As the complexity of events increases, interdisciplinary science during crisis becomes increasingly important, and scientists will face new challenges in problem-solving, communicating results, and coordinating with response managers and decision-makers. Significant advances are needed in developing best practices, a research agenda for response, and policy reforms for science during crisis.

A persistent problem in responding to a crisis event is the temptation to "fight the last war". For example, a common initial assumption is that a new oil spill is similar to one that occurred previously in the US – the signature of and response to the Exon Valdez oil spill of 1989 (a surface spill) slowed understanding of the Deepwater Horizon oil spill's (a spill 1,500 meters below the surface) potential impact. Yet every disaster is in some ways unique, and every disaster is local. Scientists, emergency managers, policy-makers, and response personnel must maintain flexibility, recognize both new and experienced voices from a variety of backgrounds and disciplines, and encourage creativity in identifying solutions and possible interventions as quickly as possible. Actions taken during crisis are likely to come under intense scrutiny, with pressure from a constant news cycle, demanding politicians, and the looming threat of litigation. Science can support legally defensible, evidence-based decisions during crisis and play an important role in informing emergency managers, policy-makers, and the public. While the threat of liability or even prosecution – such as the conviction (and later acquittal) of scientists for manslaughter in the aftermath of the deadly 2009 L'Aquila, Italy, earthquake – is a potential deterrent to scientists who wish to contribute their expertise during crisis, scientists must be ready to engage during crisis [7].

Science has played an important role during crisis for decades, and the scope of that work is broadening. The US experience is instructive. During World War II, the Office of Strategic Services (OSS) recruited scientists and engineers to provide expertise and support intelligence efforts. More recently, National Oceanic and Atmospheric Administration (NOAA) Scientific Support Coordinators have served as technical experts to support the response to oil and chemical spills in US waters [8]. Similarly, the National Weather Service (NWS) created Incident Meteorologist positions to transmit critical weather forecasts to firefighters [9]. In the public health arena, the National Institutes of Health (NIH) launched a Disaster Research Response Program (DR2P) to "create a disaster research system consisting of coordinated environmental health disaster research data collection tools and a network of trained research responders," supported by library resources coordinated by the National Library of Medicine [10]. The Centers for Disease Control and Prevention (CDC) created Global Rapid Response Teams offering technical and scientific advice in the face of global public health crises [11]. Incident management at the Department of Health and Human Services routinely includes scientists from the CDC and NIH. The Department of the Interior (DOI) established the Strategic Sciences Group (SSG), modeled after the OSS, to be deployed during crises to provide interdisciplinary scientific assessments to DOI leadership. Agencies like the US Geological Survey (USGS) coordinate with the Federal Emergency Management Agency (FEMA) to ensure scientists are on site during exercises to provide situational awareness.

Other examples exist – science is embedded in the Italian Department of Civil Protection's Augustus Method support functions, the UK's guidance documents "Emergency Preparedness" and "Emergency Response and Recovery", and Australia's Emergency

Management Manual. The Disaster Risk Management Knowledge Centre (DRMKC) fosters EU-level disaster science networks to support the European Response Coordination Centre and provide science-based advice to policy-makers. Though not an exhaustive list, these examples of organizational responses highlight the vital and growing role of science and scientists during crisis. It is to advance and improve the delivery of science during disaster events that the report "Science During Crisis: Best Practices, Research Needs, and Policy Priorities" was prepared [12].

4 ABOUT THE REPORT

In April 2017, the American Academy of Arts and Sciences held a workshop to address issues surrounding science during crisis. The Academy, founded in 1780, has served the United States as a champion of scholarship, civil dialogue, and useful knowledge. One of the nation's oldest learned societies and independent policy research centers, the Academy convenes leaders from the academic, business, arts, and government sectors to address critical challenges facing global society and provide decision-makers with authoritative and nonpartisan policy advice. The workshop on science during crisis was convened through the Academy's Public Face of Science Project, which is addressing various aspects of the complex and evolving relationship between science and the public in the United States.

The workshop engaged a diverse and interdisciplinary group of scientists, communicators and decision-makers. Workshop participants made presentations and engaged in extensive dialogue and discussion. The discussions centered on the experiences of the participants during crises and recent advances in improving the application of science for preparedness, response, and recovery. With the workshop presentations and discussions as foundation, the report provides recommendations to:

1. Identify best practices for employing, facilitating, communicating, and conducting science during a crisis;
2. Describe critical research needed to strengthen science during a crisis; and
3. Identify and prioritize policy recommendations to promote and facilitate science during a crisis.

Selected recommendations with relevance both for and beyond the United States are described below.

5 RECOMMENDATIONS FOR IMPROVING BEST PRACTICES

Best practices can advance "mission-ready" capabilities and streamline the process of employing science during crisis. This includes best practices for funding, staffing, execution, analysis, communication, and archiving of the resulting science. Such practices must reflect a range of scientific disciplines and professional organizations, meet accepted ethical standards, and protect the rights of affected persons and communities.

International, national, state, and local agencies should have available emergency funds for science during crisis. Expedited funding is necessary to enable rapid deployment and capture ephemeral and time-critical data. Dedicated funding should be set aside for research during emergency response. Administrative requirements within government agencies, universities, and other institutions should be flexible enough to enable rapid deployment of funds for science during crisis. Currently, the NSF grants for Rapid Response Research (RAPID) provide a good example. This funding mechanism allows short proposals to be processed and awarded within one to two weeks of receipt.

The emergency-response and scientific communities should expand joint training and outreach/education. Mutual understanding of well-articulated priorities, protocols, practices, and responsibilities will improve the capacity of emergency managers and scientists to coordinate activities and work safely. Some dimensions of training, such as ethics and community engagement, may require the development of new standards and best practices. Opportunities for joint training include scenario-building and emergency response exercises.

At the onset of a crisis, a central curated clearinghouse developed in advance should be activated to collect, disseminate, and coordinate relevant scientific information. Access to information during crises facilitates research. In addition, emergency managers can leverage available information to improve situational awareness, facilitate decisions, and inform the public. The optimum set of information should include existing baseline data, data collected during the crisis, decision-support tools, standardized tools for rapid data collection, models, forecasts, and preexisting research literature relevant to the event and plausible cascading consequences. Appropriate protocols should be put in place to ensure data security, particularly protection of personally identifiable information.

6 RECOMMENDATIONS FOR A RESEARCH AGENDA

Science during crisis must constantly evolve to incorporate new technologies, methods, data, and information, and to improve the delivery of usable knowledge. Supporting this process requires an interdisciplinary research agenda that takes into account both basic and applied questions regarding science during crisis. This research agenda can and should be implemented by the academic, public, private, and nongovernmental sectors.

6.1 Establishing baseline information

When crisis strikes, baseline environmental, human health, social, and economic data are critical to understanding both the short- and long-term effects of the disaster. Such data provide scientists with the ability to pre-send robust information on crisis-induced changes to decision-makers and the public. Key questions for the research agenda include:

1. What is the best way to identify and/or update baseline information needed for science during crisis in anticipation of future disasters?
2. How can the collection of baseline health data for disaster responders, including scientists, be integrated into disaster preparedness protocols?
3. What are the best methods for collecting, archiving, and sharing baseline data relevant to a crisis?

6.2 Understanding cascading consequences to document and predict the complexity of environmental and social disasters, and to improve response and rebuilding strategies

Disasters create cascading consequences for coupled human-natural systems, and understanding these consequences is essential for both emergency response and restoration of human communities, local economies, and ecosystems. Key questions include:

1. What are the environmental, health, social, and economic cascading consequences of disasters, and can they be predicted?
2. What are the consequences of repetitive disasters (such as repeated hurricanes) in one location?
3. What are the best ways to forecast cascading consequences in order to support decision-making during a crisis?
4. How has engagement between scientific institutions and affected communities advanced or hindered long-term resilience and public trust in science?

6.3 Addressing divergent scientific opinions, data, and results during crisis

During a crisis, decision-makers may be faced with studies with different or conflicting results. Such disparate findings can complicate evidence-based decision-making. Researchers should develop effective protocols and methodologies for addressing divergent scientific opinions and communicating uncertainty that may result from science during crisis. Key questions include:

1. What methods are most effective for addressing divergent scientific views during a crisis?
2. To what extent should data be proven reproducible during crisis? Do different standards apply?
3. What are the best methods for synthesizing divergent scientific findings and associated uncertainty?

6.4 Communicating science during crisis

The delivery and presentation of scientific information during a crisis – to decision-makers, the media, and the public – can significantly affect emergency response, public safety, and restoration activities. Key questions include:

1. What visualization techniques and methods of delivery or presentation are best-suited to communicating scientific information to different audiences?
2. What is the best way to: a) streamline technical communications for different audiences at different times; b) account for a variety of scientific perspectives and findings; c) address potential ethical concerns in the communication of sensitive data; and d) avoid information overload, misinterpretation, and unnecessary confusion?

6.5 Assessing how science-based decisions are made

Understanding what information is used by decision-makers and how it is used to make decisions is important for advancing the applicability of science during a crisis. Key questions include:

1. How and to what extent is scientific and technical information used in crisis decision-making?
2. What are the ethical, moral, and legal considerations that need to be considered as scientists inform decision-making processes?
3. What are the best ways to ensure science is effectively considered in crisis decision-making?

6.6 Using big data to support science during crisis

Big data sets such as those derived from social media and complex models are important complements to data collected on the ground during a crisis, and can contribute to both situational awareness and, in some cases, quality control and assurance. At the same time, reliance on big data, particularly data generated by local communities, can give rise to inherent biases in the data, given varying degrees of technological capability and access of segments of the population. Key questions include:

1. How can multiple streams of data from disparate sources (including government data, published data, grey literature, unpublished data, models, and social media) be identified and quality-assured to respond effectively and rapidly to research needs during a crisis?
2. What advances in computing and data visualization are necessary to streamline the collection, analysis, and delivery of crowd-sourced data and/or information gleaned from social media?
3. What ethical and practical challenges need to be considered when relying on big data sources, particularly those generated voluntarily by local communities?

7 POLICY RECOMMENDATIONS TO IMPROVE SCIENCE DURING CRISIS

Changes in current international, national, state, and local policies are needed to improve science during crisis. These changes will advance the conduct of science, access to and use of scientific data, the role of science in decision-making, and improve crisis response and recovery. In addition to government policies, improvements are needed in policies governing academic institutions, communities of practice, nongovernmental organizations, and private industry. Implementation of policy recommendations will vary by country, province/state, and local political institutions.

Gaps or lack of understanding between different professional cultures can lead to a mismatch between scientific activity, emergency response, and on-the-ground needs. It can also lead to a lack of institutional support for science during crisis at the regional and local level. State and provincial governments should create a Chief Science Officer position (and/or strengthen existing positions) to facilitate science during crisis. Creating a Chief Science Officer position would reduce confusion and facilitate effective conduct and application of science during crisis. The Chief Science Officer would serve as a critical liaison between national, state or provincial, and local government offices, emergency responders, and the scientific community.

Publishers of scientific journals and books should develop and implement policies that improve accessibility of scientific information during a crisis. During a crisis, access to up-to-date research is critical for the scientific community to identify gaps that need immediate attention and to find scientific solutions to pressing problems. Further, the rapid dissemination of data collected during a crisis but prior to publication is often critical for decision-making and to avoid unnecessary duplication of effort. Publishers should adopt a policy of providing free, publicly available, full-text access to journals, e-books, and databases with relevant information during and immediately following major crises. Recent advances within the biomedical community provide a potential model.

The scientific community should develop a code of conduct that addresses ethical and professional practices to which scientists engaged in science during crisis would adhere. A science during crisis code of conduct would describe scientists' distinct ethical responsibilities during a major crisis. The code of conduct should favor altruism over competition in scientific research and should recognize the primacy and rights of the communities and sovereign tribes immediately affected by the crisis. The code of conduct would recognize that science during crisis operates differently than science during non-crisis times and should be developed and agreed upon by the burgeoning science during crisis community of practice.

8 A CALL TO ACTION

Environmental and technological disasters cannot be eliminated. Each disaster and its legacy will be characterized by a unique combination of location, timing, size, duration, losses, decisions, and response. Yet risks and damage can be reduced and responses improved by the timely application of scientific knowledge. Science across all relevant disciplines will continue to play an important role in informing critical decisions and helping to guide response and recovery. The scientific community, in partnership with the emergency management community and decision-makers at all levels, has been involved in conducting, organizing, staffing, communicating, and archiving science during crisis. But further progress is needed. Best practices must be defined, a research agenda put in place, and policy reforms initiated.

Science during crisis has many long-term benefits. It can foster interdisciplinary collaborations within and among the scientific community, emergency response managers, local communities, national, state/provincial, and local governments, and the private sector. Effective engagement of local communities and citizens – particularly those who are underrepresented or highly vulnerable – can improve trust, risk perception, communication, and coordination during crisis, as well as improve long-term outcomes. The scientific community can provide more efficient and effective scientific responses to future crises.

The Academy report is a call to action for government agencies, academic institutions, professional organizations, and stakeholders who rely on and contribute to science during crisis. Future disasters will only be more frequent, severe, costly, and deadly; the communities affected by these events will need the very best science during crisis supporting them. The recommendations in the American Academy of Arts and Sciences report, if acted upon, will contribute toward that important goal.

ACKNOWLEDGEMENTS

The author would like to thank the American Academy of Arts and Sciences for the Academy's support of this effort through its Public Face of Science project, funded by the Gordon and Betty Moore Foundation and the Rita Allen Foundation, including publication of its 2019 report *Science During Crisis: Best Practices, Research Needs, and Policy Priorities*. Portions of this paper are adapted and/or excerpted from that report. Deep acknowledgement and appreciation go to Dr. Rita Colwell, co-author of *Science During Crisis*. Dr. John Randell, Director of the Academy's Science, Engineering, and Technology Programs has been an enthused and committed supporter of the overall project. I also want to thank Dr. Kris Ludwig, whose organizational and intellectual contribution to the workshop and report was significant and highly valued. Maddie Duda provided excellent research support. Brendan Roach, Mandel Presidential Fellow at the Academy, assisted with preparation of the paper, and his skilled contribution is gratefully acknowledged.

REFERENCES

[1] Swiss Re Institute, Sigma Research, Sigma 1/2018: Natural catastrophes and man-made disasters in 2017: A year of record-breaking losses. www.swissre.com/institute/research/sigma-research/sigma-2018-01.html. Accessed on: 15 May 2019.

[2] Plumlee, G., Report from ground zero: How geoscientists aid in the aftermath of environmental disasters. *Earth Magazine*, 1 October 2009. www.earthmagazine.org/article/report-ground-zero. Accessed on: 16 May 2019.

[3] European Commission, European Commission supports relief efforts in Haiti with first damage assessment: Facts and Maps. http://europa.eu/rapid/press-release_IP-10-25_en.htm?locale=en. Accessed on: 20 May 2019.

[4] Committee on Science of the National Science and Technology Council, A strategy for integrating best practices with new science to prevent disease transmission by

Aedes mosquito vectors, Executive Office of the President of the United States: Washington, DC, 2016.

[5] Machlis, G. & Ludwig, K., Science during crisis: The application of interdisciplinary and strategic science during major environmental crises. *Understanding Society and Natural Resources*, eds M.J. Manfredo, J.J. Vaske, A. Rechkemmer & E.A. Duke, Springer: Dordrecht, pp. 47–65, 2014.

[6] Mease L., Gibbs-Plessl, T., Erickson, A., Ludwig, K., Reddy, C. & Lubchenco, J., Designing a solution to enable agency-academic scientific collaboration for disasters. *Ecology and Society*, **22**(2), p. 18, 2017.

[7] Cartlidge, E., Earthquake experts convicted of manslaughter. *Science Magazine*, 22 Oct. 2012. www.sciencemag.org/news/2012/10/earthquake-experts-convicted-manslaughter. Accessed on: 16 May 2019.

[8] National Oceanic and Atmospheric Administration, Office of Response and Restoration, OR&R field staff locations and contact information. response.restoration.noaa.gov/about/orr-field-staff.html. Accessed on: 20 May 2019.

[9] National Oceanic and Atmospheric Administration, National Weather Service, A day in the life of a NWS meteorologist: Incident meteorologists. www.weather.gov/jkl/Day_In_The_Life_Day13. Accessed on: 20 May 2019.

[10] US Department of Health and Human Services, NIH Disaster Research Response (DR2), About the program. dr2.nlm.nih.gov/about. Accessed on: 20 May 2019.

[11] Centers for Disease Control and Prevention, Global Health Protection and Security, Global Health Protection and Security: CDC Global Rapid Response Team. www.cdc.gov/globalhealth/healthprotection/errb/global-rrt.htm. Accessed on: 20 May 2019.

[12] Colwell, R.R. & Machlis, G., *Science During Crisis: Best Practices, Research Needs, and Policy Priorities*, American Academy of Arts and Sciences: Cambridge, MA, 2019.

INCORPORATING CLIMATE SCIENCE INTO DISASTER MANAGEMENT PROGRAMS

ELEONORE (NORA) D. YOTSOV & DOUGLAS C. STOLZ
Port of Portland and Cross Product Atmospheric, LLC, USA

ABSTRACT

Human action (sometimes inaction) creates vulnerabilities that expose populations to impacts from disasters. The effects, especially those stemming from attributing factors such as climate change, are not often directly perceptible or understood in the context of disaster. These impacts are the most challenging to address and at the same time present an opportunity for increasing effectiveness of disaster risk reduction measures. There is much work to be done to reduce the gap between the science of climate change and disaster management. Such barriers to application include (but are not limited to) the nebulous nature of climate change itself, the perceived lack of value of prevention efforts through upfront investment and the burden whereby climate change and also the need to act now is fraught in partisan political process. There is a critical need to overcome these barriers, as the emergency response and recovery efforts are currently unable to keep up with increasing and ever worsening impacts from disasters. As humans develop and learn new information, there is often a delay between initial sense making and learning to acceptance and enculturation. There are four key steps for incorporating climate change science into the disaster risk reduction arena: 1) seek out unbiased scientific information; 2) understand the impacts and implications to develop accurate risk perception for the population; 3) reduce the existing gap by translating the science and engaging the appropriate stakeholders; and 4) apply this initiative through existing opportunities and innovations. Through history of the disaster management profession, the areas of concern expand as civilizations become more complex, interconnected and dependent on anthropogenic solutions. These impacts will only increase humanity's actions (or inactions), augmenting collective exposure and vulnerability. Understanding how current and future impacts increase vulnerability in concert with other conditions can allow the development of truly multi-disciplined disaster risk strategies.

Keywords: climate change, adaptation, disaster management, risk assessment, vulnerability, hazard, mitigation, Cuba, Tarea Vida.

1 INTRODUCTION

Today, there is no doubt that impacts to humanity from natural disasters are increasing leaving reliance on response and recovery insufficient and ineffective to adequately manage the trend. There are a variety of factors that contribute to this including population growth, social inequities such as poverty and health, increasing development in vulnerable areas, reliance on technological advances that promote protection from natural hazards based on old/inadequate data and so on.

Disaster Risk Reduction (DRR) has come to the forefront as the mechanism aimed at reducing the impact of disaster to a specific population through a series of actions embedded in the disaster management field. Incorporating climate science into DRR has been a challenge and siloed effort to date. Even though there are calls by many academics and practitioners in the field, over the past 30 years, climate change adaptation (CCA) knowledge and DRR have been mostly separate and somewhat parallel paths. Climate science provides needed knowledge to help disaster managers understand cause and effect in order to more effectively plan for and respond to situations. Not unlike the science of seismology or volcanology, climate science is a tool that is underutilized, if utilized at all, by the disaster management community. Dr. Ilan Kelman proposes that climate change should be a subset of disaster risk reduction "Rather than keeping climate change as a separate or dominating

www.witpress.com, ISSN 1743-3509 (on-line)
doi:10.2495/DMAN190101

topic, the proposal from a development perspective is to enact the 'multiple exposure' perspective by viewing climate change as one challenge amongst many" [1], [2].

Examples of development in flood zones, tsunami inundation zones, remote areas and climates not naturally able to sustain humanity are still occurring. Climate change contributes to disasters by creating conditions that can amplify the magnitude of quick onset storms, but also in creating longer duration changes that transform the environment where pre-established practice is no longer adequate. The challenge of relating climate change impacts to specific disasters is mired in politics and interacts with a variety of other factors that can mask or derail appropriate attribution. This paper addresses the need, provides a real-world example and highlights four key steps for incorporating climate science into disaster management programs.

1.1 Potential harm in neglect – NFIP as an example

The National Flood Insurance Program (NFIP) in the United States is a useful example of a well-meaning method that has created more vulnerability, due to its method of addressing a single hazard instead of including all contributing factors. The NFIP was established over 50 years ago to protect the public through insurance backing to provide financial assistance for those with limited resources recovering from floods. Rather than protect, the program created more vulnerability by allowing new development and people with financial constraints to stay in flood prone areas using risk transference rather than looking at all contributing factors related to flooding hazards. Using out-dated and inaccurate flood maps created more risk by allowing development and repetitive repairs for damaged homes, rather than looking into other drivers of floods. As a result, increases in payouts due to increased flooding and repetitive flood loss, the program has become insolvent.

The Biggert-Waters Flood Insurance Reform Act of 2012 was enacted to raise premiums to increase reflecting the "true risk" of living in high-flood areas in an effort to bail out the NFIP [3]. The U.S. Government Accountability Office (GAO) has placed the NFIP in its high-risk list. This is a result of NFIP's worsening debt in response to growing disasters and the increase in rates for homeowners who benefited from previously subsidized rates that did not previously reflect "full risk of loss". This burden falls squarely onto those who it was meant to protect [4].

In this simple example, looking at climate trends can help inform future development and limit rebuilding efforts before and after floods. While the GAO report focused on improving programmatic elements such as debt reduction, affordability and barriers to involvement, the outstanding issue is the evolving environment where development is allowed to continue. Incorporating relevant climate science information is key to understanding how the changing natural hazard risk profile will affect the human condition.

2 ADVANCES IN DISASTER MANAGEMENT

The field of Emergency or Disaster Management has made tremendous advances and evolved from a single focus fire response function to a multi-hazard professional field. In the simplest terms "emergency management is the discipline dealing with risk and risk avoidance." Traditionally a government function, in the United States this field had its start following a devastating fire in 1803 and has evolved into an all-hazards approach including all natural and manmade disasters [5]. Disaster Management has evolved from a fire response to a civil defence function focused on nuclear threats from the cold war, to expanding to natural disasters in the 1960s to the inclusion of terrorism post 2001 and today to including seismology and volcanology as pre-emptive tools to address potential hazards.

Internationally, the field includes response, recovery, finding overlap in the related fields of development, planning and humanitarian aid, where adaptation and mitigation strategies complement the similar strategies employed in disaster management.

Since Disaster Management is such a broad profession that has grown to encompass not only historical data to inform risk reduction, but also predictive modelling, assimilating relevant aspects of emerging climate science is a necessary and logical progression. Allowing for siloes to exist is no longer viable and potentially irresponsible if DRR efforts are to continue being effective.

2.1 Seismology and volcanology to inform

In the Pacific Northwest, for communities along the ring of fire, the science of seismology is rapidly being incorporated into Disaster Management practice. In only in the last 30 years, a deeper understanding of potential Cascadia Subduction Zone magnitude 9.0 earthquake impacts [6] has provided impetus for investment into development, mitigation and other related strategies. These efforts are varied and include seismically retrofitting critical infrastructure such as key bridges and the Critical Energy Infrastructure (CEI) Hub [7] as well as investment into earthquake early warning systems, such as the ShakeAlert system for the West Coast of the United States [8].

Similarly, the Pacific Northwest has a geographical distribution of volcanoes, whose hazards vary, but are also addressed through proactive methods, such as alert and warning and protection measures, such as evacuation planning [9].

The acceptance of seismology and volcanology has dynamically evolved the field of Disaster Management for communities at risk in the Pacific Northwest. By seeking out and understanding the science, disaster managers, with the assistance of the scientific community and subject matter experts have been able to translate and apply the science into effective practice to accurately address risk and proactively take action.

2.2 Displacement's increasing impact

Disaster impacts are categorized in many ways, including, but not limited to direct and indirect toll on humanity, economic loss to infrastructure, social and natural resources loss, and so on. Displacements from natural disasters are becoming more frequent and there is great interest in determining possible links to climate change – whether changing climate affects the magnitude and probability of occurrence of individual natural hazards [10]. The relatively short global observation record of extreme events as well as statistical methods used to assess attribution likelihood preclude a determination until after the event has occurred. Southeast Asia is highly prone to natural disasters, which are exacerbated by high population vulnerabilities and reliance on natural resources. In this region, those populations with some of the lowest known socioeconomic standing are situated in one of the more active tropical cyclone and riverine/inundation flood zones in the world; there is general scientific consensus that these natural phenomena will become worse/more intense in the coming decades and meanwhile rural southeast Asian populations are some of the least well equipped and apt to respond in disaster scenarios.

Still, DRR advances since the 1970s have provided protection mechanisms for many vulnerable populations in the face of natural disasters. While much work of DRR has protected lives, displacement (temporary, protracted or permanent) has been an increasing trend. Tracking disaster related displacement data started in 2008 by the Internal Displacement Monitoring Centre (IDMC). Since then, the toll displacement not only for the victims, but also host communities was largely understudied or unknown. Understanding the breadth of displacement from direct natural disaster, as well as indirect ecological change brought on by slow-onset climate driven forces, can inform disaster managers to proactively address these hazards.

In 2018, according to the IDMC, almost two thirds of the new displacements (not including protracted or permanent), an estimated 17.2 million are a result of disaster as compared to conflict [11]. Climate change can be a force multiplier for natural disasters, which increases the opportunity for displacement, thus creating cascading disasters, for not just those displaced but also host and aid communities tasked with caring for those displaced. Harnessing climate science, not just for CAA but also for DRR can be a valuable source of information advising proactive and prevention measures.

3 ADVANCES IN CLIMATE SCIENCE

3.1 Background

It is instructive to distinguish between weather and climate in a simple manner up front: weather is the specific atmospheric condition at a given place and time, whereas climate science deals specifically with variations and interactions in Earth's atmosphere, oceans, cryosphere, and biosphere over distances of up to approximately 10,000 km spatial scales and multiple decades. As such, society easily conceptualizes how day-to-day weather changes impact daily life and operations. In contrast, it is considerably more difficult for the average person to perceive changes in climate over weeks, months or even multiple years, and furthermore, how those very changes directly (and possibly indirectly) affect their livelihoods. In fact, there exists a rich history of climate research and applied operational development that has established a vast climate-science resource base. What follows next is an reasonable cross-section of presently available climate science references, including operational data and modelling systems, services and service providers, as well as information pathways that may be consulted by practitioners (referred to as, "climate information") [12] seeking to develop robust climate mitigation and adaptation strategies to be applied within the field of disaster management.

3.2 Types of climate information

Climate information that may be useful to Disaster Risk Reduction specialists can be loosely classified as historical records, future projections, and synthesized reports. For example, observations from tree rings, ice cores, coral reef deposits, subterranean bore holes in Arctic permafrost and multi-decadal air samples provide evidence of a changing climate. These types of data may be analyzed in specific ways to determine the extent of potential impacts on human life, property and infrastructure (depending on the source, these data are usually freely available to the public). In addition, such observations serve as a critical input for another form of climate intelligence – numerical climate models – which themselves are founded on the idea that current conditions can serve as the basis for future prediction of general circulation and regional temperature/precipitation patterns, etc. Finally, in the modern era of data proliferation and near-instantaneous digital communications, the general public is seemingly inundated with excess of climate information. Fortunately, both private and public entities as well as multi-national government-sanctioned agencies exist and work to consolidate and collate available research, data and documentation into concise reports for interested parties.

3.2.1 Authoritative sources of climate information

Many organizations around the world, each possibly operating at different bureaucratic levels, work collectively to address outstanding gaps in climate information delivery, essentially to inform possible gaps that exist between climate science development and practice. At the international level, the World Climate Research Program (WCRP) drives advancement in climate predictions by facilitating technical climate model intercomparison [13] as well as professional scientific workshops and conferences. The Intergovernmental Panel on Climate Change (IPCC) [14] is a body of the United Nations tasked with assessing the state-of-the-science related to climate change; the IPCC publishes its assessments periodically and meanwhile they are oft-cited in technical/policy proceedings and revered as the gold-standard of scientific climate information. Similarly, the United States (U.S.) National Research Council routinely publishes the National Climate Assessments, the most recent being the 2018 version [15], and within these pages one can gain access to regionalized climate insights and climate mitigation/adaptation strategies.

In the operational setting and using the U.S. as an example, the National Centers for Environmental Information's Climate Prediction Center (CPC) provides routine climate information updates (monthly and in some cases more frequently). Much of this information from the CPC is effectively summarized for general climate science [16] and hurricanes [17] for both situational awareness and educational purposes. Analogous organizations exist within the European Union – like the European Centres for Medium-Range Weather Forecasts (ECMWF) [18] – and they provide products that essentially cleanse, collate, and organize atmosphere/ocean observations over many decades for reference (i.e., "re-analysis"). Regional U.S. climate centers [19] exist to identify and develop sector-specific materials suitable for application in certain regions of interest. Furthermore, the U.S. National Weather Service's forecast offices maintain their own suite of climate information for localities and observation stations near critical assets and key resources.

Academic and private sector agencies provide additional subject-matter expertise and value-adding insight. Laboratories in the U.S. like the Earth Systems Research Laboratory (ESRL) house targeted research working groups, like the Physical Science Division at ESRL [20], who develop cutting-edge climate science and improve understanding of climate extremes and cascading impacts to society. Joint research institutes cultivate actionable climate information for global stakeholders; findings from their research are commonly published in the scientific peer-review literature supported by the American Meteorological Society and American Geophysical Union, etc. Lastly, organizations in the private sector develop agile, industry-specific climate information solutions that can leverage the latest innovative technologies (e.g., artificial intelligence/computer learning software) and they commonly provide these products as a service to consumers.

3.2.2 Aside on data and access

Underlying all of these sources of climate information is an enormous amount of data from computer calculations and Earth-observation platforms (which can also be utilized to "scale down" and drive specialized models of flood/storm surge/precipitation extremes or regional temperature, for example). Many, though not all, of the aforementioned authorities on climate science information will provide transparent access to their data as well as software that is designed for quick access and visualization. Collaborating with someone who is trained in the physical sciences and well-versed in technical computing is recommended, as these data are commonly archived in non-standard data formats. The trend is hosting digital data resources in web-enabled user interfaces and cloud-based data archives, thus supporting truly global information sharing for those with reasonable means of internet access [21].

3.2.3 On properly interpreting "climate information"

The urgent operational need for climate guidance should be reasonably tempered by understanding of underlying issues that affect climate information development – chief among them is uncertainty. We know from experience that the science of weather and climate prediction is imperfect, which we recognize anecdotally as differences between what was forecast vs. that which was observed for a given location, time, or even season. It is beyond the scope of this paper to detail sources of uncertainty [22], but it stems from our inability to accurately and precisely measure conditions everywhere with sufficient granularity to inform future predictions. In addition, characterizations of governing physical processes and Earth-system responses (i.e., feedbacks) to anthropogenic inputs and/or changes, are simplistic by assumption and therefore do not fully explain the process or phenomenon.

Bearing the above in mind, it is true that advances in computer technology aid in the effort to improve timeliness, accuracy, and precision in climate prediction, but the realization of a "perfect prediction" of climate is not likely to happen. Considerable effort in the field of weather and climate prediction is being focused on *the optimal means to communicate predictions along with associated error in the most effective way possible.* What this means is that triggers or thresholds for action will be based on, hypothetically for example, a 6-in-10 chance of above-normal temperatures occurring in the next 4–6 weeks somewhere within an area of 25 miles from a given location. How this type of climate information is then incorporated within emergency action plans will require inputs from subject matter experts or those that have some background experience with climate, atmospheric, and/or the Earth sciences.

3.3 Future implications for disaster management

We are generating climate information at unprecedented rates and volumes in the modern age, thereby increasing the prospects of improved accuracy and precision in climate forecasts out to several decades or more. New techniques to handle, visualize, conceptualize, and interpret this ever-growing stream of scientific intelligence for the growing base of practical consumers will be needed. To match, the science of Disaster Risk Reduction will continue to develop and support greater integration of climate information in practice. Greater spatial resolution, longer, and more-accurate climate forecasts may be the key to support breaking out risk mitigation/climate adaptation, even by hazard or at a very local level.

4 FOUR KEY STEPS AND CUBA'S TAREA VIDA

As human development learns new information, there is often a delay between the initial encounter, learning, acceptance, adoption and subsequent enculturation. There are four key steps for incorporating climate change science into the disaster risk reduction arena. Each step is listed with an example of how it was accomplished via Cuba's state strategy.

Cuba's efforts result in minimal loss of life compared to other countries in the hurricane prone Caribbean. While Cuba is considered a developing country with well-documented struggles, limited resources and infrastructure, Cuba is one of the most resilient countries in the Caribbean. So, what sets them apart from Puerto Rico, Haiti or the Dominican Republic?

Cuba's recognition of climate change impacts to humanity dates back nearly 30 years with a speech by Fidel Ruz Castro at the 1992 Earth Summit in Rio de Janeiro, Brazil. This has driven many of Cuba's efforts to address the growing hazards and to reduce vulnerabilities. "Climate change is one of the greatest challenges of these times, unleashing such phenomena as sea level rise, temperature upticks, extreme hydro-meteorological events, seasonal changes in rainfall rates, severe droughts and intense rains. If the mindset on this is not changed and dramatic measures are not taken, the future will not only hold a more expensive side, but it will also become more difficult for human survival in the face of these effects" [23]. With this in mind, Cuba set out to incorporate climate science into its disaster risk reduction strategies through a variety of policy and practitioner mechanisms.

Tarea Vida (Life Task) was approved on April 25, 2017, but had its start in 1991. Tarea Vida is the state plan for confronting climate change based on a multidisciplinary scientific basis. The plan prioritizes nearly half of its municipalities in the coastal and territorial areas that are most at risk from climate change magnification to natural disasters. It is comprised of five strategic actions and eleven tasks to proactively address impacts of climate change and protect its people. "The project will provide support in transitioning from hard disaster risk management approach to CC to a holistic approach that favors resilience through adaptation as a continuous process that maximizes the functionality of natural infrastructure along coastal zones and that is grounded on and sustained through coastal communities and informed coastal planning mechanisms" [25].

4.1 Seek

Seek out unbiased scientific information. As discussed above, climate science information is a readily available in multiple forms and to serve as an accessible resource for Disaster Management/DRR. While the body of knowledge can be overwhelming and excessively technical, there are multiple pathways of gathering this new information via online resources, in print, and via documentaries.

As with any new science, there is a period of time before a body of work can be absorbed into common knowledge and practice, meanwhile recognizing the importance of building relationships and opening dialogue channels between science groups and those who operate solely as practitioners. Cuba's tendency to consult available scientific resources is well documented. As a country with a ratio of 7.5 physicians per 1,000 people, the use of science and technology to inform policy has a long history in Cuba dating back to the pre-founding of the country [26]. Incorporating science into policy and practice has been key, even under the financial and political constraints within the country.

The Institute of Meteorology's (INSMET) role in prediction, alerting and warning is key to protecting the population. Serving in leadership roles in the World Meteorological Organization, Cuba's INSMET has a structured methodology that is well known and followed throughout the country. With offices in each province and some larger cities, INSMET provides a phased warning approach. Early warning is 72 hours in advance, followed by Special warning 66 to 48 hours in advance to be followed with localized evacuation and protection warnings, where necessary [27]. Utilizing scientific data from INSMET is only one example of how to effectively seek out scientific information.

4.2 Understand

Understand the impacts and implications to develop accurate risk perception for the population. Knowing how much each contributing factor is truly influencing disasters provides a better understanding of future mitigation and adaptation measures. Simplifying to either deny or attribute an entirety of an event to climate change impacts does not accurately help disaster managers understand what factors need to be addressed. In contrast, understanding the frequency of occurrence, maximum possible extent of affected area, and severity of events (as well as how they are measured and characterized officially) are useful lenses through which to contextualize natural hazards. Further effort should be directed towards comprehending how multiple natural hazard events occurring at once can create cascading impacts and how those hazard interactions might evolve in a changing climate.

Climate science is included at all levels of education throughout the Cuba school system, not only at the university levels, but starting at grade school. Climate information is included in various UNDP programs that operate in provinces with special focus to the specific risks. Understanding increased climate variability and trends, the Cuban government, UNDP Cuba and UNDP's Caribbean Risk Management Initiative (CRMI) created the Risk Reduction Management Center (RRMC) model. "At the heart of the model is the promotion of local level decision-making that relies on coordinated early warning systems, risk and vulnerability studies, communications systems, effective database management and mapping, GIS, and community preparedness." There are 8 provincial and 84 municipal centers. The RRMC are established to focus on localized hazards and vulnerabilities, for example, the RRMC in Santa Cruz del Sur focuses on hurricanes, flooding and storm surges, etc., while the RRMC in Santiago de Cuba additionally focuses on droughts and fires and technological hazards [28].

The general public has conceptual understanding of protection categories specific to evacuation for their location. First priority is to transfer people to lower risk and structurally safer areas in a bid to protect their safety. Second priority is to evacuate people to designated facilities including public buildings, tunnels, caves and even "vara en tierra" (traditional huts). In the city of Gibara, evacuation to the cave system outside of town is accepted practice and helped save lives when the entire town was evacuated during Hurricane Ike in 2008 [29].

4.3 Translate

Reduce the existing gap by translating the science and engaging the appropriate stakeholders. In order to effectively create programmatic elements, input from a variety of subject matter experts across multiple disciplines, such as climate science, computer science, urban planning, civil engineering, and sociology/psychology are necessary. Emphasis for such collaboration is on strengthening an all-hazards approach programs to better understand cause and effect relationships.

Since 1986, Cuba annually conducts a nationwide full-scale exercise that includes all members of government, civil society and individual members of the population. The exercise is compulsory in nature from the top down. The "Meteoro" exercise happens in May and aims at exercising all elements of hurricane response, protection, evacuation and recuperation elements. The timing of the exercise is in preparation for the hurricane seasons (June–November each year). Tarea Vida's tasks are another example of how climate science is translated into action. According to Rolber Reyes Pupo with CITMA, in Gibara alone, the following disaster risk reduction actions were taken in advance of the next hurricane [30]:

- Removal of 15 homes located in areas vulnerable to sea level rise and coastal flooding (funding for relocation strategies can be hard to come by).
- Ovidio Torres elementary school and the local hospital moved to safe places.
- New road built to link Caletones and Gibara through the settlements of Las Caobas, El Macio and Laguna Blanca aimed to reduce their coastal hazards.
- Recovery of mangroves, dunes and sand and coastal reefs as natural protection barriers.

4.4 Apply

Apply this initiative through existing opportunities and innovations. There are many pathways for disaster management, but the best approach is through the practice of DRR. Using projections from available climate models to inform sea-front infrastructure development/refurbishment design or revising existing hazard mitigation plans to include updated thresholds and triggers are basic examples of applied climate science in action.

How are these efforts applied in the case of Cuba's activity? The true application is in the ability to more effectively protect the public during hurricanes. So how does this occur? The process has been enculturated so that when there is warning of an impending hurricane, overall the population responds with well known, practiced and accepted methods. The cultural shift that occurs from the previous 3 steps, is proven in application through the relatively low mortality rate of Cuba's hurricanes vs. other Caribbean island nations, or even first world nations, like the United States.

During Hurricane Ike, Cuba conducted evacuations and protective measures for over 2.6 million people and experienced 7 direct fatalities [24]. In the United States where over 200,000 refused evacuation orders and of the 195 who died in the US, 113 alone were in Texas. Retrospective studies of communities affected by (major) hurricanes contribute that societal risk perceptions of natural hazards are often acutely related to imminent environmental cues (e.g., increasing winds and rising water levels), but also to social cues, warning messaging, and personal preference or inherent risk tolerance; these factors collectively lead behavioral response and protective-decision making [31]. Nearly 30% of respondents to a post-hurricane Ike inquiry cited the highest importance level of peer communications in evacuation decision making [32], thus alluding to the importance of enculturated disaster preparedness practice. In Cuba, strong social networks work in tandem with well-practiced and accepted methods.

5 DISCUSSION

We recognize that socioeconomic, political, geographical, or even other artificial barriers might need to be overcome as part of risk reduction initiatives geared to the dynamic, natural process of climate change. A main goal of this paper is to establish that disaster risk reduction principles and climate science information can be leveraged simultaneously to promote better outcomes while constantly grappling with ever-changing community-wide risk factors and vulnerabilities. To mitigate some of that uncertainty, an effective general framework could involve the steps of 1) seek, 2) understand, 3) translate, and 4) apply information in practice. Using Cuba's Tarea Vida as a quintessential example, successful mitigation practice arises from widespread acknowledgment of the impact of climate change and subsequent enculturation of the ideals of disaster risk reduction.

It is possible that availability, accessibility and applicability climate science information will co-evolve with the burgeoning field of disaster risk reduction. In a perfect world, dialogue between practitioners and scientists will become more common place; such open discussion could see practitioners express their targeted needs for guidance and science experts reciprocating by informing practitioners of the current state-of-the-art in addition to providing distilled meaning of available climate science information. It is these kinds of proactive collaborations that can, and will over time, engender a conscious educational paradigm shift from reactive toward predictive approaches to disaster risk reduction. As other sciences have been successfully incorporated into disaster management programs, climate science cannot remain siloed but must be incorporated to assist with the evolution and efficacy of the field.

ACKNOWLEDGEMENT

The authors would like to thank M.D Ricardo Suarez Bustamante, Comprehensive Expert in Science, Technology and the Environment (CITMA) in Baracoa, Cuba for his insights into Cuba's Tarea Vida strategy.

REFERENCES

[1] Kelman, I., Gaillard, J. & Mercer, J., Climate change's role in disaster risk reduction's future: Beyond vulnerability and resilience. *International Journal of Disaster Risk Science*, **6**(1), pp. 21–27, 2015.

[2] Mall, R., Srivastava, R., Banerjee, T., Mishra, O., Bhatt, D. & Sonkar, G., Disaster risk reduction including climate change adaptation over South Asia: Challenges and ways forward. *International Journal of Disaster Risk Science*, **10**(1), pp. 14–27, 2018.

[3] Fema.gov, Biggert Waters Flood Insurance Reform Act of 2012: Impact of National Flood Insurance Program (NFIP) Changes, 2019. www.fema.gov/media-library-data/20130726-1909-25045-0554/bw12_sec_205_207_factsheet4_13_2013.pdf. Accessed on: 29 Mar. 2019.

[4] Gao.gov, High Risk: National Flood Insurance Program, 2019. www.gao.gov/highrisk/national_flood_insurance/why_did_study#t=1. Accessed on: 29 Mar. 2019.

[5] Haddow, G., Bullock, J. & Coppola, D., *Introduction to Emergency Management*, pp. 1–2, 2017.

[6] Oregon Department of Geology and Mineral Industries, DOGAMI open file report series. www.oregongeology.org/pubs/ofr/p-O-18-02.htm. Accessed on: 15 May 2019.

[7] Wang, Y., Steven, B. & Scott, M., Earthquake risk study Oregon's critical energy infrastructure hub, Oregon.gov, 2013. www.oregon.gov/energy/safety-resiliency/Documents/2013%20Earthquake%20Risk%20Study%20in%20Oregon's%20Critical%20Energy%20Infrastructure%20Hub.pd. Accessed on: 15 May 2019.

[8] ShakeAlert®, Earthquake early warning. www.shakealert.org. Accessed on: 15 May 2019.

[9] USGS, Program VH, Cascades Volcano Observatory. https://volcanoes.usgs.gov/observatories/cvo/cascade_volcanoes.html. Accessed on: 15 May 2019.

[10] Stott, P.A. et al., Attribution of extreme weather and climate-related events. *Wiley Interdisciplinary Reviews: Climate Change*, 7, pp. 23–41, 2016.

[11] Internal Displacement Monitoring Centre, Global report on internal displacement (GRID) 2019. www.internal-displacement.org/global-report/grid2019/. Accessed on: 29 May 2019.

[12] NOAA, Climate information. www.ncdc.noaa.gov/climate-information.

[13] A short introduction to climate models – CMIP & CMIP6. www.wcrp-climate.org/wgcm-cmip/cmip-video. Accessed on: 21 May 2019.

[14] IPCC, About the IPCC. www.ipcc.ch/about/. Accessed on: 21 May 2019.

[15] NCA, Fourth National Climate Assessment – Volume II: Impacts, Risk, and Adaptation in the United States. https://nca2018.globalchange.gov. Accessed on: 21 May 2019.

[16] Climate.gov., Science and Information for a Climate-Smart Nation. www.climate.gov. Accessed on: 21 May 2019.

[17] National Hurricane Center and Central Pacific Hurricane Center, www.nhc.noaa.gov/?atlc. Accessed on: 21 May 2019.

[18] Advancing Global NWP through International Collaboration, https://www.ecmwf.int. Accessed on: 21 May 2019.

[19] Regional Climate Centers, www.ncdc.noaa.gov/customer-support/partnerships/regional-climate-centers. Accessed on: 21 May 2019.

[20] Physical Sciences Division, Physical Science for Predicting Extremes. www.esrl.noaa.gov/psd/. Accessed on: 21 May 2019.

[21] NOAA National Centers for Environmental Information: Data Access, www.ncdc.noaa.gov/data-access. Accessed on: 21 May 2019.

[22] Eyring, V. et al., Overview of the coupled model intercomparison project Phase 6 (CMIP6) experimental design and organization. *Geoscientific Model Development*, **9**, pp. 1937–1958, 2016.

[23] Ministerio de Ciencia, Tecnología y Medio Ambiente (Cuba). www.ecured.cu/Ministerio_de_Ciencia_Tecnología_y_Medio_Ambiente. Accessed on: 22 Mar. 2019.

[24] Civil Defense Cuba, Editor's note quote from Division General Ramon Pardo Guerra, Chief of the National Civil Defense Headquarters, p. 1, 2018.

[25] Green Climate Fund, Coastal adaptation to climate change in Cuba through ecosystem based adaptation. Republic of Cuba, United Nations Development Programme (UNDP), p. 9, 2018.

[26] World Bank Database, Physicians per 1,000 people. https://data.worldbank.org/indicator/SH.MED.PHYS.ZS?end=1974&locations=CU&start=1974&view=map&year=2014&year_high_desc=false. Accessed on: 22 Mar. 2019.

[27] Davila, W., Highly powerful hurricanes: Protecting the population and its assets in Cuba. *Civil Defense Cuba*, **1**, p. 5, 2018.

[28] UNDP, A Cuban model for a resilient Caribbean. www.undp.org/content/undp/en/home/presscenter/articles/2015/02/25/a-cuban-model-for-a-resilient-caribbean.html. Accessed on: 22 Mar. 2019.

[29] *Gibara Response to Hurricane Ike and Matthew Interview with M.D. Bustamante*, Baracoa, Cuba, 2018.

[30] ¡ahora!, Redacción. Tarea Vida with Remarkable Results in Holguín. www.ahora.cu/en/holguin/1967-tarea-vida-with-remarkable-results-in-holguin. Accessed on: 31 Mar. 2019.

[31] Huang, S.-K., Lindell, M.K., Prater, C.S., Wu, H.-C. & Siebeneck, L.K., Household evacuation decision making in response to Hurricane Ike. *Natural Hazards Review*, **13**(4), pp. 283–296, 2012.

[32] Morrs, R.E. & Hayden, M.H., Storm surge and "certain death": Interviews with Texastavb coastal residents following Hurricane Ike. *Weather, Climate, and Society*, **2**, pp. 174–189, 2010.

APPLYING THE STAPLEE CRITERIA TO DEVELOP NATURAL HAZARDS MITIGATION ACTIONS: CASE STUDY AND LESSONS LEARNED IN NORTHERN PUERTO RICO

JAVIER VÉLEZ AROCHO[1], CARLOS MAYSONET[2] & JOSÉ L. VALENZUELA[3]
[1]EcoStahlia Consultores Ambientales LLC, Puerto Rico
[2]Autonomous Municipality of Vega Alta, Puerto Rico
[3]Central Recovery and Reconstruction Office of Puerto Rico (COR3), Puerto Rico

ABSTRACT

A key strategy to identify risks associated with natural disasters is the use of appropriate criteria that allow protection of life and property from future hazard events. With the effects of climate change increasing it is important to effectively identify the vulnerability of communities, as well as properties of the municipalities that are exposed to natural hazards. Using the correct criteria could provide a base for the development and implementation of mitigation measures aimed at reducing the loss of life and property. Implementing these measures could help reduce the economic and social impact of the natural hazards that affect communities in Puerto Rico. The use of inadequate planning in the design of mitigation activities may not be enough nor sustainable in the long term, when addressing natural hazards in regions like the Caribbean. Hurricanes, earthquakes, tsunamis, droughts, flooding and coastal erosion have already claimed the lives of hundreds of people and throughout the last decade, have caused over $100 billion in damages across the region. Based on this scenario, a case study is featured using the United States Federal Emergency Agency's (FEMA) STAPLEE Criteria. STAPLEE is an acronym for the seven criteria used to conduct a feasibility review. These criteria are: Social, Technical, Administrative, Political, Legal, Economic, and Environmental feasibility. After describing the method, the paper focuses on the reliability of the process and the results obtained in a coastal municipality in northern Puerto Rico. Twenty-three mitigation actions were developed to address the most pressing natural hazards affecting the municipality. The use of the criteria addresses the challenge developing the appropriate mitigation actions at the local level while complying with the archipelago-wide approach developed by the state government of Puerto Rico.

Keywords: multi-hazard mitigation in Puerto Rico, FEMA, community resilience, climate change, planning, coastal hazards.

1 INTRODUCTION

On 20 September 2017 at 10:15 a.m., the worst natural disaster on record to affect the archipelago of Puerto Rico, and the islands of Dominica and US Virgin Island made landfall causing catastrophic destruction and the loss of thousands of lives in these countries. According to the United States Federal Emergency Management Agency (FEMA), total losses from the hurricane were estimated at over US $91 billion, and it is considered the third costliest tropical storm on record [1]. The main island of Puerto Rico suffered major infrastructure damage and a major humanitarian crisis; most of the island's population suffered from flooding and a lack of resources, compounded by a slow relief process. The storm caused the worst electrical blackout in US history, and in June 2018, thousands of homes and businesses were still without power [2]. At the peak of the storm, the maximum sustained winds reached 175 mph (280 km/h) and dropped over 30 inches of rain in a period of 24 hours. The hurricane caused approximately 25 landslides per square mile, damaging state, and municipal roads across the island affecting the recovery efforts for months (Fig. 2) [3].

WIT Transactions on The Built Environment, Vol 190, © 2019 WIT Press
www.witpress.com, ISSN 1743-3509 (on-line)
doi:10.2495/DMAN190111

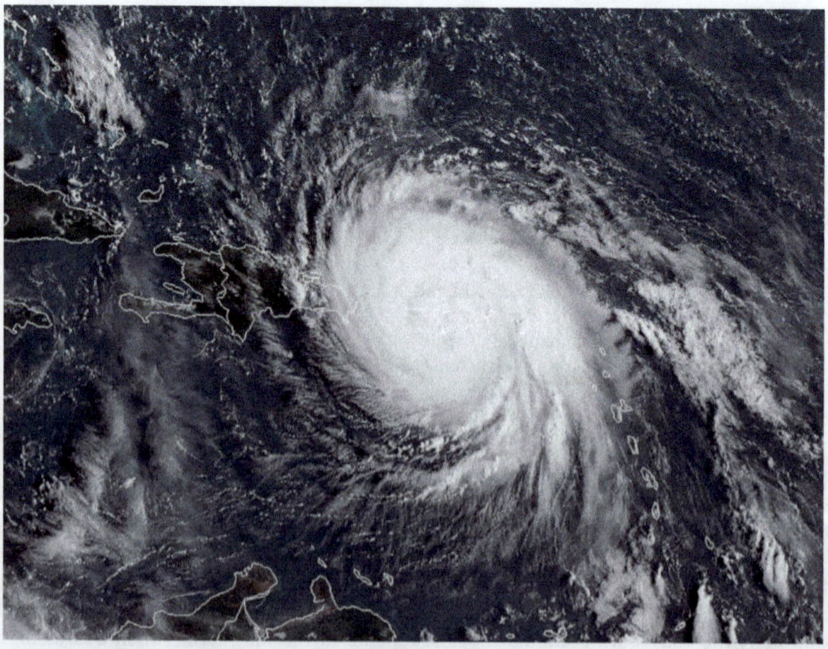

Figure 1: Satellite image of Hurricane María over the archipelago of Puerto Rico. *(Source: NASA.)*

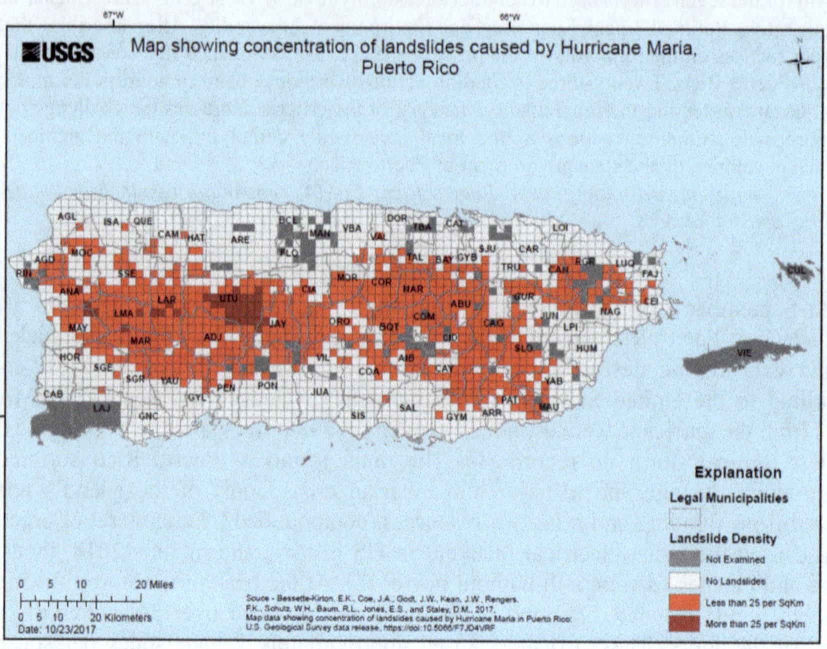

Figure 2: Map showing concentration of landslides caused by Hurricane María. *(Source: USGS.)*

According to the authors the hurricane's wind, storm surge, and rain disrupted most of the island already weak infrastructure that was damaged by Hurricane Irma two weeks before Hurricane María. The system impacted all 78 municipalities damaging dams, bridges, coastal barriers, highways, and critical buildings including police departments, hospitals, fire departments, shelters, schools, among others. The passing of the tropical disturbance presented the state and local governments with a unique opportunity to develop strategies aimed to create more resilient communities facing natural hazards like hurricanes, severe droughts, heavy rains, earthquakes, and coastal erosion (Fig. 3).

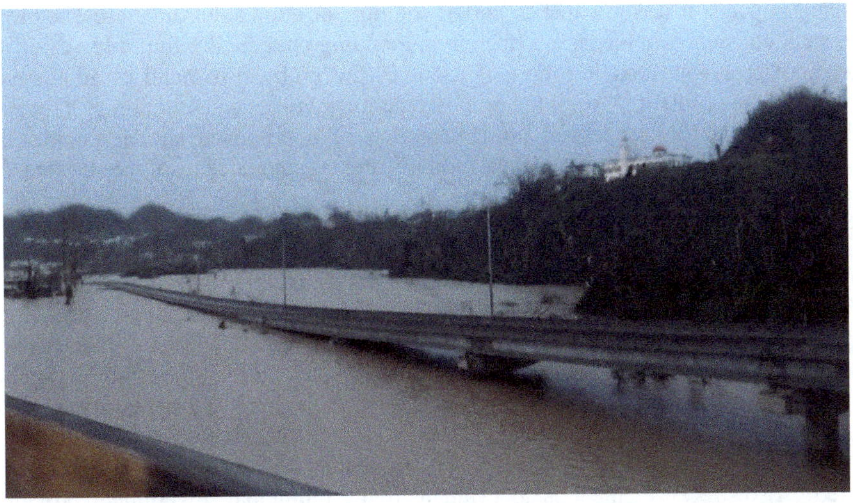

Figure 3: The flooded interchange between state road PR#2 and expressway PR#22 in the town of Vega Alta.

2 APPLYING THE STAPPLEE CRITERIA FOR LOCAL STRATEGIES

In 2003 the United States Federal Emergency Management Agency (FEMA) created a process known as STAPLEE. The acronym stands for Social, Technical, Administrative, Political, Legal, Economic, and Environmental, and it is being used by communities in the United States and the territory of Puerto Rico to explore the opportunities and constraints of each proposed mitigation actions as part of a more comprehensive plan to address all known natural hazards. This planning tool will produce an outcome to support and assist local governments and communities in determining priorities for hazard mitigation [4]. Not all processes are the same as every community has different needs or infrastructure conditions. According to the federal agency, when applying STAPLEE, it is vital to consider important questions relevant to each criterion. The criteria are defined as followed.

2.1 STAPLEE: Social

From the local point of view, the local government, community, and other stakeholders – considering each planning situation – must support the overall implementation strategy and specific mitigation actions. Therefore, evaluating the projects in terms of community acceptance to avoid unwanted results. For example, obtaining feedback to determine if the proposed action adversely affects any segment of the population, disrupts established neighborhoods, breaks up voting districts or cause the relocation of lower-income people.

Other important variables include community values, cultural resources, and if the proposed actions will be in harmony with social, cultural, and religious beliefs and customs.

A key component in the development of a mitigation strategy aimed to increase resilience of a community is the technical component of the proposed action.

2.2 STAPLEE: Technical

During the planning phase is critical to determine if the proposed action is technically feasible by examining whether the action will help to reduce losses in the long term, it has minimal secondary impacts, if it is a whole or partial solution, or not a solution at all. The proposed action shall consider whether it is effective in avoiding or reducing future losses, if it may create more problems than it solves, if it solves the problem at hand or addresses only symptoms of the problem. Also, if the proposed action involves construction, is it technically feasible to build. The successful implementation of a proposed action requires proper assessment of the management, staffing, funding, and maintenance resources needed.

2.3 STAPLEE: Administrative

During the planning phase, the community representatives shall assess carefully the Administrative evaluation criteria to determine the staffing required, funding, and maintenance requirements for the mitigation action. This review will help in determining if the community or local government has the personnel and administrative capabilities necessary to implement the action or whether outside help will be necessary. During the process, local representatives are required to assess if the local government has the capability (staff, technical experts, and/or funding) to implement the action, or can it be readily obtained? Also, a key element is to evaluate if the municipal government provides the necessary maintenance to a proposed action. Around the world, politics have a profound impact in the implementation of initiatives, projects, or ideas where funding is required. During the planning phase and discussion of the proposed project, looking into the local politics is important to improve the possibilities of success.

2.4 STAPLEE: Political

The involved personnel should understand how the community and state political leadership – as per their particular planning situation – feels about issues related to the environment, economic development, safety, and emergency management. Through years, Puerto Rico has seen important projects fail because of a lack of political acceptance or will. It is important to ensure that a designated member of the planning team consults with the board of supervisors, mayor, city council, administrator, manager, or other political offices of local governments. Also, the process of mitigating political issues may help avoid political pitfalls. It is recommended to identify whether there is local political support to implement and maintain the proposed action, if politicians have participated in the planning process, who are the key stakeholders, and is there enough public support to ensure the success of proposed actions.

2.5 STAPLEE: Legal

One key component of the stakeholder's meetings is to determine whether the community has the legal authority to implement the action, or whether new laws or regulations are needed. The personnel will identify the unit of government undertaking the mitigation action, and include an analysis of the interrelationships with local, regional, state, and federal government. Sometimes, it will be required to enable legislation to allow the local government to take the proposed action. It has been identified that the legal authority plays a large role later in the process when the community determines how to implement mitigation activities and to what extent mitigation can be enforced. Having a legal counsel is very important to answer questions regarding jurisdiction to implement a proposed activity. Specially is there a technical, scientific, or legal basis for the mitigation action, or if there are laws, ordinances, and resolutions in place or are any amendments to current laws, ordinances, or resolutions necessary.

2.6 STAPLEE: Economic

It is well known that economic prosperity ebbs and flows, so when it comes to mitigation actions, if funding is available, communities are more likely to implement them. However, the flip side is also a reality, so if mitigation actions require indebtedness, then the actions often remain unimplemented. In recent times, as Puerto Rico faces great economic challenges due to strict financial requirements by the Oversight Management Board (PROMESA), all economic considerations must include the current economic base and projected growth. It is very important to consider an outside source of funds to implement a mitigation action which is helpful for those with budgetary constraints. During the planning phase, staffers need to consider if the funds are currently available to implement the action. Also, it is critical to consider what benefits will the action provide to the community or the region, as well if the associated costs seem reasonable and potential benefits. Furthermore, some proposed actions can put a burden on the tax base, affecting future investment due to compromised future earnings.

2.7 STAPLEE: Environmental

The last part of the method covers potential environmental impacts from the proposed mitigation actions. Most municipalities desire sustainable and environmentally healthy communities, and, when using federal funds, there are various statutes that need to be considered, such as the National Environmental Policy Act (NEPA). When considering proposed actions, it is very important to evaluate possible negative environmental consequences to assets, such as, threatened and endangered species, wetlands, environmental justice, and other protected natural, cultural, or religious resources.

When working with stakeholders it is vital to include health departments, conservation commissions, environmental or water resource agencies, building officials, historical preservation groups, environmental groups, and wildlife management agencies. The idea is to assess the potential effects of the proposed action on the environment (land, water, residents, and endangered species) or if the action complies with local, state, and federal environmental laws. However, mitigation actions may benefit the environment. For instance, acquisition and relocation of structures out of the floodplain, sediment and erosion control actions, and stream corridor and wetland restoration projects, all offer benefits to land, species, or other environmental aspects.

Once the process of identifying potential mitigation actions, the rating of such proposals will help selecting those with better possibilities of being funded or implemented. The process is known as relative-rating where quantitative values are assigned to determine priority (low, medium, or high). The process usually includes a template to assign values to proposed actions to help in the decision process [5].

3 THE MUNICIPALITY OF VEGA ALTA MULTI-HAZARD MITIGATION PLAN 2019

The Multi-Hazard Mitigation Plan of the Autonomous Municipality of Vega Alta [6] was prepared and adopted on 22 May 2012, following the provisions of 44 CFR Parts 201 and 206 and in compliance with the "Disaster Mitigation Act" of the year 2000. As of May 2019, the Plan is being revised by the Municipal Review Committee with the assistance of the Central Office for Recovery, Reconstruction and Resilience (COR3), ATKINS Global® and EcoStahlia Environmental Consultants, LLC [7]. The plan outlines that once the revision is completed, the local government will issue an Executive Order adopting the new mitigation actions to be implemented. After the plan is adopted, it will be sent to the Regional Director of FEMA, with the concurrence of the Agency for Emergency Management and Disaster Management of the Commonwealth of Puerto Rico (AEME) for final approval.

4 METHODOLOGY

During a three month period, a series of workshops and public meetings were organized with the assistance of the Municipal Government of Vega Alta, the Central Office for Recovery, Reconstruction and Resilience (COR3), ATKINS Global® and EcoStahlia Environmental Consultants, LLC. Power Point® presentations, and tables based on the STAPLEE process were used to collect specific information on how a proposed action met the communities' needs. After each presentation, question and answer sessions were recorded to allow the attendees to classify the proposed actions as high, medium or low priority. Responses were annotated for further analysis. Each proposed mitigation project was evaluated following the STAPLEE criteria. The actions were considered for natural and man-made hazards including coastal erosion, hurricanes, droughts, landslides, fires, flooding, and climate change. The process provided stakeholders with different levels of knowledge of the issues the opportunity to offer facts in order to minimize bias; for example, photos of flooded areas. Also, responses to the information and questions from the staff were used to obtain data that was used to prepare maps to educate others of specific hazards or changes within their areas. The STAPLEE methodology, using the relative-rating method (high, medium and low priority), provided the grounds to select the most important mitigation strategies to be implemented in Vega Alta. Feedback was obtained from members of the Municipal Review Committee as well as from residents of the eight wards of the City of Vega Alta (Fig. 4). The results from the committee members were compared with those obtained from public meetings to adjust any difference or to propose new strategies based on the needs identified by residents for a specific area. Variables like time, cost vs. benefits ratio, potential support from the state or federal agencies as well as complexity of the proposed actions were analyzed to obtain a priority list with projects aimed to be completed in a five-year period. In order to allow more residents to comment on the proposed mitigation strategies, the draft document was made available by having a hard copy located in the town's public library. An email address was offered to receive any comments from residents of Vega Alta or neighboring towns (Fig. 5).

5 RESULTS AND DISCUSSION

According to the Federal Emergency Management Agency, any proposed mitigation strategy shall include a section that identifies and analyzes a comprehensive range of specific mitigation actions and projects being considered to reduce the effects of each hazard, with particular emphasis on new and existing buildings and infrastructure (Requirement §201.6(c)(3)(ii)) [8], [9]. The plan shall include a mitigation strategy that provides the

Worksheet #4 **Evaluate Alternative Mitigation Actions** **step 2**

1. *Fill in the goal and its corresponding objective. Use a separate worksheet for each objective. The considerations under each criterion are suggested ones to use; you can revise these to reflect your own considerations (see Table 2-1).*
2. *Fill in the alternative actions that address the specific objectives the planning team identified in Worksheet #1.*
3. ***Scoring:*** *For each consideration, indicate a plus (+) for favorable, and a negative (-) for less favorable.*

When you complete the scoring, negatives will indicate gaps or shortcomings in the particular action, which can be noted in the Comments section. For considerations that do not apply, fill in N/A for not applicable. Only leave a blank if you do not know an answer. In this case, make a note in the Comments section of the "expert" or source to consult to help you evaluate the criterion.

Goal: ______________________________

Objective: ______________________________

STAPLEE Criteria	S (Social)		T (Technical)			A (Administrative)			P (Political)			L (Legal)			E (Economic)				E (Environmental)				
Considerations → for Alternative Actions ↓	Community Acceptance	Effect on Segment of Population	Technical Feasibility	Long-term Solution	Secondary Impacts	Staffing	Funding Allocated	Maintenance/ Operations	Political Support	Local Champion	Public Support	State Authority	Existing Local Authority	Potential Legal Challenge	Benefit of Action	Cost of Action	Contributes to Economic Goals	Outside Funding Required	Effect on Land/ Water	Effect on Endangered Species	Effect on HAZMAT/ Waste Sites	Consistent with Community Environmental Goals	Consistent with Federal Laws

Figure 4: STAPLEE criteria worksheet template.

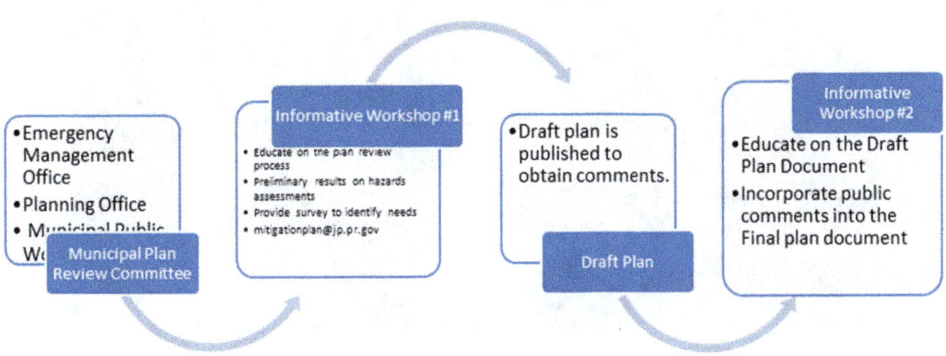

Figure 5: Description of the public comments process for the Vega Alta Multi-Hazard Plan.

jurisdiction's blueprint for reducing potential losses identified in the risk assessment, based on existing authorities, policies, programs and resources, and its ability to expand on and improve these existing tools. Thirty residents participated in the public meetings. The review committee did not receive comments or questions by email. During the discussion process 24 mitigation actions were proposed by the Municipal Review Committee, and stakeholders for adoption. Some of the proposed mitigation actions included retaining walls, raising road levels, and improving stormwater drainage structures. These projects covered flooding, coastal erosion due to climate change, coastal flooding due to tsunamis and hurricanes, and landslides. Mitigation strategies also included public education, property protection, non-structural projects like watershed protection plans, retrofitting emergency buildings and existing infrastructure maintenance. As examples, structural projects included installing better drainage systems to manage storm waters at downtown Vega Alta, and non-structural projects included the development of watershed management plans to protect the Honda Creek which crosses the center of the city. Based on federal guidelines, the criteria to establish the most important projects included location of the proposed action, hazard to be mitigated, priority, lead agency, funding source, completion date, and status as of 2019 (Fig. 6). With the assistance from two contractors (Atkins Global and EcoStahlia), the Municipal Mitigation Review Committee proceeded to analyze the proposed actions taking into consideration the STAPLEE criteria for the establishment of viability. As part of the analysis, the committee compared the location of critical infrastructure and how it was going to be protected by the proposed mitigation action. For both, the federal, and state governments, critical infrastructure includes hospitals, police and fire departments, power generation plants, sewer treatment facilities, and potable water plants.

During the discussion, the stakeholders brought their concerns for potential impacts to community integrity, and permanent disruption of daily activities. Many residents asked

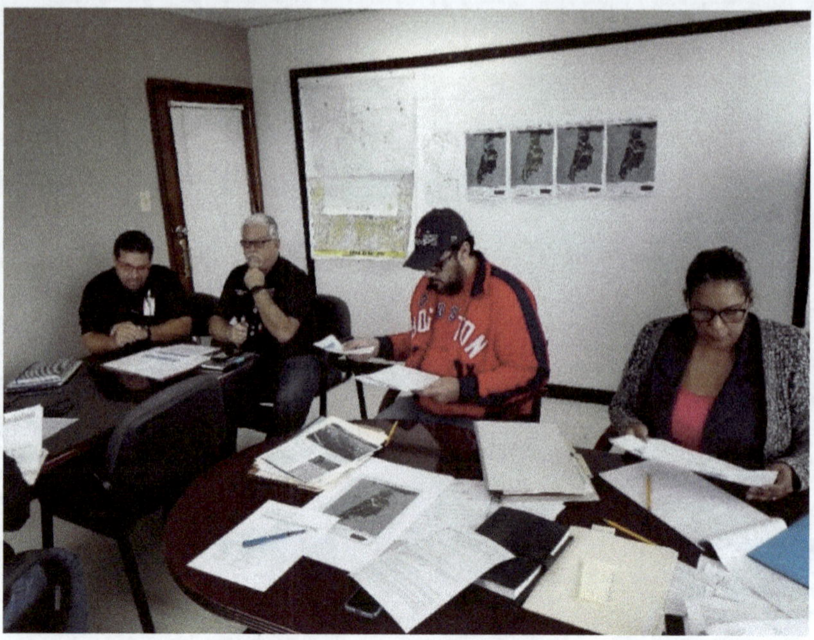

Figure 6: Staff of the Municipal Review Committee assessing some of the proposed actions.

questions regarding the availability of funds considering the financial struggle Puerto Rico currently faces with PROMESA [10]. A recurrent element in the analysis was the commitment by both the state and federal governments to allocate the necessary funds to specific mitigation strategies as the costs of implementing the plan will exceed the $80 million dollars. An example of a proposed action includes the elevation of 2 km of the state road #647 estimated in approximately $4 million dollars. Residents understand that the local government has limited resources and depend on external financial support to implement the more complex mitigation strategies. Nevertheless, most stakeholders were fully aware of the need for strategies aimed to keep hazard problems from getting worse. In the municipality of Vega Alta, flooding and landslides are considered major hazards for thousands of residents due to the existence of many surface water bodies, including the Cibuco River and Quebrada Honda, both prone to major flooding during tropical storms and hurricanes. Compared to previous plans, the 2019 revision includes non-structural mitigation strategies including the design of landscape projects instead of concrete channels or levees to minimize the impact to water bodies.

The updated plan also includes public education and awareness activities that are used to advise residents, elected officials, business owners, potential property buyers, and visitors about hazards, hazardous areas, and mitigation techniques they can use to protect themselves and their property. Public campaigns to encourage the acquisition of flood insurance by local residents were included in the plan. Although public education and outreach strategies may not result in a quantifiable reduction of damages, there is a relationship for the probable future and the cost of each measure that were considered when mitigation actions were planned. Once the plan is adopted by the municipality, the use of decision-making tools like the Analytic-Hierarchy Process (AHP) may help the community deal with the complex decision process of implementing these strategies (Table 1) [11].

6 CONCLUSIONS

Although local capability for mitigation can vary significantly between communities, developing and implementing a sound Multi-Hazard Mitigation Plan provides as described in Section 5, a great opportunity to establish policies and performance standards that address identified hazards. Also, according to the authors, establishes the base for more resilient communities capable of recovering after major natural hazards events (Fig. 7). In the development of multi-jurisdictional hazard mitigation plans, local governments with limited capacity or capability may use the planning process to develop cooperative agreements, mutual aid agreements, or service agreements that enhance their capacity to undertake mitigation activities. The Municipal Government of Vega Alta, Puerto Rico supported by the Central Recovery and Reconstruction Office of Puerto Rico (COR3), ATKINS Global® and EcoStahlia Environmental Consultants, LLC, updated their 2012 Multi-Hazard Mitigation Plan using FEMA's STAPLEE criteria as one of the methodologies to identify potential mitigation strategies to address natural hazards in a five-year period. Although a low participation from the communities was observed, the planning process identified valuable information as well as complex challenges for three key stakeholders; local, state, and federal government. New approaches to address natural hazards like flooding, climate change, and coastal erosion were presented by different members of the community, offering opportunities to foster resilience without compromising the economy and the environment. However, the forecast from the Center for a New Economy points to a complex economic future presenting a major challenge to local, state, and federal administrators to identify the necessary financial resources to implement many of the actions presented in the plan [12].

Table 1: Example of table prepared by the Municipal Committee describing proposed mitigation actions.

Category	Sector Strategy/activity	Hazard	Priority	Lead agency	Funding source	Completion date	2019 status
Proposed mitigation actions							
P-1	**Cerro Gordo** Debris removal from the creek bordering Cerro Gordo Community	Flooding and pollution	High	DRNA OPM MAVA	State and Federal	2024	Partial debris removal has been completed
P-2	**Highway PR2** Maintenance to the storm water system	Flooding	High	DTOP-AC OPM del MAVA	State and Federal	Continuous	On-going effort by MAVA without support form state government
P-3	**Santa Ana Community** H-H study to determine water flow impacting road	Flooding	Medium	OPM MAVA	Municipal	2024	Has not started
P-4	**Urb. Extensión Santa Ana** Increase road elevation to control flood level	This approach is too expensive and the inconveniences to residents was considered a major issue. The flooding problems in the community have been associated with the lack of maintenance to the Honda Creek and potential storm water discharges from the San Juan Cement Processing Plant.					
P-5	**Morán Community, and Breñas** Sink holes improvement and clearing	Flooding	Medium	DRNA-OPM MAVA	State and Municipal	2024	Has not started

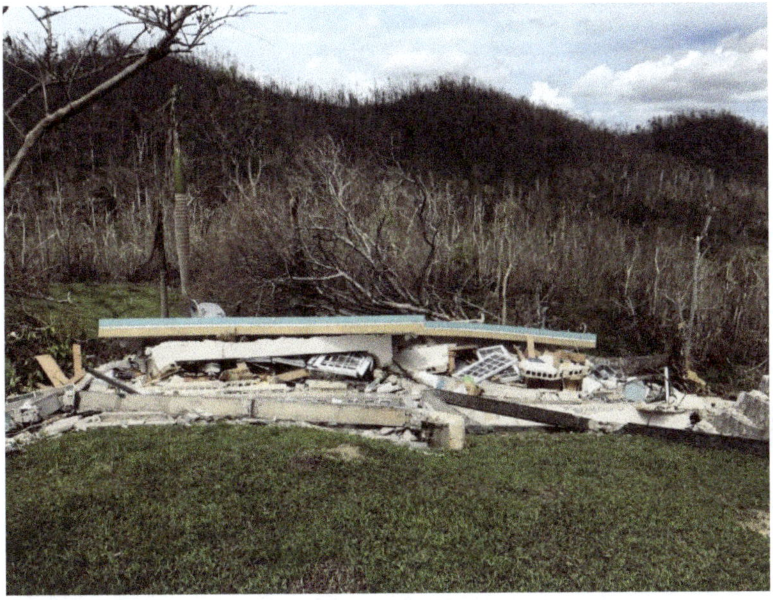

Figure 7: In some parts of the island, winds from Hurricane María destroyed concrete structures entirely.

REFERENCES

[1] NOAA, Office of Coastal Management. https://coast.noaa.gov/states/fast-facts/hurricane-costs.html. Accessed on: 20 May 2019.

[2] Giusti, C., Puerto Rico issues new data on Hurricane Maria deaths. *NBC News*, 13 Jun. 2018.

[3] USGS Landslide Hazards Program, Preliminary locations of landslide impacts from Hurricane Maria, Puerto Rico.

[4] Federal Emergency Management Agency, State and local mitigation planning how-to guide: Developing the Mitigation Plan – Identifying mitigation actions and implementation strategies, 2003. www.fema.gov/fima/planning_howto3.shtm. Accessed on: 21 May 2019.

[5] https://emilms.fema.gov/IS318/MP0403010t.htm. Accessed on: 15 May 2019.

[6] 2012 Multi-Hazard Mitigation Plan for the Municipality of Vega Alta.

[7] 2019 Multi-Hazard Mitigation Plan for the Municipality of Vega Alta.

[8] Federal Emergency Management Agency, FEMA Multi-Hazard Mitigation Planning Guidance – Disaster Mitigation Act 2000, 137 pp.

[9] www.ahcancal.org. Accessed on: 25 May 2019.

[10] https://oversightboard.pr.gov/. Accessed on: 27 May 2019.

[11] www.dii.unisi.it/~mocenni/Note_AHP.pdf. Accessed on: 27 May 2019.

[12] https://grupocne.org/2018/10/24/puerto-ricos-unfinished-business-after-hurricane-maria/. Accessed on: 30 Jun. 2019.

SEISMIC EMERGENCY PLANNING IN THE MUNICIPALITIES OF ELCHE AND ALICANTE, SPAIN: FIRST STEP FOR DISASTER MANAGEMENT

JOSE ANTONIO HUESCA-TORTOSA[1], NOELIA AGEA-MEDINA[2], SERGIO MOLINA-PALACIOS[3], JUAN JOSE GALIANA-MERINO[4], JULIO ROSA-HERRANZ[4] & JUAN LUIS SOLER-LLORENS[3]
[1]Department of Architectural Constructions, Polytechnic School, University of Alicante, Spain
[2]MIES Ramóm Margalef, University of Alicante, Spain
[3]Department of Earth Sciences and Environment, Faculty of Sciences, University of Alicante, Spain
[4]Department of Physics, Systems Engineering and Signal Theory, Polytechnic School, University of Alicante, Spain

ABSTRACT

The south and south-east of Spain are the regions with a higher seismic hazard in Spain. However, although a regional normative focused on the importance of developing seismic emergency planning in many of the municipalities of the Valencian Community was established in 2011, only Elche and Alicante have started to compute the seismic risk and it is planned that their emergency plans will be finished before the end of 2019. The seismic hazard update in the region has shown that the main earthquake scenarios, which will hit both cities, correspond to the Crevillente and the Bajo Segura faults (also responsible of damaging historical earthquakes). The main goal of the developed emergency planning (PAM) is to provide a fast, effective and coordinate response from the public and private stakeholders when a damaging earthquake happen. Assuring, therefore, the maximum protection to the inhabitants and infrastructures in the urban area. The basic functions of the PAM are: a) To establish clearly the organizational and functional structure for intervention in emergencies due to earthquakes that affect the territory; b) To assure the coordination between the emergency agencies at the national, regional and urban level; c) To map a seismic risk zonation that can be used to plan the intervention and locate non-damage infrastructures to be used in the emergency; d) To Increase the population resilience through emergency procedure and education.

Keywords: emergency plan, seismic risk, seismic resilience, emergency management, disaster management.

1 INTRODUCTION

Great loss of human life, structural damage, and social and economic upheaval have occurred repeatedly in recent history due to such natural hazards as earthquakes, hurricanes, landslides, floods and tsunamis. Although earthquake disasters are a minority in comparison to other natural catastrophes, they are responsible of a 77% of fatalities and a 34% of overall losses. This is the reason why public authorities have to improve the planning and seismic policy for the earthquake-prone countries. This is the only way of reducing fatalities and losses.

Spain is a low to moderate seismicity country with historical damaging earthquakes as the 1829 Torrevieja earthquake (south-east of Spain) and the 1884 Andalucia earthquake (south of Spain), both with estimated magnitude higher than 6.0 [1]. Additionally, the M5.1, 2011 Lorca earthquake was the first one causing fatalities since the implementation of modern earthquake-resistant codes in Spain. Nine fatalities, thousands of displaced persons, significant damage to relatively recent buildings and elevated economic losses were the sad budget of this event. In this case, failures on construction conception and the poor performance of non-structural elements were behind this disaster [2].

On April 29, 2011, the government of the autonomous Valencian region approved the *"Plan Especial frente al Riesgo Sísmico"* (special plan against seismic risk) through the Order 44/2011. This Order promotes that, at least, 183 municipalities have to prepare their management and emergency plans against the inherent regional seismic risk. Amongst others, the objectives of those plans should not only include a detailed seismic hazard evaluation but also the analysis of the vulnerability of the existing building stock and the computation of earthquake loss scenarios in order to better prepare for emergency situations. However, currently, none of the municipalities have completed its emergency plan and only the municipalities of Elche and Alicante have given the first steps in order to have it ready before the end of 2019.

The mitigation policy to be established within a seismic emergency planning for any municipalities can be delineated by the following actions:

a) Define an organizational and functional structure that can intervene when an earthquake happens.
b) Take into consideration the coordination with other seismic emergency planning at a regional and national level.
c) Compute the seismic risk in the municipality and establish areas in terms of safeness that can be used in the emergency.
d) Settle the preparedness measures (including education).
e) Establish a database of any infrastructure agencies that can be available to act if an emergency starts.

Therefore, the goal of this paper is to summarize the steps given in Alicante and Elche towards an efficient emergency planning.

2 SEISMIC EMERGENCY PLANNING IN SPAIN

In Spain, since 1995 (according to BOE of May 25, 1995) there is a Basic Civil Protection Planning Directive against the Seismic Risk that was modified in 2004 (according to BOE of October 2, 2004) and which is implemented with the State Plan (March 2010), which is characterized as the Master Plan. Therefore, it establishes the general, organizational and functional aspects of the planning to be specified in the operational planning (coordination and support plans) and in specific action procedures.

This State Plan for Civil Protection against Seismic Risk aims to establish the organization and procedures of action of those State services and, where appropriate, other public and private entities, which are necessary to ensure an effective response to the different seismic situations that may affect the Spanish State.

From this Basic Directive and from the State Plan (Master Plan), the Special Plans are prepared for the seismic risk by those Autonomous Communities in whose territory there are areas where the seismic hazard, in terms of EMS-98 intensity is equal to or greater than VI, for a return period of 500 years, in accordance with the provisions of the Basic Civil Protection Directive against Seismic Risk (Table 1).

All the Autonomous Communities obliged to prepare their Special Plan for Seismic Risk have the same approved by the National Civil Protection Commission, and some of them also have also approved their respective update. This is the case of the Murcia autonomous community which was updated after the 2011 Lorca earthquake.

One of the most important result of these regional seismic emergency planning is that they allow to define the municipalities in which it is compulsory to develop a specific plan. This is done also using the corresponding threshold value of the seismic hazard obtained for each municipality (intensity VI or higher).

The Valencian Community (named Valencia in Table 1) is the case study of this paper because although the regional plan was approved in 2011, currently none of the municipalities have approved their specific plans and only Elche and Alicante have started its development (Fig. 1).

Table 1: Summary of seismic risk emergency plans approved and updated.

Autonomous community	Approval date	Update date
Cataluña	05.06.2002	
Baleares	01.12.2004	
Murcia	19.07.2006	29.10.2015
País vasco	10.07.2007	
Andalucia	16.12.2008	
Extremadura	28.04.2009	
Canarias	03.12.2009	12.12.2017
Aragón	03.12.2009	
Galicia	03.12.2009	
Valencia	01.03.2011	
Navarra	21.07.2011	
Castilla-La Mancha	10.09.2018	

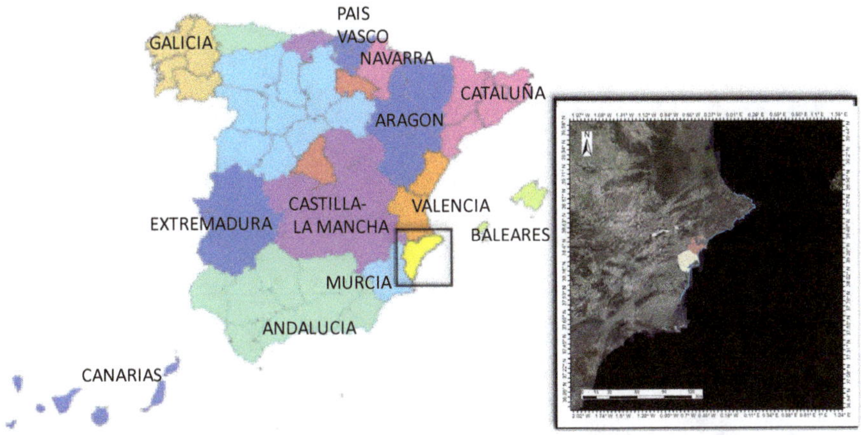

Figure 1: Autonomous regions with a seismic risk emergency plan approved. A detail of the Alicante province and the location of the municipalities of Elche (yellow) and Alicante (red).

3 DEVELOPING A SEISMIC EMERGENCY PLAN FOR THE MUNICIPALITIES OF ELCHE AND ALICANTE

3.1 Seismic risk analysis

A detailed seismic risk analysis has been carried out for the municipalities of Elche and Alicante using several scenarios that can hit both cities [3]. The Crevillente Fault will be the responsible of the two main earthquakes (Mw 5.5 and 6.5) that can affect severely the municipalities in terms of damage and losses. This fault runs along to the Internal and External Betic Zones contact, representing the former limit between the Eurasian and African plates. The CF fault zone and associated fold is 60 km long; the fault presents reverse kinematics (with a minor sinistral component) from the Tortonian [4]. This fault is also responsible of moderate earthquakes in the region, such as the 1787 Elche earthquake, with intensity VI in the EMS-92 scale, and the 1958 Fortuna earthquake (Mw 4.0 and intensity VI) and the 2018 Albatera earthquake with a Mw 4.2, widely felt in the city of Elche and Alicante. Besides, the maximum magnitude (Mw) from length using empirical relationships is 6.79 (6.67–6.79) [5].

Fig. 2 shows the computed ground motion in terms of PGA. As we can see, the ground motion decreases from north to south in Elche although in Alicante the ground motion is lower, due to the higher distance to the rupture, the variations in the soil conditions also introduce important variations in the PGA in the municipality. The PGA has a maximum of 0.23 g and 0.41 g in Elche for a Mw 5.5 and 6.5 respectively. On the other hand, the maximum PGA ranges from 0.11 g to 0.24 g in Alicante.

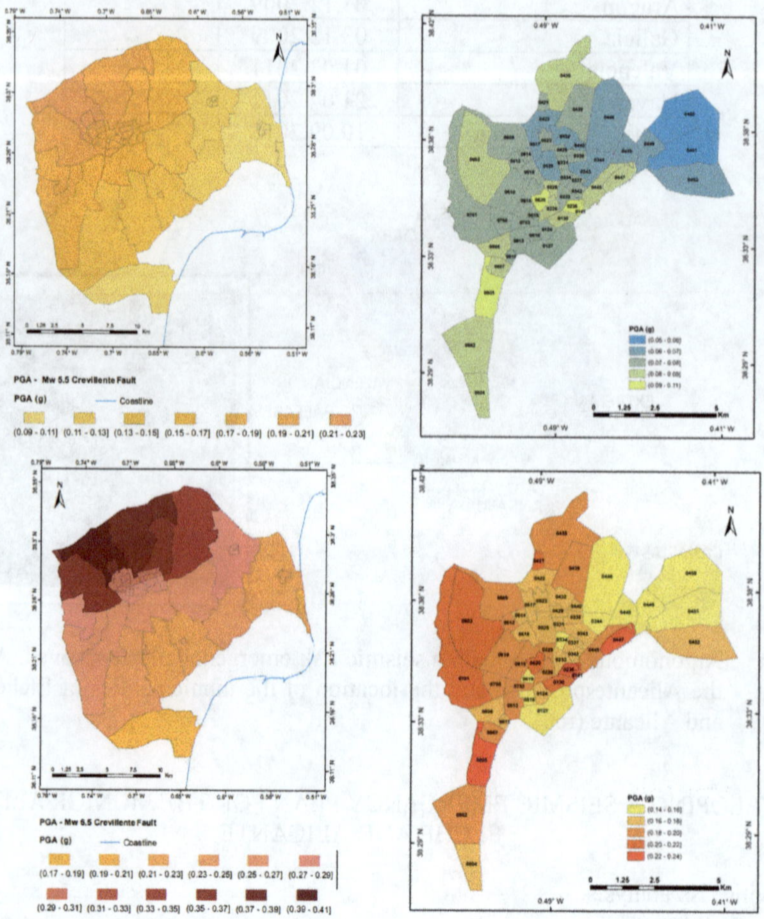

Figure 2: Ground motion scenarios of a magnitude 5.5 (top) and 6.5 (bottom) at the Crevillente Fault for Elche (left) and Alicante (right). *(Source: Molina et al. [3].)*

As a summary, they found that 13% of the building stock in Elche and 0.7% in Alicante would be inhabitable after a Mw 5.5 earthquake (74% in Elche and 18% in Alicante for a Mw 6.5) [3]. The homeless will range from 0.4% in Alicante to 17% in Elche for a Mw 5.5 and 8 to 82% for a Mw 6.5. The people injured (from slight injuries to even death) also ranges from 0.03% in Alicante to a 0.8% in Elche for a Mw 5.5 and from 1.7 to a 7% for a Mw 6.5. The economic losses will increase from 0.6% of the constructed value in Alicante for a Mw 5.5 to 45% of the constructed value in Elche for a Mw 6.5. Table 2 summarizes these results in terms of absolute values, and Fig. 3 represents the mean damage ratio (MDR in percentage) in each of the geounits corresponding to both municipalities. At the top, we can compare the impact for the magnitude 5.5 (left) and 6.5 (right) so we can see that some districts of the urban area are widely affected in both cases although the impact is obviously higher in the magnitude 6.5 (MDR of 68 to 88%) and lower in the magnitude 5.5 (MDR of 15 to 22%).

Table 2: Summary of the seismic risk results for both municipalities.

Scenario	Municipality	Uninhabitable buildings	Homeless	People injured	Economic losses (millions €)	Mean damage ratio (%)
5.5	Elche	4576	40,013	1900	2300	10.3
	Alicante	178	1300	96	228	0.8
6.5	Elche	25,534	190,085	15,800	13,500	63.0
	Alicante	4362	25,784	5304	6190	16.6

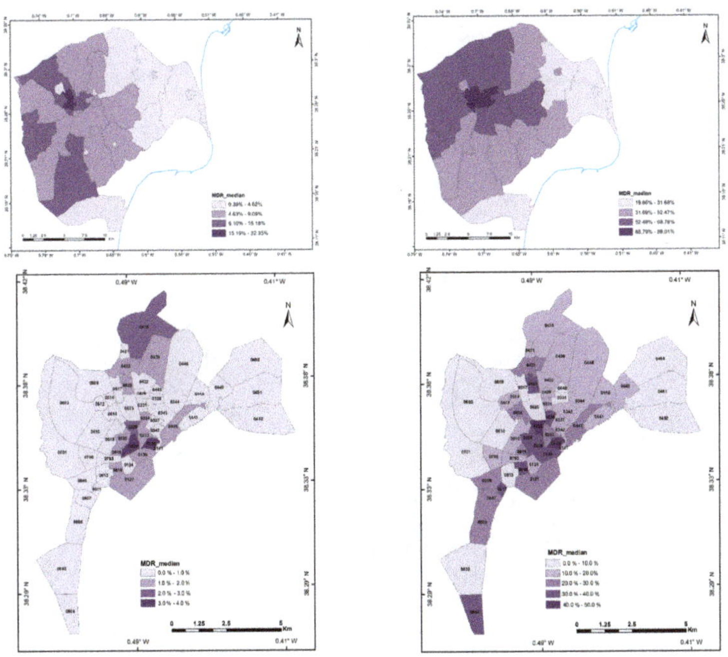

Figure 3: Impact of the magnitude 5.5 and 6.5 (Crevillente Fault) in terms of Mean Damage Ratio in Elche (top) and Alicante (bottom). *(Source: Molina et al. [3]).*

Regarding the municipality of Alicante (Fig. 3 bottom) we observe the same behavior although as we saw with the ground motion the MDR distribution is quite heterogeneous due to the soil effect and vulnerability distribution in the municipality. For both magnitudes, the old urban area has the highest MDR, ranging from 3–4% for Mw 5.5 to 40–50% for Mw 6.5.

From the previous results, it was observed that even the Mw 5.5 which cause important damages in the municipality of Elche affect also the municipality of Alicante and the oldest districts of both cities with buildings constructed without any seismic regulations are the most affected [3]. Additionally, soil effects also have an important effect on damage distribution.

3.2 Effectiveness and functionality

The organizational structure of both municipalities of the province of Alicante, follow the scheme of the Basic Directive and State Emergency Plan for this special risk, as well as that of the Special Plan for the Seismic Risk of the Valencian Community. Identifying three levels of organization for the emergency: Strategic level (CECOPAL), Tactical Level (PMA) and Operational Level (BASIC UNITS).

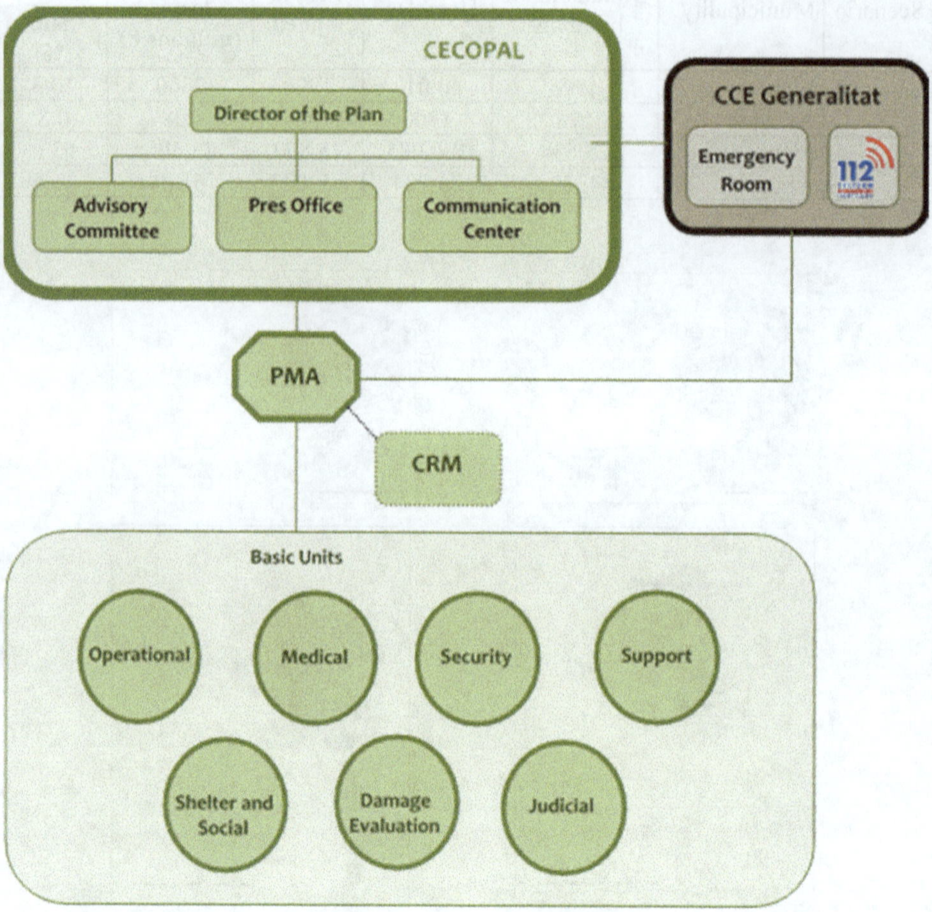

Figure 4: Functional organization schemes for emergency management against seismic risk in the municipalities.

In the first level the CECOPAL (Municipal Operational Coordination Center) is organized with the Director of the Plan in charge, together with the Advisory Committee (Councilors and Headquarters of the Services / Areas affected, and a Panel of Experts), the Press Office and the Communication Center.

On a second level and depending on the severity and type of emergency, the PMA (Advanced Command Post) is made up with the leaders of the Basic Units mobilized by the Plan Management and in constant communication with the CECOPAL

Finally, the third level is composed by the Basic Units of services and people involved from the early stages of the emergency.

It is a very probable fact that both municipalities have to organize themselves, not only among themselves, but also in a broader scope with other municipalities also affected by the same earthquake. And in this way, it is very important that between municipalities there is a system of response and organization, on another scale, operational and effective. On this matter, we propose to take it into account in the development of the Municipal Action Plans and in the future revision of the Special Plan of the Valencian Community against seismic risk. Where a coordinated, operational and effective intermunicipal plan could be constituted.

3.3 Resilience

In the wider sense, resilience incorporates technical, organization, social, economic and environmental issues. The current goal of minimizing casualties and economic and functionality loss is extended to the requirement for the affected community or system to return to "normal" conditions within the shortest possible time. For both municipalities we have established some procedures developed to increase the population resilience:

a) A leaflet with procedure about what to do before, during and after an earthquake will be include to the seismic emergency planning so each municipality will be able to distribute it between the population and include it in its web page.
b) For each municipality, the urban planners will select "secure areas" as meeting points. These places will be marked with specific signs and the population will be instructed to safely walk towards these areas if an earthquake happens. Unfortunately, many of the injuries to the population during the 2011 Lorca earthquake happened because they stood close to the buildings so they were hit by falling object.
c) Greater control and surveillance over the non-structural elements that can affect, with the fall to the public highway, the safety of the population and the functionality of the evacuation routes.
d) The municipality will establish a set of conferences and educational programs on earthquake protection devoted to schools and population. The enhancement of the information of the population to seismic risk may serve a better response on how and what to do if it happens.
e) Finally, the urban planner will also use the microzonation results in order to establish local normatives to avoid the soil-structure resonance by limiting the number of stories according to the predominant period of the soil and the fundamental period of the designed buildings.
f) With the revision of some constructive details provided by the national seismic-resistant norm, perhaps some damage due to affection between structures could be reduced.
g) The realization of joint exercises between municipalities, which, probably due to their proximity, can be affected by the same earthquake, could contribute to a better knowledge of the resources and technical and human resources, and to an efficiency in the operability between them.

4 CONCLUSIONS

Risk management planning for seismic disaster is an integral part of the municipality policies aiming at creating a resilient community. Some initiatives have to be taken in order to increase the local communities' preparedness level, for example, divulgative workshop to the population, meetings with the civil protection and authorities at a local and regional levels, pilot exercises, etc. Although there are many issues to be solved, the seismic emergency planning of Alicante and Elche are great steps forward because they have made possible the updating of procedures, the reactivation of many processes related to earthquake preparedness and the establishment of a starting point in terms of resilience improvement.

ACKNOWLEDGEMENTS

The present research has been funded by the Ministerio de Economia, Industria y Competitividad (CGL2016-77688-R AEI/FEDER,UE), the Generalitat Valenciana (AICO/2016/098) and the cooperation and funding of the Elche and Alicante municipalities.

REFERENCES

[1] Molina, S. et al., Seismic risk scenarios for the urban area of Almoradi (Southeast Spain). *Proceedings of the 8th International Workshop on Seismic Microzoning and Risk Reduction*, 2009.

[2] Navarro, M., García-Jerez, A., Alcalá, F.J., Vidal, F. & Enomoto, T., Local site effect microzonation of Lorca town (SE Spain). *Bulletin of Earthquake Engineering*, **12**, pp. 1933–1959, 2013.

[3] Molina S. et al., Seismic damage scenarios in the municipalities of Elche and Alicante (Spain): A first step to the emergency planning. *International Journal of Safety and Security Eng*ineering, **1–2**, 2019 (in press).

[4] Martin-Rojas, I., Alfaro, P. & Estevez, A., 3D geometry of growth strata in a fault-propagation fold: insights into space–time evolution of the Crevillente Fault (Abanilla-Alicante sector), Betic Cordillera, Spain. *International Journal of Earth Sciences*, **104**(5), pp. 1387–1404, 2015.

[5] Stirling, M., Rhoades, D. & Berryman, K., Comparison of earthquake scaling relations derived from data of the instrumental and preinstrumental era. *Bulletin of the Seismic Society of Am*erica, **92**(2), pp. 812–830, 2002.

RISK COMMUNICATION IN ORDER TO FACILITATE COMMUNITY RESILIENCE AGAINST A LARGE-SCALE FLOOD

TAKEYASU SUZUKI
Disaster and Environmentally Sustainable Administration Research Center, University of Yamanashi, Japan

ABSTRACT

Due to global abnormal weather, large-scale floods that exceed the planned scale flood have occurred in Japan in recent years. The necessity of wide-area evacuation beyond municipal boundaries is required in order to prevent further victims, because drowning and isolation occurred due to recent large-scale floods. The author applied the risk communication method proposed by the author to the Riverside District (about 1,400 households with a population of about 4,000), Chuo City, Yamanashi Prefecture, Japan which is close to the river bank of the large river and is one of the most dangerous districts out of the inundation area of the Kofu Basin. The northern half of the district is in the zone where houses are swept away by streams of water when bank breakage occurs. The risk communication was designed by setting implementation items at each of five processes "C-A-U-S-E", incorporating workshops, questionnaire surveys or presenting evacuation simulation results. Through three years of risk communication activities, local residents were aware of and understood the flood risk which exists in the community, found a solution on its own, accepted proposals for wide-area evacuation, and finally they formulated the community disaster management plan for the wide-area evacuation. This paper introduces all processes of this risk communication and endogenous activities by the residents and systematically summarizes achievements as the risk communication method.

Keywords: risk communication, community resilience, community disaster management plan wide-area evacuation, flood.

1 INTRODUCTION

The number of typhoons frequenting Japan, including the amount of precipitation, has appeared to increase in recent years because of the global weather anomaly [1]. Moreover, whereas both the national and local governments have strengthened and implemented strict laws on disaster mitigation, preparedness and response, people's awareness of self-help and mutual help during a disaster has weakened, thereby raising the tendency to rely on administrative aid for disaster management [2]. Imminent dangers associated with a typhoon landing, such as river flooding, sediment disasters, and tsunamis, could be avoided through strategic evacuation management planning and implementation.

This highlight of this study is dealing with the impact of a large-scale flood scenario. In 1959, approximately 5,098 human casualties, the largest in Japan's history on typhoon damage, were recorded on the landing of the Isewan Typhoon. In turn, the typhoon impact paved a way for the introduction of several countermeasures, including the Disaster Countermeasure Basic Act, the River Act, and the Flood Control Act, among others. Following their successful implementation, which resulted in a reduction in the number of human casualties in recent years, these countermeasures have been continuously developed and improved up to the present time. In line with an earlier premise, the scale of the damage caused by flooding due to heavy rainfall has likewise widened, to the extent that floods induced by mountain rivers (which normally contain debris and sediment) have seemingly become frequent. From an environmental perspective, disasters are also triggered by harmful activities or a predisposition against nature and society, normally by us.

WIT Transactions on The Built Environment, Vol 190, © 2019 WIT Press
www.witpress.com, ISSN 1743-3509 (on-line)
doi:10.2495/DMAN190131

The heavy rains experienced today tend to surpass both the structural and non-structural countermeasures, with the accompanying fear that the extent of this damage will only intensify in future. Structural measures are indispensable, yet they require a great deal of time to develop. On the other hand, non-structural measures, such as people's awareness of disaster management, are easy to establish, but nonetheless require strengthening and improvement. At present (i) realization of an early warning system for incoming disasters and (ii) evacuation schemes are urgent demands.

2 CURRENT STATUS OF WIDE-AREA EVACUATION

The 2015 Kanto and Tohoku heavy rains resulted in massive flooding of the Kinugawa River and 40 km^2 or one-third of the area of Joso City in Ibaraki Prefecture, leaving two human casualties. At the height of the flood, more than 4,000 people were stranded in the flooded area and later rescued by helicopters and boats [3]. A survey conducted by Irie [4] indicated that the largest number of evacuees, accounting for 35% of the total, was headed outside Joso City via car transport (89% of all related evacuation means). In terms of motive, 41% of the evacuees were "family and friends prompted". Moreover, most of those affected indicated that their reason to remain indoors was to maintain a semblance of normality, believing that the heavy rain would not inundate, or that it was difficult to move "considering the elderly". The reason "neighbors are not evacuating" rated high as well, accounting for 12% of the survey responses.

The July 2018 Western Japan heavy rain disaster caused the Oda River, Suematsu River, and Takama River to overflow in Mabi-cho, Kurashiki City, Okayama Prefecture. Approximately 27% or 27 km^2 of Mabi-cho, was flooded leaving 51 human casualties, of which 45 (88%) were elderly (over 65 years of age) [5]. At least 42 people needed evacuation aid. The evacuation rate during floods in Japan has not yet reached 10%. This implies that during large-scale floods, those who cannot evacuate by themselves become casualties.

Typically, such large-scale flooding causes houses to collapse and other properties or structures to get washed away from break points of rivers. Evacuation should not only be judged by the depth of inundation but also by the presence of a dike nearby, where banks may break and intensify water flow. Fig. 1(a) shows the damage near the break point of Joso City during the 2015 Kanto Tohoku heavy rainfall. Similarly, Fig. 1(b) illustrates the extent of damage caused by the 2018 Western Japan heavy rainfall in Mabi-cho.

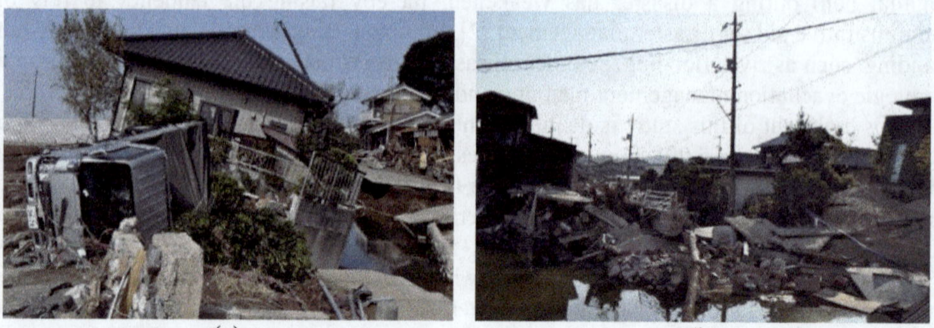

(a) (b)

Figure 1: Damage to houses and properties near river banks or break points caused by large-scale flooding. (a) Joso City at the height of the 2015 Kanto Tohoku heavy rain disaster; and (b) Mabi-cho, Kurashiki City during the 2018 Western Japan heavy rain disaster.

As mentioned earlier, a wide-area scheme is necessary to incorporate early evacuation outside the municipalities before the incoming disaster, based on lessons learned from the flooding in Joso City and Mabi-cho. Such a scheme should prioritize those needing immediate evacuation, with transportation readied by local municipalities toward welfare facilities coupled with the support of neighbouring communities [6]. In other words, coordination between residents and governments is an essential element in the evacuation scheme. Moreover, a wide-area evacuation of community residents can be realized, provided they willingly intend to evacuate. Such intentions can be strengthened by a platform encouraging residents to evacuate through the support of families, friends, and neighbours, and the local government will provide control and guidance in terms of transport and safe routes. In addition, the success of evacuation is dictated by the strength of coordination and communication between municipalities, especially when transferring evacuees to public shelters or welfare facilities [6].

The present study has developed a risk communication method mainly characterized by the CAUSE, for training on the creation of a disaster prevention system for local governments and community residents [8]. This study has also conducted demonstrative research. The focal objectives herein are basically aligned with introducing efforts on risk communication implemented in recent years for the wide-area evacuation of people from the Kofu Basin in case of an expected maximum flood level.

3 FLOOD RISK IN THE KOFU BASIN

Residents who do not evacuate even when normal evacuation information is issued will impede the success of a well-organized wide-area evacuation scheme. A wide-area evacuation plan is defined as a strategy that spans several municipalities and is organized by prefectures. Nevertheless, scheme proposals from both prefectural and municipal governments will not be readily accepted by community residents unless residents are convinced of the necessity to evacuate. As such, a more efficient community disaster management plan on wide-area evacuation could be formulated by considering the proactive activities of the residents, so that the intent of municipality support as well as the coordination scheme between municipalities, prefectures, and residents can be clarified. This study asserts that an effective formula should be created in a bottom-up structure, where community residents play an active role in establishing evacuation plans.

Fig. 2 shows the location of the Kofu Basin in Yamanashi Prefecture. The Eurasian Plate and the North American Plate collide in the east and west respectively, and the highest mountain range in Japan is formed to the west of the basin. Meanwhile, the Philippine Sea Plate collides with the two plates from the south, and subducts under the Eurasian Plate and the North American Plate. The Kofu Basin is located at the collision center of the three plates and has a mysterious structure with an inverted triangle. Additionally, it is located in the Mt. Fuji volcanic belt, with Mt. Fuji to its south. Aesthetically, it is surrounded by beautiful mountain greenery and hot springs. However, the collapsed earth located in the north of the basin due to volcanic activities is deeply deposited in the subsurface of the basin. On the basin perimeter, fans are formed by the supply of debris flow deposits from mountainous rivers. During heavy rainfall, sediment and water from the surrounding mountains gather in the basin. Particularly because rivers drain flood water to the center of the basin, crops in the land could not be harvested. Since the Middle Ages, dikes have been purposely constructed and flood control schemes have been implemented to move the river channel to the edge of the basin, in an effort to turn the land into a suitable area for crop cultivation.

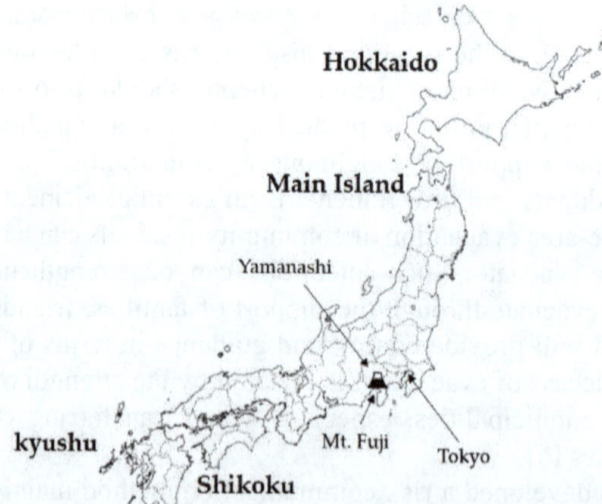

Figure 2: Japanese Archipelago and location of Yamanashi Prefecture.

Fig. 3 shows the main rivers and possible inundation on the Kofu Basin. The inundation area, due to expected maximum rainfall (a probability of 1 in every 1,000 years), is demonstrated on the hazard map according to the categorization of the Ministry of Land, Infrastructure, Transport, and Tourism (MLIT), and the inundation area of Mabi-cho, Kurashiki City, Okayama is also shown on the same scale. In comparison, Kofu Basin has a larger inundation area (specifically, more than 10 times larger than that of Mabi-cho), which indicates that the evacuation distance exceeds 10 km, depending on the location in the basin; therefore, evacuation by car is more suitable. For example, out of a total population of 22,000 people, 51 died during the July 2018 heavy rainfall in Mabi-cho, representing a mortality rate of 0.23%. If such a rate is applied to the inundation area in the Kofu Basin with approximately 300,000 people, the death toll would be an estimate of 690. However, given the low evacuation rate performance of Yamanashi Prefecture in recent years, this figure is underrepresented.

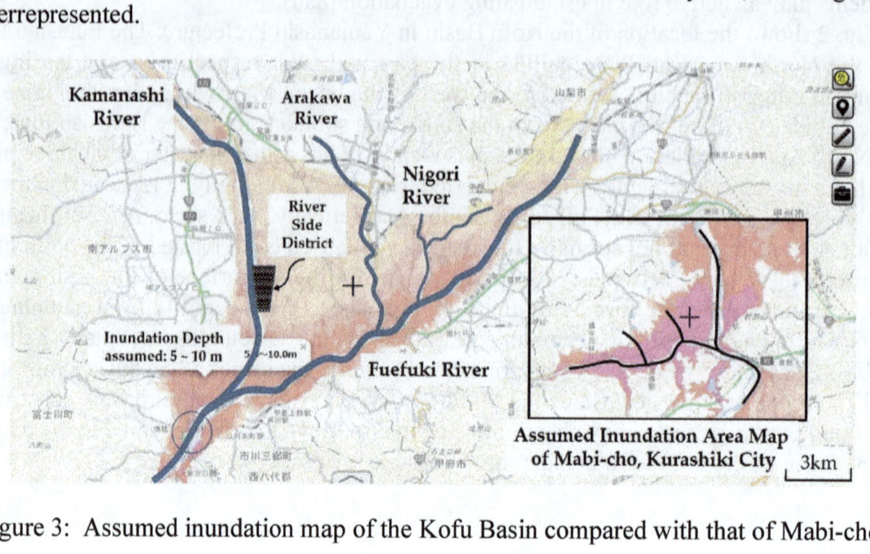

Figure 3: Assumed inundation map of the Kofu Basin compared with that of Mabi-cho.

4 FACILITATING COMMUNITY DISASTER MANAGEMENT PLAN

4.1 CAUSE model

The CAUSE model was proposed by Rowan as a risk communication method aimed at educating regional crisis managers [7]. CAUSE literally represents Confidence, Awareness, Understanding, Satisfaction with the proposed solution, and Enactment, which are also the essential stages of risk communication. Here, the crisis manager is assumed to be in an administrative job, such as a police officer or a fireman, whose communication counterpart is the general population. That is, crisis managers need to learn what people do at each stage of the CAUSE model to provide them with risk awareness, understand their content, accept the solutions presented by the risk managers, and put them into action.

Although the CAUSE model proposed by Rowan is an educational process for local crisis managers to communicate with the general population, the CAUSE model developed in this study is a risk communication method that improves the disaster response ability of the municipalities and the community resilience of the residents. Here, S (together with Satisfaction) includes the stage of the solution, where participants propose solutions or decide on solutions by themselves [8].

4.2 Community disaster management plan

Japan has established the Disaster Countermeasure Basic Act as a comprehensive and long-term plan at the national level and a regional disaster management plan for prefectural and municipal governments at the local level, and has implemented disaster management activities at each level.

However, in the 2011 Great East Japan earthquake, it was strongly recognized that disaster countermeasures after a large-scale wide-area disaster work well with the mutual cooperation of self-help, mutual help and public help. On the basis of the lessons learned, some provisions concerning self-help and mutual help were added in the Disaster Countermeasure Basic Act in 2013. At that time, from the point of view of the promotion of disaster management activity by mutual help in the local community, a community disaster management plan system regarding voluntary disaster management activities conducted by residents and businesses (community residents, etc.) of certain districts in municipalities was formulated.

4.3 The first stage of risk communication

The Riverside District in Fig. 3 is the name of a community indicating a so-called Riverside Town in Chuo City, Yamanashi Prefecture. It is located on the left bank of the Kamanashi River, and was once a water reservoir sandwiched between a dike and the left bank of Kamanashi River. The Usuinuma swamp was formed after the flood of the Kamanashi River in 1907. Reclamation of the swamp began in 1959, and residential area construction has been carried out as the largest residential district (a future population of 7,000) in the Kofu Basin. Nearly 1,400 households and 4,000 residents live in the area. Residential land started being sold from the north area, represented by three residents' associations: the 1st Association of the North, the 2nd Association of the Central, and the 3rd Association of the South.

In 2015, the author received a request from the 3rd Residential Association for risk communication, which has since been initiated to support the formulation of a wide-area evacuation plan with no casualties [9]. During the initial stage of "Awareness", a questionnaire survey on flood risk in the district was conducted (with an estimated recovery rate of 65%) targeting approximately 1400 households in the entire Riverside District. The results of the survey were shown in Fig. 4(a) and (b). When asked if you are interested in the flood in Joso City, 88% of residents replied "have strong interest" or "somewhat interested" as shown Fig. 4(a)). Next, in response to the question of whether there is a high risk of suffering similar damage as Joso City in this district, more than half of the residents answered "extremely high" or "high" as shown in Fig. 4(b). Through the questionnaire survey, community residents were made aware of the commonness of damage caused by floods in this district and Joso City (Awareness).

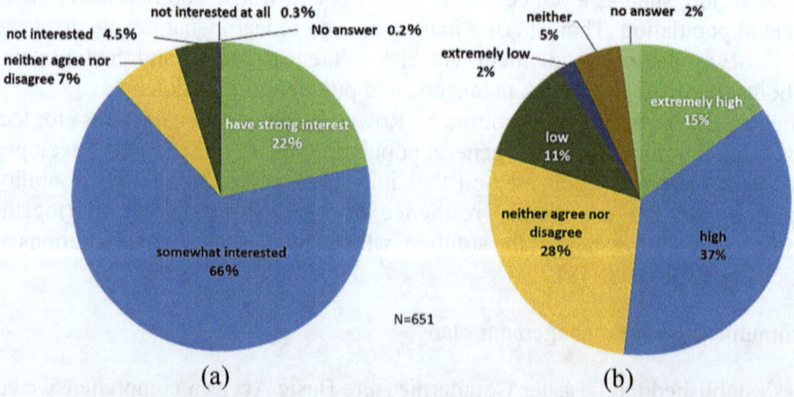

Figure 4: Results of questionnaire survey conducted at the stage of "Awareness".

In this questionnaire survey, some questions were asked about evacuation of persons who need help in evacuation. In response to the question of whether you know the persons who need help in evacuation living in the neighbourhood, the percentage of those who answered that they were grasping was 32% at the 1st Residents' Association, 21% at the 2nd Residents' Association, and 14% at the 3rd Residents' Association, respectively. We asked the respondents who replied they were grasping what are the issues solved in the evacuation of persons who need help for wide-area evacuations. The answer to the question is summarized in Fig. 5. Thus, the residents are aware that means of transportation to shelters is the most important issue.

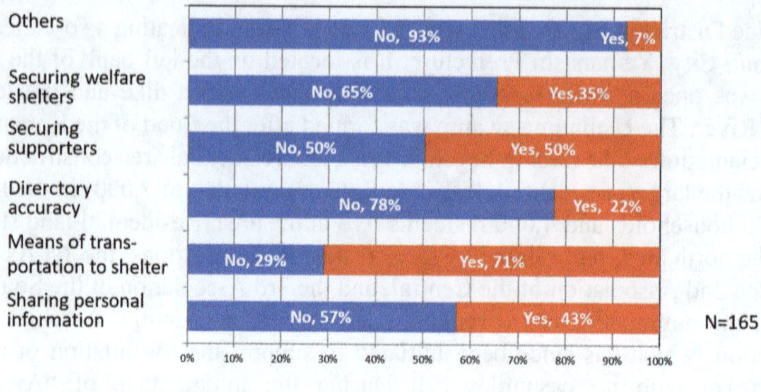

Figure 5: Summary of questionnaire survey on issues which should be solved in wide-area evacuation for persons who need help in evacuation.

The next stage of "Understanding" was designed to promote understanding so that many district residents could participate in activities for evacuation of the area. Within the district, it will be necessary for community residents to mutually discuss wide-area evacuation and support to persons who need help each other in the neighbourhood. Therefore, the author thought that the distribution of the above-mentioned questionnaire results was effective. The results of the questionnaire survey are summarized as easy-to-understand reports such as adding large graphs, letters, and explanations of graphs. Based on this report, the author reported the results to the representatives of the three Residents' Associations and held a meeting to exchange views. As a result, the 3rd Residents' Association decided to copy the report by the number of households, and the chairman determined to explain to the group leaders in the leader meeting and to instruct the group leaders to inform all households of each group by the circulation board.

The report made the chairman of the 1st and 2nd Residents' Associations who had hesitated to start efforts to establish an evacuation support system for persons who need help. As a result, the report was to be informed in the same way at all of the 1st through 3rd Residents' Associations. The results of the questionnaire were shared with the many neighbouring residents, and it would provide a favourable environment for future efforts. Thus, residents shared the flood risk of the district and understood the necessity of an evacuation support system, especially for those needing help during evacuation (Understanding).

The author proposed the establishment of a system in which neighbours support those who need help for evacuation. The representatives of the 3rd Residents' Association agreed with the construction of the evacuation support system and asked the author for guidance on the specific construction method. Therefore, the author developed and proposed two types of assistance styles so that the supporter group can determine evacuation support activities as a timeline without a professional facilitator.

The first assistance style was used in order for supporters to grasp the required degree of support by asking the person who need help in evacuation about the communication ability and walking ability, and whether family support can be given. The next assistance style was used to summarize the role of each supporter as a timeline in the process of taking the person who need help to a temporary evacuation site. The 3rd Residents' Association accepted the method (Satisfaction), and a support system for six persons who need help for evacuation was immediately established. Fig. 6 shows the build-up of support system for the persons who need help for evacuation.

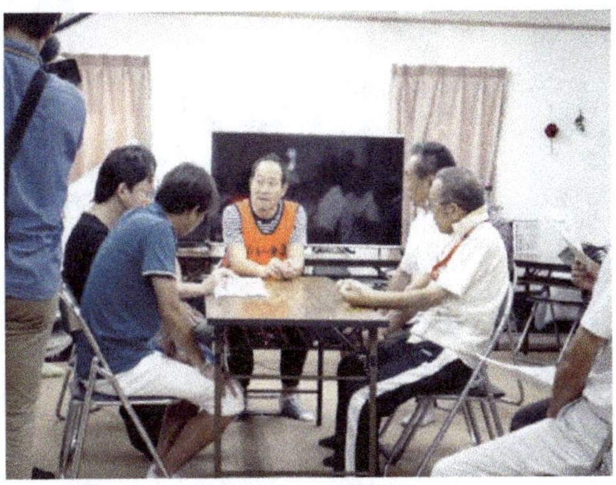

Figure 6: Build-up of support system for persons who need help for evacuation.

Alternatively, district residents suggested that one should hang a towel on the second floor as a sign to inform completion of evacuation. It was decided to implement these suggestions and white towels were distributed to each household. (Satisfaction and Solution).

Therefore, a wide-area evacuation plan, in which all the district residents began evacuation outside the district after evacuating those needing help, was formulated by the 3rd Residents' Association in March, 2018 (Enactment) [9]. Subsequently, representatives of the 1st and 2nd Residents' Associations participated in this risk communication, learned, and joined the activities of the 3rd Residents' Association in the succeeding year.

4.4 The second stage of risk communication

In 2018, another process of the CAUSE model was applied to support the community disaster management plan of the entire Riverside District (from the 1st through the 3rd Residents' Associations). At the meeting of the representatives of the three residents' associations of the Riverside District held in August 2018, the author was informed that both the 1st and the 2nd Residents' Associations had finished establishing a support system for persons who need help in evacuation. At the meeting, the author introduced the results of the agent simulation of the evacuation from the district by car at the "Awareness" stage. In this simulation, the district was divided into a plurality of blocks in order to show the effectiveness of time difference evacuation in which time differences were made by giving an order for each block. When evacuations were started all at once, it was indicated that the intersection would become a bottleneck and traffic congestion would occur. Although some representatives stated that time difference evacuation was effective, some residents did not follow the rules of timed evacuation, and they said that they would start evacuation first.

Therefore, the author cut out screen shots near the bottleneck intersection from the evacuation simulation results, created the materials shown in Fig. 7 to explain the troubled situations that occur at various locations during simultaneous evacuation. As the stage of "Understanding", a questionnaire survey was conducted for all households in the district (using explanatory materials through screenshots of evacuation simulation by cars) to enable residents to understand the necessity of evacuation by cars, with a time difference in each block divided in the district.

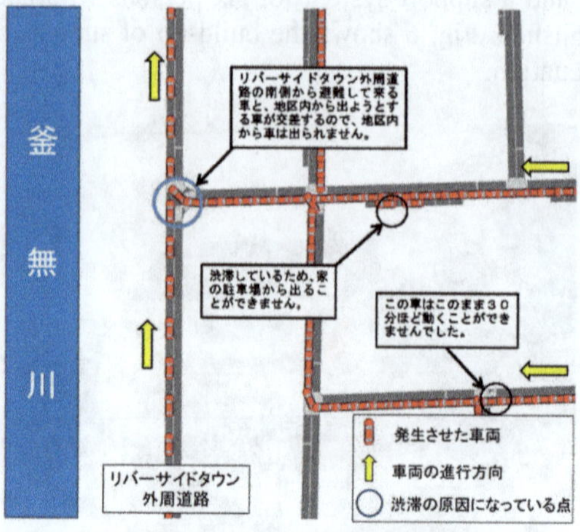

Figure 7: Explanatory material through screenshot of evacuation simulation.

As a result, 91% of the answers from 557 people to the question of "what is the problem during evacuation with cars simultaneously?" was "the occurrence of traffic congestion". Apart from that, 47% of "restricted evacuation route" and 35% of "occurrence of traffic accident" were selected, so the district residents understood that traffic regulation was necessary. Fig. 8 shows the result of the answer to the question "Do you follow the instruction when the time difference evacuation instruction is issued from the residents' association?". The responses "follow" and "may follow" accounted for 65% and it was confirmed that the author's proposal on time-lag evacuation was accepted by many residents.

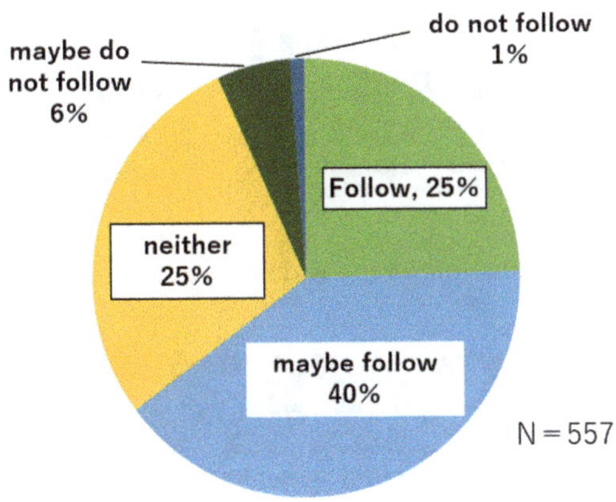

Figure 8: Result of the answer to the question "Do you follow the instruction when the time difference evacuation instruction is issued from the residents' association?".

In the Riverside District in Chuo City, Yamanashi Prefecture, the community disaster management plan for wide-area evacuation was formulated in the entire district in May 2019 (1,400 households of the 1st to 3rd Residents' Associations with 4,000 people) at the final stage of "Enactment". Fig. 9 is a schematic representation of the wide-area evacuation plan for the Riverside District. Fig. 10 is the "My Timeline" of evacuation behaviour (and preparation) distributed to each household. When the authors presented such a timeline in the form of dividing the evacuation behaviour as shown in Fig. 10 into 10 stages, the residents added some ideas to finally create the timeline shown in Fig. 10. The timelines were printed on B5 size glossy paper in black and red two-colour printing and were distributed to all the households. According to the tabulation results, the recovery rate of collection slips was 65%, where the timeline had already been created at 80%. Thus, more than 52% of all households in the district were involved in the creation of the timelines.

5 CONCLUDING REMARKS

The author proposed the implementation of a risk communication approach by using the CAUSE model to evacuate community residents. In the Riverside District in Chuo City, the author proposed and implemented new processes based on the CAUSE model and implemented these twice for wide-area evacuation plan development. The first process covered the evacuation plan of the 3rd Residents' Association, and the second process expanded it to the entire Riverside District (1,400 households 4,000 people). As a result, the community disaster management plan of the whole district on the wide-area evacuation plan was formulated.

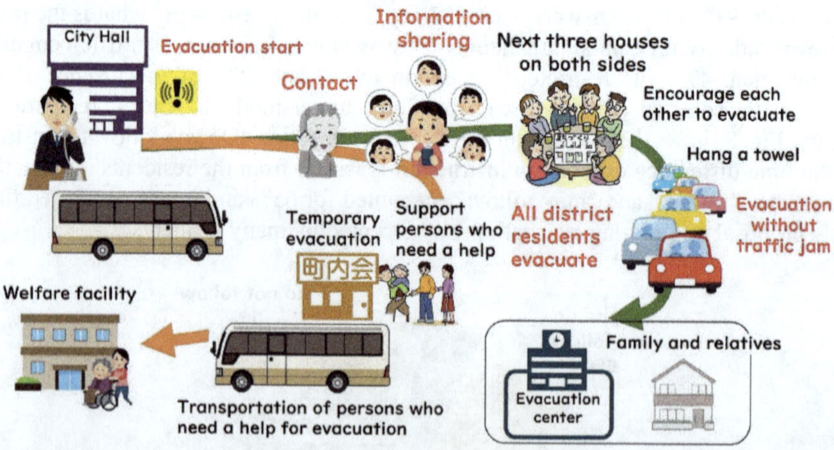

Figure 9: Schematic representation of the wide-area evacuation plan of Riverside District.

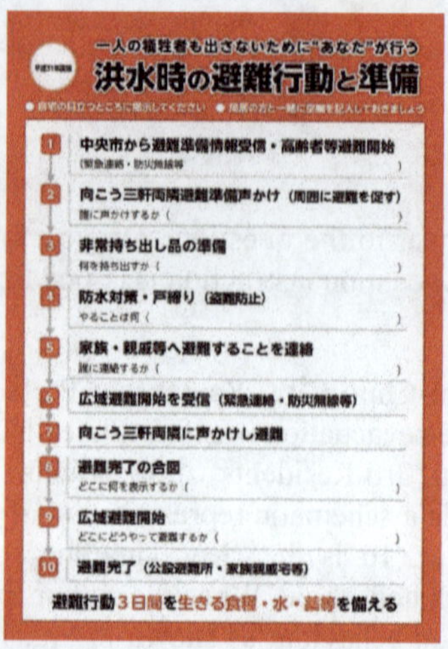

Figure 10: My Timeline for each household printed by Residents' Associations.

Through three years of risk communication activities, local residents were aware of and understood the flood risk which exists in the community, found a solution on its own, accepted proposals for wide-area evacuation, and finally they formulated the community disaster management plan for the wide-area evacuation as an enactment.

ACKNOWLEDGEMENTS

The authors express their deep gratitude to the Ministry of Land, Infrastructure, Transport and Tourism and to the Kofu River National Highway Office for their funding and support of this research. Above all, the authors express their great appreciation to the residents of Riverside District for their cooperation in the questionnaire survey and in the creation of my timeline, and to the representatives of the district for distributing and retrieving the questionnaires.

REFERENCES

[1] Cabinet Office of Japan, Disaster management in Japan. www.bousai.go.jp/1info/pdf/saigaipamphlet_je.pdf. Accessed on: 10 May 2019.

[2] Murosaki, Y. & Tominaga, Y., *Chapter 5 Mutual Help in Creation of People to Confront Disasters*, Minerva Shobo: Kyoto, Japan, pp. 77–86, 2018. (In Japanese.)

[3] Joso City Flood Control Verification Committee, Verification report on disaster response to flood in Joso City due to Kinugawa River flood, 2015. (In Japanese.)

[4] Irie, S., How did citizens in Joso City evacuate when the Kinugawa River broke down? *Broadcast Research and Survey*, pp. 36–65, 2016. (In Japanese.)

[5] Okayama Prefecture, Verification report on the July 2018 flood disaster: Verification committee of the July 2018 heavy rain disaster. www.pref.okayama.jp/uploaded/life/601705_5031910 _misc.pdf. Accessed on: 10 May 2019.

[6] Suzuki, T., System creation and information sharing environment aiming for wide-area cooperation at the time of large-scale disaster. *City Planning Review*, **64**(6), pp. 64–67, 2018. (In Japanese.)

[7] Rowan, K., Botan, C.H., Kreps, G.L., Samoilenko, S. & Farnsworth, K., Risk communication education for local emergency managers: Using the CAUSE model for research, education, and outreach. *Handbook of Risk and Crisis Communication*, eds R.L. Heath & H.D. O'Hair, Taylor and Francis: London, pp. 168–191, 2009.

[8] Suzuki, T., *Wisdom, Technique, Mechanism to Protect Life from Great Disaster*, Shizuoka Academic Publishing: Shizuoka, pp. 154–196, 2014. (In Japanese.)

[9] Suzuki, T., Watanabe, T. & Okuyama, S., Community disaster management plan to implement extensive evacuation without a single victim against flooding. *Journal of Community Disaster Management Society (C-Bosai)*, **13**, pp. 35–50, 2018. (In Japanese.)

STUDY OF THE INUNDATION ANALYSIS OF FLASH FLOODS IN URBAN AREAS FOR RAINFALL IMPACT FORECASTING

SUK HO LEE, DONG HO KANG, KYUNG SU CHU & BYUNG SIK KIM
Department of Urban and Environmental Disaster Prevention Engineering,
Kangwon National University, Republic of Korea

ABSTRACT

Due to climate change, changes in weather such as heavy rains and typhoons have caused various disasters. In addition, the scale of damage is also increasing, which requires quantitative analysis. The purpose of this study is to analyze the impact of rainfall in a specific area and to analyze the secondary damage caused by flash flooding during heavy rains and to use it in forecasting. In order to calculate the depth of flooding due to heavy rain, a rainfall depth of 0–300 mm is increased by 20 mm intervals to produce flooding depth data according to rainfall and, using this, the rainfall-immersion depth relationship curve was developed. Using the developed curve equation, the rainfall (limit rainfall) causing the specific submersion depth (10, 20, 50 cm) was calculated, and the rainfall flood forecasting was performed in the target area based on the calculated threshold rainfall. The target areas were divided into grids of 1 km × 1 km for the Sadangcheon basin, including the vicinity of Sadang Station, which was flooded due to heavy rains in 2011. The target of the second disaster was limited to urban flooding caused by flash floods in the Sadangcheon basin and model coupling techniques of the rainfall-leakage model (S-RAT) and the flood-campaign model (FLO-2D) were used to analyze urban flooding. The targets of the disaster were categorized into people, vehicles, and facilities, and the rainfall (threshold rainfall) that could cause damage to each target was calculated. In addition, the damage stage was divided into four stages by using the rainfall intensity (rainfall impact level). Based on the heavy rains that occurred in the Sadangcheon basin in July 2011, the results were compared with the forecast results due to the inundation status of the Sadang Station and the rainfall impact level.
Keywords: S-RAT, FLO-2D, coupling technique, threshold rainfall, heavy rain impact level.

1 INTRODUCTION

Recently, various disasters occur due to the change of weather due to climate change, and the damage scale is increasing. Meteorological phenomena and socio-economic impacts According to the inertia analysis, the most frequent and largest damages are the disasters. Meteorological phenomena that cause meteorological disasters are heavy rains and typhoons. In addition, the most common weather factor between heavy rain and typhoon is rainfall. Therefore, natural disasters in our country occur most frequently due to rainfall, and thus, we can minimize the damage to disasters by predicting and preparing for them in advance. Currently, the Meteorological Agency uses the ensemble prediction technique to predict future rainfall information. Ensemble prediction is a system that complements the limitations of deterministic prediction of a single numerical forecast and predicts the future probabilistically by performing several models with different initial conditions, physical processes, boundary conditions, etc. Using this, the Korea Meteorological Administration currently conducts forecasts for rainfall in various forms such as short-term, mid-term, long-term forecasts, neighborhood forecasts, national forecasts, and special reports. The biggest drawback of current forecasts, however, is that heavy rainfall forecasts are being made without considering regional characteristics because they only predict the absolute value of rainfall. Of course, there are additional forecasts for protecting facilities, paying attention to flooding, and preparing for flooding. To this end, the World Meteorological Organization has

WIT Transactions on The Built Environment, Vol 190, © 2019 WIT Press
www.witpress.com, ISSN 1743-3509 (on-line)
doi:10.2495/DMAN190141

already identified the impact of disasters and established guidelines for forecasting services. Emphasis is placed on the importance of forecasts for weather agencies in each country. Weather forecasting countries, including the United Kingdom and the United States, have already implemented partial impact forecasts (Yeh [1]). The Flood Forecasting Centre (FFC) in the UK has created a user manual for forecasting flood impacts and has created a flood risk matrix to divide the flood risk stages into four stages [2]. In addition, in the United Kingdom, grid-based flood impact forecasts are carried out and grid-based impact forecasts are carried out using the G2G (grid to grid) model, which is a distributed model, to simulate flooding (Cole [3], Price et al. [4], Cranston et al.[5]).

In Korea, research for the impact forecast is underway. Kim et al. [6] explained the characteristics of impact forecasts and analyzed the current status and cases of impact forecasts in advanced countries and Lee [7] estimated the marginal rainfall causing flood damage, focusing on flood damage cases in Gangnam area.

Rainfall is also important in estimating rainfall for forecasting impacts, but rainfall is largely dependent on topography, i.e. the characteristics of the region (rivers, mountains, urban areas), land use, and soil. Depending on the region's drainage management system, various secondary damages can occur, such as urban flooding, landslides and flooding. Even for the same runoff, the impact of the runoff may vary between regions and time periods. Therefore, if the characteristics of the secondary and tertiary disasters caused by precipitation are identified, it is possible to predict the impact on actual damages, not the forecasts limited to rainfall.

The purpose of this study is to analyze the impact of rainfall in a specific area and to forecast the damage caused by flooding during the secondary damage caused by actual rainfall. In 2011, the target areas were divided into 1 km × 1 km grids for three areas of Sadang-dong and Seocho-dong, which were affected by flooding due to torrential rains, to determine the limit rainfall causing specific flooding in each area. In order to estimate the Threshold Rainfall, the model coupling technique of rainfall-runoff model S-RAT (Kim et al. [8]) and flood overflow model FLO-2D [9] was used. Based on the estimated rainfall, the forecasting stage according to rainfall was divided into four stages. In fact, the intensive rainfall scenario that occurred around Sadang-dong and Seocho-dong in 2011 was applied. Inundation cases were compared and analyzed.

2 RESEARCH METHOD

This study is to develop a method of estimating the rainfall impact that causes constant flooding in each region and classifying the risk impact from heavy rainfall over time. The lowest mark is defined as the starting point of flooding in the grid where heavy rain damage occurred among the target areas, and the runoff amount is calculated at the lowest mark, and the amount of runoff is used as input data of the flood scope model to conduct inundation analysis to develop the depth-high water flow relationship curve. The developed rainfall-submersion curve is used to produce marginal rainfall that causes a specific submersion depth. The critical grid for the critical rainfall was 1 km × 1 km, but in the runoff analysis, the watershed was calculated by dividing the basin based on the lowest elevation point in the 1 km × 1 km grid, and the flooding depth was calculated by applying the calculated runoff to the immersion model. Using the simulation results, the rainfall-submerged depth curve was calculated using the maximum submerged depth in the 1 km × 1 km grid. Therefore, the target grid of marginal rainfall is 1 km × 1 km, and the range applied to rainfall-flow and flooding simulation is the entire flood basin including the target grid. In addition, the threshold rainfall of each grid is calculated using the developed curve equation and the results are compared and analyzed using the rainfall scenario. The research procedure is shown in Fig. 1.

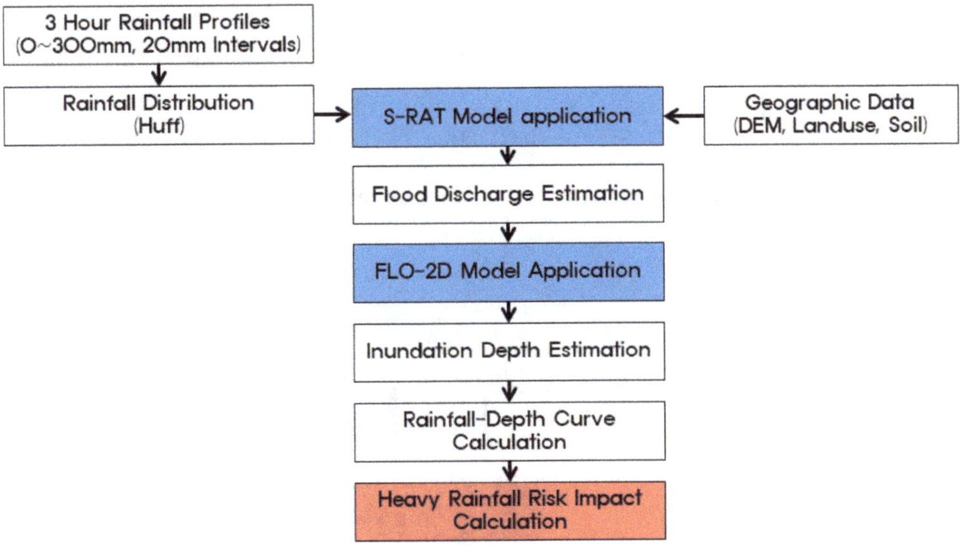

Figure 1: Study flow chart.

3 THEORETICAL BACKGROUND

3.1 S-RAT

The S-RAT (Spatial Runoff Assessment Tool) model is a distributed rainfall-runoff model developed by Kim et al. [8]. It is designed to simulate the spatial and temporal runoff changes in the watershed by calculating the balance. Most distributed hydrologic models also rely on GIS-related commercial packages, such as Arc-related software or IDRISH, to extract topographical parameters to be entered in the model, but S-RAT has its own parameters extracted and simplified input. The S-RAT model used the SCS curve number (CN) method to estimate the permeation and direct runoff for each grid. To do this, the soil map and land use are input and the CN value grid data is generated and calculated

$$S(i,j) = 254(100/CN(i,j) - 1), \quad (1)$$

where $S(i,j)$ is the potential reserve; $CN(i,j)$ is CN value per grid

$$\frac{P_n[t,(i,j)]}{P[t,(i,j)]} = \frac{F[t,(i,j)]}{HS(i,j)}, \quad (2)$$

where $F[t,(i,j)]$ is the infiltration capacity of the infiltration reservoir (water content) (mm); $HS(i,j)$ is capacity of infiltration storage tank

$$I[t(i,j)] = P[t,(i,j)] - P_n[t,(i,j)], \quad (3)$$

$$\mathrm{W[t,(i,j)]} = \frac{F[t,(i,j)]}{HS}, \quad (4)$$

$$\mathrm{I[t(i,j)] - W[t,(i,j)]} = \frac{dF[t,(i,j)]}{dt}, \tag{5}$$

where W[t, (I, j)] is subsurface spill ; $P_n[t,(i,j)]$ (mm) is direct outflow, H_s is a conceptual parameter as a dimensionless constant. Eqns (3)–(6) are used to calculate the governing equation of mass storage of the infiltration reservoir. Eqn (7) can be interpreted using the fourth-order Runge–Kutta method

$$\frac{dF[t,(i,j)]}{dt} = -\frac{F[t,(i,j)]}{HS} - E[t(i,j)] + \mathrm{P[t,(i,j)]}\left\{1 - \frac{F[\mathrm{t,(i,j)}]}{HS(\mathrm{i,j})}\right\}. \tag{6}$$

Fig. 2 shows a conceptual diagram of the grid water balance calculation of this model.

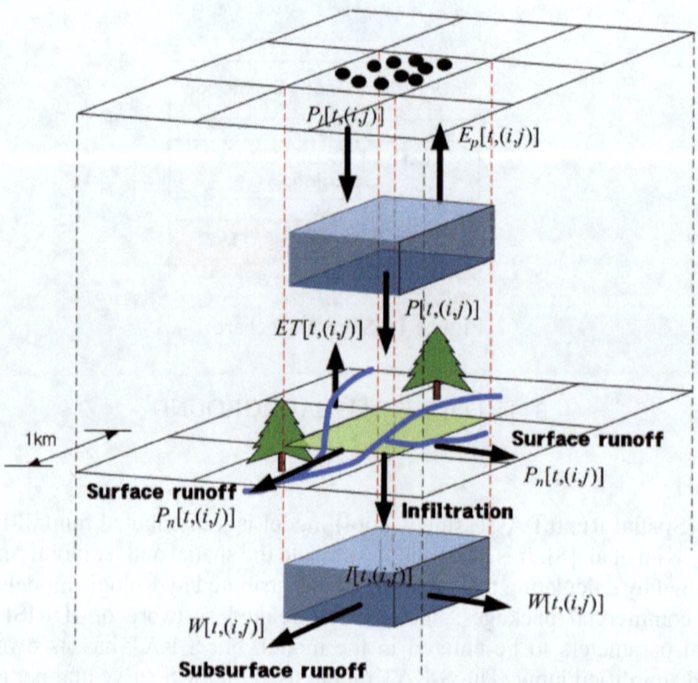

Figure 2: Conceptual diagram of grid water balance [8].

3.2 FLO-2D

The FLO-2D model was first developed in 1988 to identify insurance flooding areas in the US state of Colorado [9]. The FLO-2D model reproduces the tracing of the flood while preserving the volume. Basically, starting with surface flood simulations, components can be added to the simulation for various topographical requirements, flow obstructions in buildings, bridges, dikes, etc. in urban areas, and losses in flow paths. The FLO-2D model is certified by the US Federal Emergency Management Agency (FEMA), so it is highly reliable, and GDS, MAPPER ++, etc. can be used to automatically distinguish flooded areas. In addition, the results are processed as a graph, so it is easy to check space and time. The flow equation of FLO-2D is same as eqn (7), and it is based on continuous equation and momentum equation

$$\frac{\partial h}{\partial t} + \frac{\partial hV}{\partial x} = i,$$

$$S_f = S_0 - \frac{\partial h}{\partial x} - \frac{V}{g}\frac{\partial V}{\partial x} - \frac{1}{g}\frac{\partial V}{\partial x} = 0, \tag{7}$$

where h is the depth of the flow, V is the average velocity of one of the eight direction flows (x-directions) in the starting lattice, and i is the excess rainfall intensity. S_f is based on the Manning equation with a friction gradient.

Fig. 3 flows from eight flow directions at the top right are differentially distributed to adjacent grids according to the elevation difference. The distributed flow rate is distributed along the elevation difference with adjacent grids, moving along a constant pathway.

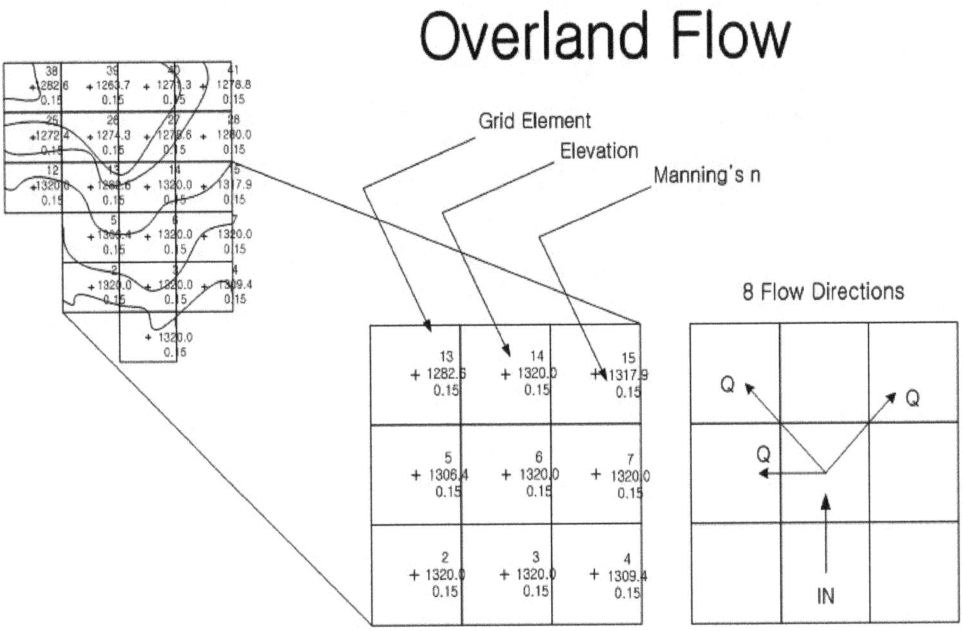

Figure 3: Discharge flux across grid element boundaries [9].

4 APPLICATION AND RESULTS

4.1 Target area

The area of this study was about 300 mm of heavy rainfall from 01:00 to 23:00 on 27 July 2011 at Sadangcheon, located in Dongjak-gu, Seoul, Korea. In order to analyze the damage, the submerged area was divided into grids of 1 km × 1 km (Fig. 4).

4.2 Construction of input data

The data needed in the rainfall-runoff model are rainfall and terrain data (DEM, Landuse, Soil map). The 500 year probability rainfall of 3 hours in Seoul rainfall station is 243 mm [10]. Therefore, a total of 15 types of rainfall scenario were established by dividing 20 to 300 mm into 20 mm units. In order to distribute the total amount of rainfall in time series,

Huff rainfall distribution method was used to convert the time series into rainfall data format [11]. we used the second quartile, which is considered to reflect the rainfall pattern of Korea, and the third quartile, which is the median of the quartile, to consider the extreme situation. The results of the third quartile rainfall scenario for the 3 hour sustainment time are shown in Fig. 5.

In order to calculate the surface flow direction and surface discharge of the target grid, subwatersheds including target grids were divided and spatial information of DEM, Landuse, and Soil map with 30 m × 30 m resolution was constructed. The spatial information deployed is as shown in Fig. 6.

Data required for flood analysis using FLO-2D are the flood scope and the DEM. The runoff is calculated using the rainfall-flow model of the flood overflow flow, and the DEM uses the same spatial data as the DEM used in the rainfall-flow model.

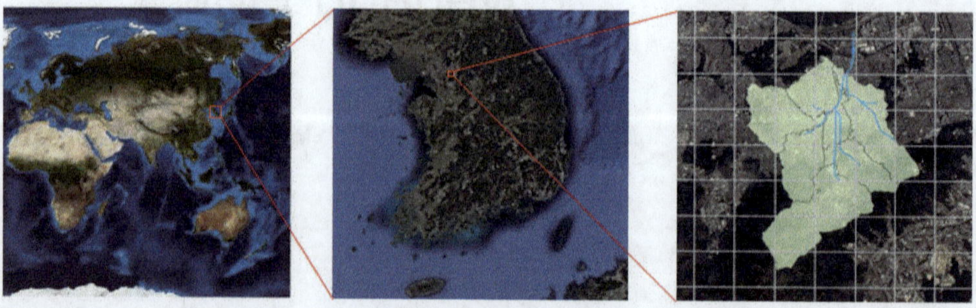

Figure 4: Study area.

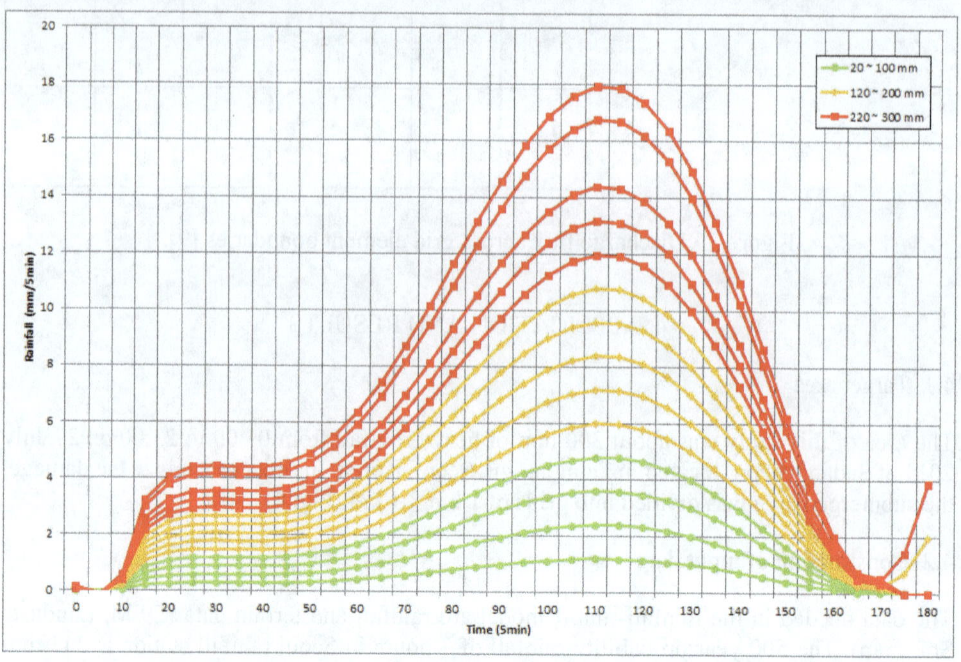

Figure 5: Rainfall scenarios with third quartile in the duration of 180 min.

DEM	Land use	Soil
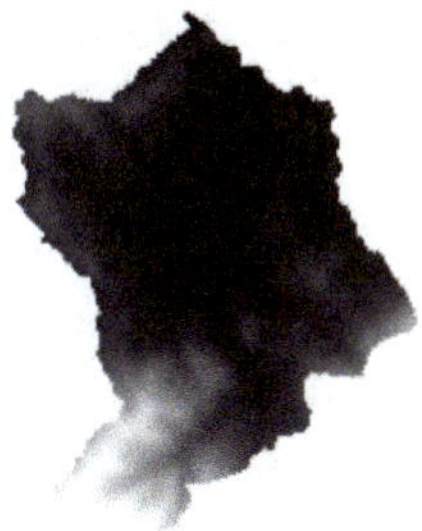	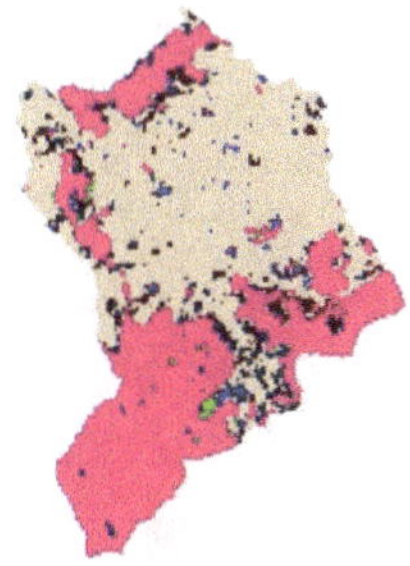	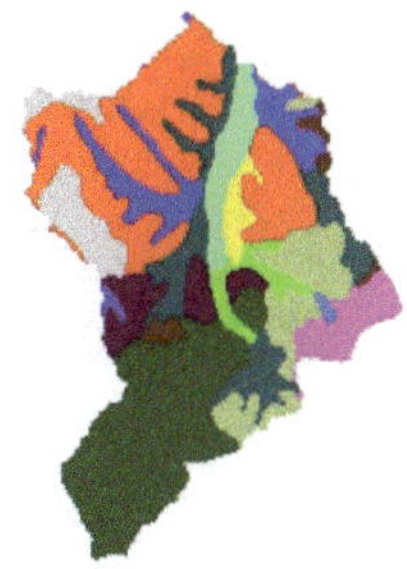

Figure 6: Topographic data.

4.3 Application of rainfall-spill model (S-RAT)

Using the set rainfall for each scenario, the S-RAT model is used. Rainfall-flow analysis of five basins was conducted. The resolution of the subwatershed is 30 m × 30 m, so the flow rate can be checked for each grid. The basic unit for impact prediction is 1 km × 1 km, and the reference point for application of the flooding model within the grid is defined as the lowest elevation point at the reference grid (1 km × 1 km). In the case of the S-RAT model, once the watershed rainfall-runoff simulation is completed, the flow rate of the grid can be immediately identified on any grid. Fig. 7 is a grid of rivers forming during rainfall in the Sadangcheon basin. Calculate the amount of runoff from each grid using 15 types of rainfall in Fig. 5. The calculated discharge amount becomes the discharge flow rate from the flood control model and is used as the input value of the flood analysis. The release rate of No. 4, the final exit point of the basin, is as shown in Fig. 8.

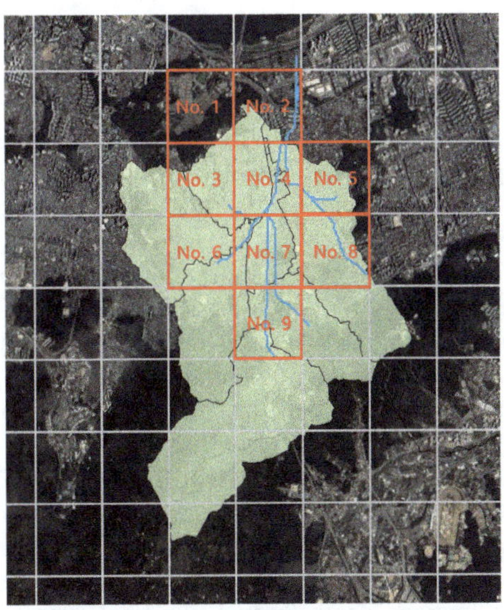

Figure 7: Basin for runoff model.

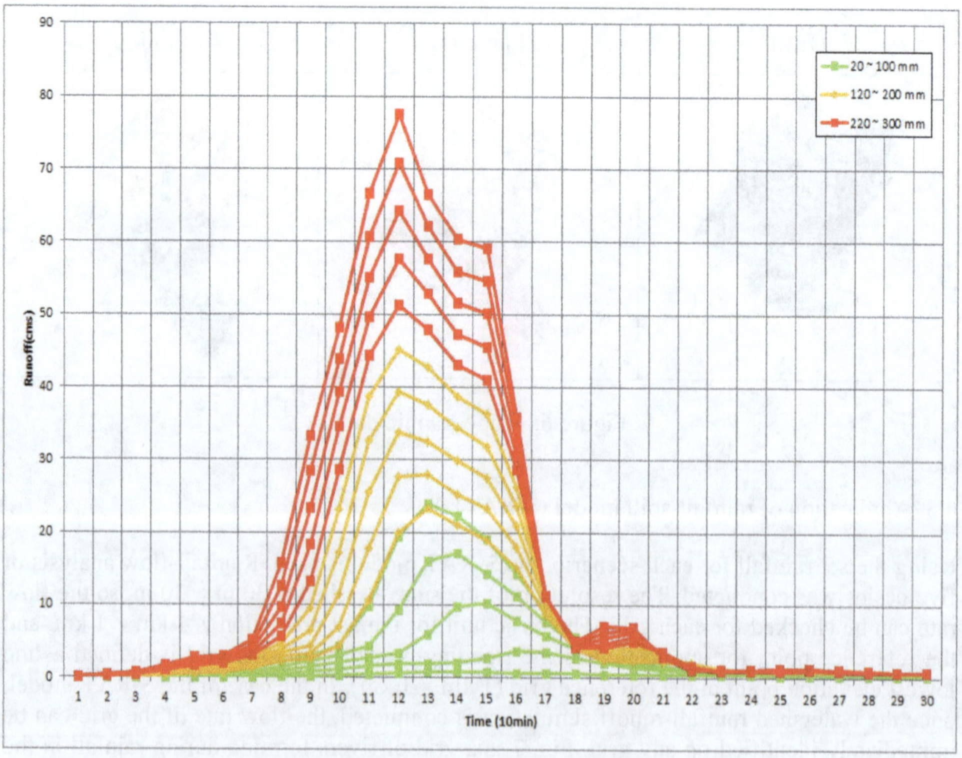

Figure 8: Result of runoff in study area.

4.4 Flood campaign model (FLO-2D) application

In order to simulate the depth of flooding, the runoff value from the analysis point calculated above was distributed to the minimum elevation of each grid over time. For more accurate simulation of flooding in urban areas, the flow rate through the sewer network from the surface runoff calculated by the rainfall-runoff model is used as an input to the flood overflow model (except for underground runoff). In the case of immersion analysis for forecasting the impact of the UK, the flooding capacity of five years was regarded as the flood protection capacity, and the immersion analysis was carried out using the flow rate excluding the flood protection capacity of five years from the runoff. According to the frequency of Korea's sewage system, design is currently underway based on the target rainfall for anti-disaster performance by the Ministry of Public Administration and Security, but the existing pipe network has been designed and constructed at frequencies between 5 and 15 years. In addition, the flooding around the Sadang station, which is the study area, also lacked the water supply capacity of the network, but it was also a factor that prevented the smooth water supply of the network due to manhole residues such as soil and leaves. Therefore, in this study, immersion analysis was carried out considering only surface runoff except ground runoff through sewer pipe network. Fig. 9 shows the rainfall-submerged depth curves of nine grids in the Sadangcheon basin, the analysis area, and shows the relationship between rainfall for each scenario and the submerged depth through the final submerged analysis. Using the recording curve produced in Fig. 8, the limit rainfall is calculated according to the flood depth.

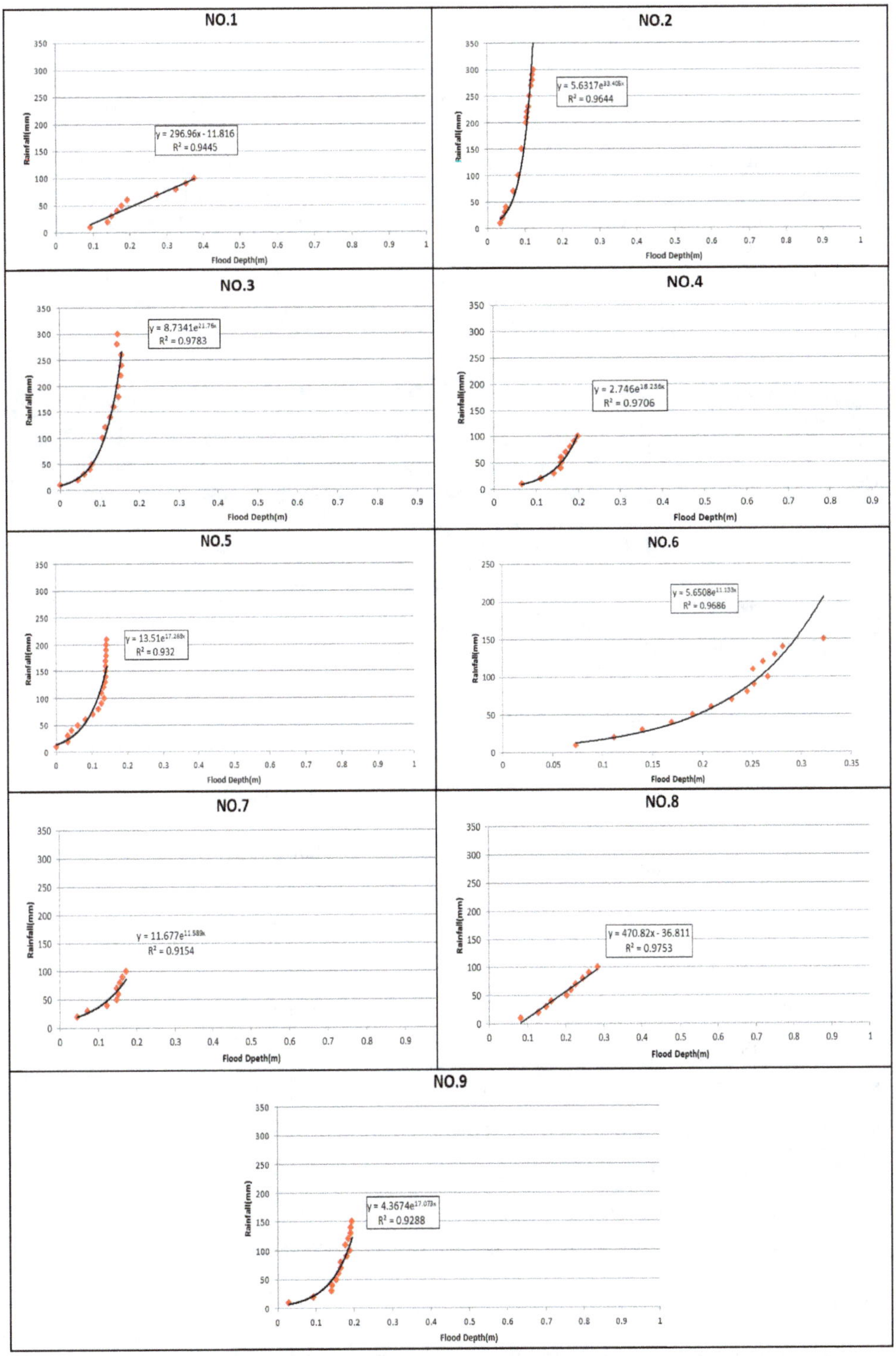

Figure 9: Rainfall-depth curve.

4.5 Estimation of threshold rainfall

In order to forecast the impact of flooding due to rainfall, it is necessary to determine who will be affected by flooding and the depth of flooding that will be affected. In this study, the subjects of damage were defined as three cases: life, vehicle, and building.

Considering the relevant data, the rainfall impact level was set to four levels. The first stage is 0–10 cm, which is considered to be inconvenient for walking, the second stage is 10–20 cm, which is the improper height of passenger cars, and The third step is 20–50 cm considering the height of the installation waterproof plate, and the fourth step is determined to be more than 50 cm causing the flooding of the facility. And the rainfall-flood depth curve of Fig. 10 was used to estimate the marginal rainfall that induces submerged depths representing the boundary of each rainfall impact level (Table 1).

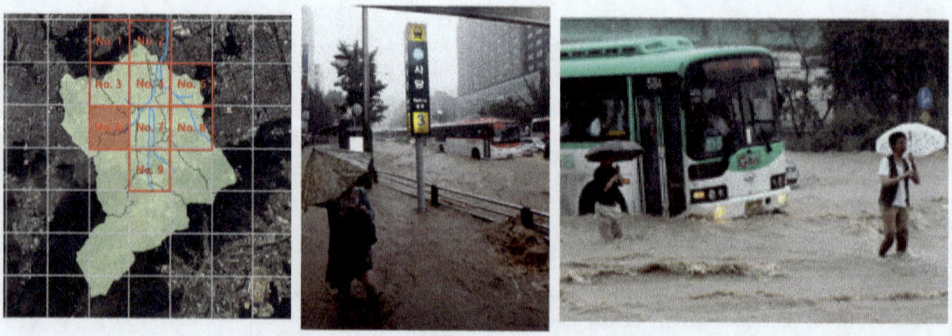

Figure 10: Study area and real case (No. 6).

Table 1: Calculation of critical rainfall and impact level.

Grid	Rainfall-depth curve	Critical rainfall/impact level						
		<	10 cm	~	20 cm	~	50 cm	<
No. 1	$y = 296.46x + 188.92$		17 mm		105 mm		–	
No. 2	$y = 5.6317e^{33.405x}$		76 mm		427 mm		–	
No. 3	$y = 8.7341e^{21.76x}$		52 mm		200 mm		–	
No. 4	$y = 1355.9x + 84.598$		37 mm		119 mm		–	
No. 5	$y = 13.51e^{17.269x}$	Level 1	10 mm	Level 2	57 mm	Level 3	199 mm	Level 4
No. 6	$y = 521.13x + 93.267$		23 mm		78 mm		244 mm	
No. 7	$y = 1018.2x + 208.32$		24 mm		133 mm		–	
No. 8	$y = 500.17x + 164.89$		159 mm		–		–	
No. 9	$y = 4.3674e^{17.073x}$		32 mm		49 mm		72 mm	

4.6 Study area application

Based on the total rainfall, a comparative analysis was performed using the actual rainfall in the area of analysis. On 26–29 July 2011, Seoul suffered 34,152 victims, including 22 deaths and 39 injuries. During this period, the heavy rains, which occurred from 01:00–23:00 on the 27th July, were about 300 mm, which caused large flooding damage in the areas of Sadang-dong and Seocho-dong. Therefore, a 24 hour rainfall impact forecast was performed assuming the rainfall data during this period as a predicted rainfall scenario. The forecasting time was every 1 hour, and the rainfall impact level was calculated by comparing the marginal rainfall corresponding to the life, vehicle, and building based on the rainfall after 3 hours from the reference time. In the case of Sadang-dong Sadang Station (grid No. 6), flooding impact level 2 started from 03:00 and maximum flooding depth of 30 cm (three levels of heavy rain impact level) occurred after 19:00. As seen in Fig. 10, it affected walking and vehicle movements around Sadang Station.

Table 2: Result of rainfall impact level (No. 6).

Time	01:00	02:00	03:00	04:00	05:00	06:00	07:00	08:00	09:00	10:00	11:00	12:00
Rainfall (mm)	0.98	14.71	42.14	77.42	60.16	62.90	59.88	115.6	159.3	140.4	85.75	29.15
Depth (cm)	0	9	18	24	21	22	21	27	30	29	24	15
Impact level	–	1	2	3	3	3	3	3	3	3	3	2
Time	13:00	14:00	15:00	16:00	17:00	18:00	19:00	20:00	21:00	22:00	23:00	–
Rainfall (mm)	19.70	10.48	14.49	6.35	7.85	7.55	0.00	2.82	1.11	0.00	0.98	–
Depth (cm)	11	6	8	1	3	3	0	0	0	0	0	–
Impact level	2	1	1	1	1	1	–	–	–	–	–	–

5 CONCLUSION

Even though the same rainfall occurs, the depth of flooding in each region varies according to the topographic conditions and flood protection ability of the region. Therefore, if you know in advance the rainfall that causes a certain flooding depth in a particular area, you can use the predicted rainfall to proactively predict damage. In this study, for the prediction of heavy rain effects, we investigated the method of forecasting the damage effect using flooding depths in urban areas caused by heavy rains. Damage targets due to flooding were divided into population, traffic, and facilities, and the damage criteria for flooding were investigated and analyzed to create four-step Impact Levels according to the damage status, and the threshold rainfall causing marginal flooding at each stage was determined. Rainfall impact forecasts were carried out using real rainfall in the affected areas of Seodang-dong in Sadang-dong, assuming that the real rainfall was the predicted rainfall. Based on the immersion depth of each time, the rainfall impact level was assigned by comparing with the threshold rainfall and compared with the rainfall impact level and actual flood damage cases. As a result of the comparison, it was confirmed that the results of immersion analysis with time showed similar patterns according to the impact level. In many studies of disasters, risk is largely determined by three conditions: disaster, exposure and vulnerability. To analyze the risks of heavy rain effects and forecast their impacts, we analyze disasters (inundation depths) caused by heavy rains, estimate exposure and vulnerability by considering the spatial and spatial distribution of population, traffic, and facilities in each region. The final impact level should be calculated.

Up to now, the rainfall impact thresholds have been assigned based on the submerged depth only. Therefore, additional studies should be conducted on the values of 10, 20, and 50 cm, which are the depths of heavy rain impact limits for each level. In addition, it is also necessary to study how to consider infrastructure such as people, vehicles, and facilities in places where the same flooding is caused.

ACKNOWLEDGEMENTS

This work was funded by the Korea Meteorological Administration Research and Development Program under Grant KMI[2018-03010]. This work was supported by Korea Environment Industry and Technology Institute (KEITI) through Advanced Water Management Research Program, funded by Korea Ministry of Environment (MOE) (83091). This work was financially supported by Ministry of the Interior and Safety as "Human Resource Development Project in Disaster Management".

REFERENCES

[1] Yeh, S.W., A suggestion for expanding impact prediction services. *Meteorological Technology and Policy*, **10**(1), pp. 6–17, 2017.

[2] Flood Forecasting Centre, *Flood Guidance Statement User Guide*, 2017.

[3] Cole, S., Flood forecasting at national scales: Some UK experiences. *National Flood Management Conference*, Dublin, 2018.

[4] Price, D. et al., Operational use of a grid-based model for flood forecasting. *Water Management*, **165**(2), pp. 65–77, 2012.

[5] Cranston, M. et al., Countrywide flood forecasting in Scotland: Challenges for hydrometeorological model uncertainty and prediction. *Weather Radar and Hydrology*, eds R.J. Moore, S.J. Cole & A.J. Illingworth., IAHS Publication 351, pp. 538–543, 2012.

[6] Kim, H.M., Min, K.R., Kim, I.G., Lim, B.H., Youn, M.J. & Kim, S.B., Paradigm shift to impact-based forecasting and warning services for natural hazard response. *Korea Society of Innovation*, **12**(3), pp.161–178, 2017.

[7] Lee, B.J., Analysis on inundation characteristics for flood impact forecasting in Gangnam drainage basin. *Korean Meteorological Society, Atmosphere*, **27**(2), pp. 189–197, 2017.

[8] Kim, B.S., Yoon, S.K., Hong, S.J. & Kwon, H.H., Development of grid-based conceptual hydrologic model. *Korea Water Resources Association*, **42**(7), pp. 667–679, 2010.

[9] FLO-2D Manual, 2009.

[10] Ministry of Land, Infrastructure and Transport, Korea Precipitation Frequency Data Server, 210.92.123.136, 2011.

[11] Huff, F.A., Time distribution of rainfall in heavy storms. *Water Resources Research*, **3**(4), pp. 1007–1019, 1967.

PERCEPTIONS OF 9/11 AMONG COLLEGE-AGED STUDENTS, 2017–2019

AUDREY HEFFRON CASSERLEIGH & REBECCA S. L. ROGERS
Emergency Management and Homeland Security Program, Florida State University, USA

ABSTRACT

As Millennials have begun to age out of experiencing 9/11 in the US and having tangible memories of the attack and its aftermath, a natural scepticism has grown surrounding the details of the event. The purpose of this survey was to understand perceptions of young adults (N = 297) as they comprehend or remember the events of 9/11 and details surrounding the attacks themselves. This survey seeks to understand the current perceptions of the events as they occurred by a Millennial student population. Independent variables include: (1) members of family in the military; (2) citizenship; (3) education; and (4) age at time of event. Dependent variables explore the following: perceptions of why the event occurred; who perpetrated the event; the involvement of the US Government; and truth and trust of media reporting. This is the first two years of a ten year longitudinal study. All survey respondents were between the ages of 20 and 22 at the time the survey was administered and enrolled in the college course "Introduction to Terrorism". Preliminary results indicate that a majority of respondents have inaccurate perceptions of the event and exhibit a high distrust of the US Governments' role in the attacks on 9/11 and how they came to be.

Keywords: Millennials, terrorism, 9/11, Government.

1 INTRODUCTION

This study is focused on understanding the current perceptions of the events of 11 September 2001 as they occurred by a Millennial student population at Florida State University (FSU). A literature review examining distrust of institutions, the influence of social media, and conspiracy theories will be presented followed by six hypotheses made by the researchers. Then the methods will be explained with sections on data collection, independent variables, dependent variables, and data analysis. Next, the results will be presented narratively and with appropriate tables, including notes on each specific hypotheses. The paper will close with a conclusion and reference page.

2 LITERATURE REVIEW

The current literature has a breadth of information regarding the attacks of 9/11 and how they have influenced current security in the USA and abroad. However, there exists a noticeable gap in the literature when it comes to the perceptions of the events by different populations. The following sections will examine the current body of knowledge surrounding the distrust of institutions (especially by youth populations), the influence of social media, and conspiracy theories.

2.1 Distrust of institutions

Current literature and research reveals that Millennials express low levels of confidence in nearly every American institution (Economic Innovation Group [1]). Millennials are born between the years of 1981 and 1996, with the youngest Millennials currently in their late teen years, and the oldest in their early 30s (Mitchell [2]).

Specifically, the report finds, "corporate America, Governors, and the news media inspire the lowest levels of confidence, with only one-fifth of Millennials placing a lot or a great deal

www.witpress.com, ISSN 1743-3509 (on-line)
doi:10.2495/DMAN190151

of stock in them" (Mitchell [2]). Of 1,200 Millennials polled in a study by the Economic Innovation Group, they responded as having the least amount of confidence (defined as "some" or "very little") in the Federal Government (72%), News Media (73%), Governors (72%) and Corporate America (72%) (Economic Innovation Group [1]). Interestingly, colleges, universities and the military are the only institutions that garner the confidence of the majority of Millennials (Economic Innovation Group [1]). Millennials distrust of US Government is shown again in a Harvard study that asked young Americans (aged between 18 and 29 years old) how confident they were in the US judicial system (Institute of Politics [3]). Distrust in the US judicial system was 49%; more specifically 35% said they had "not much confidence" and 14% reported they had "no confidence" whatsoever (Institute of Politics [3]).

2.2 Influence of social media

One of the most striking differences between Millennials and older generations is that Millennials officially get more news from social media than watching actual news outlets or reading newspapers or other online news sources. A Pew Research Centre [2] study noted that 61% of respondents receive their news from Facebook and only 37% receive their news from traditional news sources such as television programming and online newspapers. This is in stark contrast to previous generations who utilize social media significantly less, with only 39% of Baby Boomers (those born after World War II) utilizing Facebook as a news source (Miller et al. [4]). This could be an element contributing to disjointed perceptions of events between Millennials and older generations.

This use of social media as a primary source for information can be fraught with problems including: (1) low accountability of journalists and publications; (2) a lack of fact based relevance; and (3) possible influence peddling (Shearer and Gottfried [5]). Social media is conversely aware of the influence it can have on its audience. Facebook, Twitter, and YouTube have experienced a 15% increase in market influence between 2016 and 2017 (Shearer and Gottfried [5]).

Research also indicates Millennials are expressing unprecedented levels of social distrust. When asked the following question, "Generally speaking, would you say that most people can be trusted or that you can't be too careful in dealing with people", only 19% of Millennials say most people can be trusted, compared with 40% of Baby-Boomers (Pew Research Center [6]). Millennials comfort with disbelief of facts related to the attacks on September 11th, 2001 can be partially explained by distrust in Government and mainstream media reporting, combined with an increased acceptance of conspiracy theories.

2.3 Conspiracy theories

Sunstein and Vermeule [7] define conspiracy theories as, "an effort to explain some event or practice by reference to the machinations of powerful people, who attempt to conceal their role". Similarly, Uscinski [8] define a conspiracy as a "secret arrangement between two or more actors to usurp political or economic power, violate established rights, hoard vital secrets, or unlawfully alter government institutions". They continue by stating that "a key point is that conspiracies speak to actual events that have occurred or are occurring" (Uscinski [8]).

Recent polls show that conspiratorial beliefs are not only common, but that most Americans believe in one conspiracy theory or another (Miller et al. [4]). Conspiracy theories surrounding 9/11 are prevalent, and, "...given the advances in information technology and social media, as well as individuals' tendencies to sort themselves into attitude-consistent silos, even ideas with little basis in fact have the potential to quickly spread unchecked" (Miller et al. [4]). Uscinski et al. [9] writes, "Many scholars have suggested that beliefs in specific conspiracy theories are the product of an underlying predisposition toward viewing events and circumstances as the product of conspiracy".

One of the most prominent conspiracy theories is the belief that the JFK assassination was coordinated by the US Government. In a 2001 poll, the Zogby Organization found that 68% of US citizens support the JFK assassination conspiracy (Kurtz [10]). Similar to conspiracies surrounding 9/11, the foundation of this conspiracy is a mistrust of the American Government and the belief in "widespread and systematic cover-up of critical evidence by various Government agencies" (Kurtz [10]).

Lasting conspiracy theories, such as the moon-landing hoax, have long-term consequences. One study found that exposure to information about the moon-landing conspiracy "resulted in greater endorsement of belief in moon landing conspiracy theories" (Jolley [11]). Exposure to conspiracy theories and belief in them can influence socio-political behaviour and result in widespread "negative attitudes towards powerful groups" and be a "significant predictor of prejudices" towards various dominant groups (Jolley [11]).

Of note, "Those who subscribe to conspiracy theories may create serious risks, including risks of violence" and the "existence of such theories raises significant challenges for policy and law" (Sunstein and Vermeule [7]). Some of the most common conspiracy theories surrounding 9/11 include: the crash in Shanksville, Pennsylvania was a missile and not an airplane, planned stock trades took place before the attacks to ensure certain individuals profited from the attacks, and that jet fuel cannot melt steel meaning the towers fell from a controlled demolition. Perceptions of 9/11 events, and the prevalence of alternate theories, could heavily influence future security environments.

3 HYPOTHESES

The researchers in this study are embedded in a Millennial-rich environment while working on a large University campus with a diverse student population. The lead researcher is a terrorism expert with over 20 years of teaching in the field. Although it has been almost 20 years since the attacks, researchers, writers, filmmakers, and students seem to have taken more interest in the events that took place. This past year, was the first year that students who turned 18 had not been alive for 9/11 and the researchers considered how this could impact the perception of those events.

The following hypotheses were formulated based on the current literature, the expertise of the lead researcher in the field, and guided the design of the study:

H1: A majority of college age students believe the US Government was involved in the 9/11 attacks in some way.
H2: College age students that have served in the military will believe the US Government had no knowledge of the 9/11 attacks.
H3: Male students are more likely to distrust current facts surrounding the events of 9/11.
H4: Female students will be more likely to believe the number of deaths were in line with those reported by the media.
H5: Over time, age is going to influence the perceived role of the US Government in the attacks of 9/11.
H6: Over time, age is going to influence the perception of those responsible for perpetrating the attacks.

3.1 Hypothesis connections

3.1.1 *H1* → *H5* and *H6*

As time continues, college aged students will become further and further removed from the 9/11 event which could influence how their "age" influences their perceptions of the US Government and perpetrators.

3.1.2 *H2* → *H3* and *H4*

Over time, the number of students who have served in the military may increase or decrease, influencing the beliefs of male and female students. More specifically, a greater percentage of male than female students at FSU have served in the military. This could have an impact on their perceptions of the 9/11 event.

4 METHOD

The following section will explain the method used by the researchers to conduct this research. Information regarding data collection, independent variables, dependent variables, and data analysis will be presented.

4.1 Data collection

4.1.1 Population and setting

In order to collect the data used in this inquiry, the researchers administered a survey titled "Perceptions of 9/11" on the first day of a large seminar class titled "Introduction to Terrorism". This class was chosen based because of its convenience for sampling, the age range of students, the high number of students consistently registered for the course, and the relative inexperience the students in the course have with the subject-matter. All surveys are anonymous and sorted by the research assistant each time they are disseminated. Students have the option to not complete the survey and ask any clarifying questions while taking the survey in class.

4.1.2 Sample

The goal is to have approximately 100 students complete the survey each semester over the course of 10 years to eventually develop a complex longitudinal study. The results in this paper are from the first year and a half, or three semesters, of data, with N = 297.

4.2 Independent variables

The independent variables were meant to provide a baseline, but also attempted to distinguish differences in a relatively homogenous population.

4.2.1 Ethnicity

In any given semester, minorities (any ethnicity other than Caucasian) present as less than 5% of the entire class. While ethnocentricities are not currently surveyed in the independent variables, this is a possible modification for future studies and is important to note before presenting the results.

4.2.2 Age of respondents

This longitudinal survey captures the age of the respondent at the time of the survey, and the age of the respondent during 9/11, resulting in the provision of both stagnant and variable data. Age at time of survey will likely remain constant over time as most college age students are between 18 and 22 years of age. Currently the average age of all respondents is 21 at the time of the survey.

Eventually, age at time of 9/11 will move from a positive to a null number. In a few years, college age students will not yet have been born when the 9/11 event occurred. The average age of the respondents during the 9/11 event is 4.5 years of age, suggesting a limited observational ability. It can be reasonably assumed age 4.5 was too young to have full situational awareness during the 9/11 event and its aftermath.

4.2.3 Gender of respondents

Gender was coded in as male, female, and other. Of the N = 297 respondents 140 identified as male, 152 identified as female, 1 identified as other, and 4 declined to answer the question. Of the respondents who chose to identify their gender in a binary manner (either male or female) 48% were male and 52% were female, representing a balanced response.

4.2.4 College level of students

This survey was administered to an upper level undergraduate course, registered at the 4,000 level, the highest level in the undergraduate suite of classes. FSU, where the class and survey were administered, is a very large, public university in the southeast United States. Total undergraduate enrolment as of Spring 2019 at FSU is 31,257. The independent variable that asked for years in college yielded a range of answers from 0.5 to 5, with the average years in college calculated at 2.9. Since this survey was administered in an upper division course, this average seems appropriately reflective of the experience of the respondents as juniors or seniors in college.

4.3 Dependent variables

The survey questions were developed by the lead researcher and research assistant and were based on the main factors they hypothesized would impact a student's perception of the event. The current literature and the expertise of the lead researcher were considered when developing the survey questions. The survey tool gave respondents the option to mark multiple answers, allowing them to pick more than one in each of the dependent variable areas.

4.3.1 Who perpetrated the event?

The first category of dependent variable asked the respondents about who they believed perpetrated 9/11. They were able to choose multiple options including "Terrorists", "The US Government", "Foreign Governments", or "Other". These variables were coded as 9/11 Perp-Ter, 9/11 Perp-US Govt, 9/11 Perp-Foreign Govt, 9/11 Perp-Other.

4.3.2 Why the attacks occurred

The second category of dependent variable examined the reason 9/11 happened. Respondents were allowed to select multiple options including "Terrorists wanted to target America", "the President needed an excuse to go to war", "The President wanted to re-elected", and "Other". These variables were coded as 9/11 Due to: Terrorists, 9/11 Due to: War Excuse, 9/11 Due to: Re-election, 9/11 Due to: Other.

4.3.3 Death perceptions of the attacks

The third category of dependent variables sought to examine perceptions of deaths in 9/11. The respondents were asked if they believed the deaths were "As was reported by the US Government", "Higher than was reported", "Lower than was reported", "Zero deaths", or

"Other". These variables were coded as 9/11 Deaths: Reported-US Govt, 9/11 Deaths: Higher, 9/11 Deaths: Lower, 9/11 Deaths: Zero, 9/11 Deaths: Other.

4.3.4 The role of the US Government

The fourth category of dependent variables sought to understand the role the US Government played in 9/11, as understood by the respondents. The survey asked if the US Government had, "No prior knowledge", "Some prior knowledge", "Some prior knowledge, but did nothing", "Some prior knowledge and encouraged it", "The US Government perpetrated 9/11", and "Not sure". These variables were coded as, US Govt: No prior knowledge, US Govt: Some prior knowledge, US Govt: Prior knowledge/did nothing, US Govt: Prior knowledge/encouraged it, US Govt: Did 9/11, US Govt: Not sure.

An example of the survey questionnaire is shown in Fig. 1.

4.4 Data analysis

Because the data is only representative of one and a half years of a 10 year study, the researchers used basic statistical analysis to answer each of the hypothesized responses. Each

I believe the 9/11 event was perpetrated by:

a. Terrorists
b. US Government
c. Foreign Governments
d. Other

I believe the 9/11 attacks happened because:

a. Terrorists wanted to target the US
b. The US Governments needed an excuse to go to war
c. The US President at the time wanted to get re-elected
d. Other

I believe the direct deaths from 9/11 were:

a. 2,996 people, as was reported
b. A higher number than was reported
c. A lower number than was reported
d. Zero people
e. Other

I believe the US Government:

a. Had no prior knowledge of 9/11
b. Had some prior knowledge of 9/11
c. Had prior knowledge of 9/11 but did nothing about it
d. Had prior knowledge of 9/11 and encouraged it
e. Conducted the 9/11 event
f. Not sure
g. Other

Figure 1: Perceptions of 9/11 survey example.

survey was analysed by asking whether the respondent answered "Yes" or "No" to each of the question answers. If a respondent answered that the 9/11 event was perpetrated by terrorists, "perpetrated by terrorists" would receive a "Y" and "perpetrated by US Government", "perpetrated by Foreign Governments", and "perpetrated by other" would be marked "N". From here, individual charts were created to tabulate the results of each question asked and each answer received. A simple percentage was calculated to determine how each student responded to the survey (i.e. "__% of students believe that 9/11 was perpetrated by terrorists"). The goal is to use these baseline percentages to track patterns and changes that occur over the years as students age further and further away from the events on 9/11.

5 RESULTS

The first question that truly gets at the heart of any 9/11 conspiracy belief is: "Who perpetrated the 9/11 attacks?" By asking the respondents who was culpable the plan was to identify schisms in perceptions of responsibility (Table 1).

This initial question and the results seem in line with mainstream thinking that 9/11 was perpetrated by terrorists. These dependent variables show no statistical significance when measured against any of the independent variables including age, gender, or exposure to service in the military.

The second set of questions gets at motivation by asking why the 9/11 event occurred. The results in Table 2 are in line with mainstream thinking that excludes any internal motivation on the part of US leadership.

Interestingly, while most respondents did not choose the popular conspiracy theory that President Bush wanted to be elected, we do begin to see a possible eschewing of mainstream beliefs in the selection of the "Other" category. Respondents were given an open answer opportunity at the end of the survey, but the open ended answers predominately reflected questions that were already asked. For example, one respondent wrote, "I believe it was a

Table 1: "I believe the 9/11 event was perpetrated by…". Where $N \neq 297$ some respondents did not answer or answers were unclear.

Responses	Perpetrated by terrorists (1a)	Perpetrated by US Government (1b)	Perpetrated by Foreign Governments (1c)	Perpetrated by Others (1d)
N = Yes	281	31	37	9
N = No	15	266	260	288
Percentage Yes	94.6%	10.5%	12.45%	3%
Percentage No	5.4%	89.5%	87.55%	97%

Table 2: "I believe the 9/11 attacks happened because…".

Responses	Terrorists wanted to target the US (2a)	The US Government needed an excuse to go to war (2b)	The US President at the time wanted to get re-elected (2c)	Other (2d)
N = Yes	258	51	9	19
N = No	39	246	288	278
Percentage Yes	86.8%	17.2%	3%	6%
Percentage No	13.2%	82.8%	97%	94%

combination of President Bush wanting to get re-elected and foreign terrorists supported by Foreign Governments. I think they knew about each other". When the variables 2b, 2c, and 2d are combined it reveals that 26.2% of the respondents believed there was an internal influencing factor that led to the events on 9/11.

When asked about the number of death attributed to the 9/11 event students were asked to choose one of the following answers. In some cases multiple answers were selection so N = 308 for this DV.

Table 3 reveals that respondents have mistrust about the number of death reported, with 44% indicated they believe there were a higher number of deaths than was reported. Of greatest relevance is that 48% of the respondents don't believe the numbers as they were reported. This may tie back to the research on distrust in the media (Miller et al. [4], Tang et al. [12]). Is it that Millennials distrust the media reporting? That they feel the Government was dishonest about the number of deaths? Or something else? This is something the researchers want to try and further understand in future surveys.

Table 3: "I believe the direct deaths from 9/11 were…".

Responses	2,996 people, as was reported (3a)	A higher number than was reported (3b)	A lower number than was reported (3c)	Zero people (3d)	Other (3e)
N = Yes	154	135	13	0	6
Percentage Yes	50%	44%	4%	0%	2%

The fourth category of dependent variables begins to get at the knowledge or participation by the US on the 9/11 event.

Table 4 begins to reveal perceptions of culpability of the part of the US Government. 84.2% of the respondents do not believe the US Government was unaware that 9/11 was going to happen. However, when asked the reverse, if they believe the US Government had some prior knowledge, only 39.4% of the respondents answered in the affirmative. When asked specifically about knowledge of the attacks before they happened, the respondents had even less support for the idea of the Government having prior knowledge. What becomes more interesting is when variables are grouped into larger influence categories. When variables 4a (39.4%), 4b (26.6%), 4c (3.4%), and 4d (3.3%) are combined, we see that 72.7% of the respondents believed the US Government had some prior knowledge of the 9/11 event.

5.1 Specific hypotheses

The results regarding ***H1:*** A majority of college age students believe the US Government was involved in the 9/11 attacks in some way, were found to be a positive number. Over 70% of the respondents felt the US Government had some role in the 9/11 event.

The second hypothesis, ***H2:*** College age students that have served in the military will believe the US Government had no knowledge of the 9/11 attacks was not proven, because the numbers of prior service member in the survey pool was insignificant.

With regard to ***H3:*** Male students are more likely to distrust current facts surrounding the events of 9/11 it turns out there is no statistical difference between the perceptions of male versus the perceptions of females. Both genders indicated a high distrust of facts regarding number of dead, and both genders equally believed the US Government had played a role in

Table 4: "I believe the US Government…".

Responses	Had no prior knowledge of 9/11 (4a)	Had some prior knowledge of 9/11 (4b)	Had prior knowledge of 9/11 but did nothing about it (4c)	Had prior knowledge of 9/11, and encouraged it (4d)	Conducted the 9/11 event (4e)	Not sure (4f)	Other (4g)
N = Yes	47	117	79	10	10	23	8
N = No	250	180	218	287	287	274	289
Percentage Yes	15.8%	39.4%	26.6%	3.4%	3.3%	7.7%	2.6%
Percentage No	84.2%	60.6%	73.4%	96.6%	96.7%	92.3%	97.4%

the 9/11 attacks. Females were just as likely to distrust the facts, like number of reported dead, as males, lending no support to ***H4:*** Female Students will be more likely to pick the number of deaths as reported.

The two hypotheses that are designed to evaluate change over time cannot yet be evaluated. More longitudinal data will be required to examine ***H5:*** Over time, age is going to influence the perceived role of the US Government and ***H6:*** Over time, age is going to influence perception of perpetrators.

6 CONCLUSION

As Millennials grow up further away from the events of 9/11, the disbelief of facts surrounding the event are expected to grow. As the study continues, the researchers expect to see more disconnect between the facts that were released and the perception of those facts by the Millennial generation (and eventually Gen Z). This preliminary analysis shows that there is valuable analysis that can be done to understand the distrust of Government and media by younger generations.

The data aggregated in this paper is only a small sample of what will eventually be a larger pool of responses. Future analysis will evaluate multi collinear probabilities looking for more significant relationships between the variables.

REFERENCES

[1] Economic Innovation Group, The Millennial economy: Findings from a new EY and EIG national survey of Millennials, EIG: Washington DC, 2016.

[2] Mitchell, A., *Millennials and Political News*, Pew Research Center, 2015.

[3] Institute of Politics, No front-runner among prospective republican candidates, Hillary Clinton in control of Democratic Primary, Harvard youth poll finds, Harvard Kennedy School: Boston, 2016.

[4] Miller, J.M., Saunders, K.L. & Farhart, C.E., Conspiracy endorsement as motivated reasoning: The moderating roles of political knowledge and trust. *American Journal of Political Science*, **60**(4), pp. 824–844, 2015.

[5] Shearer, E. & Gottfried, J., *News Use Across Social Media Platforms 2017*, Pew Research Center, 2017.

[6] Pew Research Center, Millennials in adulthood: Detached from institutions, networked with friends, 2014. www.pewsocialtrends.org/2014/03/07/millennials-in-adulthood/.

[7] Sunstein, C. & Vermeule, A., Conspiracy theories: Causes and cures. *Journal of Political Philosophy*, **17**(2), pp. 202–227, 2008.

[8] Uscinski, J.E., *American Conspiracy Theories*, Oxford University Press: Oxford, 2014.

[9] Uscinski, J.E., Klofstad, C. & Atkinson, M.D., What drives conspiratorial beliefs? The role of informational cues and predispositions. *Political Research Quarterly*, **69**(1), pp. 57–71, 2016.

[10] Kurtz, M.L., *The JFK Assassination Debates: Lone Gunman Versus Conspiracy*, University Press of Kansas, 2006.

[11] Jolley, D., The detrimental nature of conspiracy theories. *Psychology Postgraduate Affairs Group Quarterly*, **88**, pp. 35–39, 2013.

[12] Tang, J., Hu, X. & Liu, H., Is distrust the negation of trust? The value of distrust in social media. *Conference Proceedings of Hypertext 2014*, Santiago, Chile, 2014.

LINK BETWEEN TERRORISM AND SOCIAL, ECONOMIC AND SECURITY-POLITICAL FACTORS

JAN BŘEŇ[1], TOMÁŠ ZEMAN[1] & RUDOLF URBAN[2]
[1]University of Defence, Czech Republic
[2]The College of Regional Development and Banking Institute, Ambis, Czech Republic

ABSTRACT

Terrorism is formulated as a planned use of violence targeting a wide range public. The aim of terrorism is to attract attention and cause fear through which specific political, religious or ideological intentions are achieved. An integral part of the issue of terrorism is not only the consequences of committed terrorist acts which lead to subsequent security measures but also the cause of terrorist activities which determine the reasons why people are motivated for these activities. The immediate causes of terrorist attacks vary on a case-by-case basis so their determination is not generally possible. However, it is possible to identify and analyze factors, which create preconditions for the emergence of terrorism. Some publications suggest that poor structural social conditions, economic deprivation and security-political instability situations create frustration, which in turn makes terrorism more likely. The paper deals with the social factors (social inequality, standard of living, level of citizen's education), economic factors (GDP, unemployment, inflation) and security-political factors (corruption, criminality, political instability, government ineffectiveness, war and violent conflict) which potentially generate future terrorist activities. The main aim is to find out correlations between these factors and terrorism. In order to calculate results we gathered data (relevant indexes and indicators, which express individual social/economic/security-political factors) in 162 countries in the year 2017. Using Spearman's correlation coefficient as the statistical method, we made comprehensive statements about the link between individual social/economic/security-political factors and terrorism. Many previous analysis, studies and publications have focused on this issue but there are different statements about the causes of terrorism. This paper confirms some of these statements – that social inequality, GDP, current war conflict, corruption and political instability have increased the terrorist threat throughout the world.
Keywords: factors, economic, factors, security-political, social, statistics.

1 INTRODUCTION

There are many factors in society, which motivate people to terrorist ideas and then to practical actions. Most of these factors come from social, economic and security-political area. It is possible to identify features or characteristics in these areas, which are common to a wide range of terrorist actors.

A publication by Ola [1] shows that citizen's social inequality leads to support and spread of terrorism in different countries in the world. High social inequalities produce isolation, poverty and aggression that may occur in frequent violent conflicts and terrorism. Government expenditures to social welfare of citizens are associated with reduction in terrorism. This is also confirmed by Lai's research [2]. Study by Azam and Thelen [3] shows there is positively link between level of citizen's education and terrorism. Considering the influence of education on terrorism, the findings of Drakos and Gofas [4] and Kurrild-Klitgaard et al. [5] do not indicate that education is significantly associated with terrorist attacks. Research by Krueger and Maleckova [6] points out that poor economic conditions of people do not affect the generation of terrorism to such extend. Piazza [7] in his research is convinced about very close link between citizens standard of living and the number of terrorist attacks despite of previous statement. Findings of Azam and Delacroix [8] also suggest that personal economic development significantly reduces the genesis of terrorism.

WIT Transactions on The Built Environment, Vol 190, © 2019 WIT Press
www.witpress.com, ISSN 1743-3509 (on-line)
doi:10.2495/DMAN190161

Regarding to the link between economic performance and terrorism, the existing evidences are ambiguous. Publication by Blomberg and Hess [9] provides results that level of economic performance of state is associated with a higher number of terrorist attacks. Krueger and Laitin [10] note that there is no systematic link between economic performance of state and the evolution of terrorism. Their findings do not suggest that economic change translates into higher terrorist activity and further indicate that economic success exerts no independent effect of on terrorist attacks. Unemployment in general is a highly statistically significant predictor of terrorism. Goldstein study [11], which extensively analyses economic factors related to the risk of terrorism highlights unemployment, is an important aspect of terrorism causes. Piazza [12] focused on consumer prices fluctuations in relation to terrorist activities. The rise of prices is an indicator of positive correlation between inflation and terrorist activities. This was not confirmed by study of Campos and Gassebner [13]. Also study by Dural and Jahangir [14] does not confirm positive correlation. Even their conclusion is very different – increasing terrorism leads to decreasing inflation.

Corruption is other factor where is no consensus. A publication by Boussiga and Ghdamsi [15] reveals a long-term correlation relationship between corruption and terrorism. Simpson [16] found completely different results – there is no statistically significant relationship between those two variables. A publication by Odehnal and Sedlacik [17] points to dominant position of political instability as a determinant of terrorist activity. Li [18] in his publication that domestic political instability is actively entering and influencing terrorism. The findings also suggest several important policy implications. Democracy does not have a singularly positive effect on terrorism as is often claimed and found. By improving citizen satisfaction, electoral participation, and political efficacy, democratic governments can reduce the number of terrorist incidents within their border. Asongu et al. [19] confirms the fact government ineffectiveness has a major negative impact of the dynamics of terrorist activities. Freytag et al. [20] contests previous statement and their study shows that government ineffectiveness does not influence terrorism activities. There is no doubt about the strong link between factor of criminality and terrorism. The positively relationship is confirmed by Stanojoska's publication [21], which analyses the link between criminality, organized crime and terrorism. According to her statement, the connection between terrorisms and organized crime sometimes is very close and sometimes is even invisible. Some terrorist organizations started using organized crime acts; some organized crime networks started using terrorist acts. National and international violence conflicts (including wars) are one of the most important determinants, which generate terrorist activities according to Plamper and Neumayer [22].

Related to these analyses, studies and publications there are different statements about link between related factors from social/economic/security-political areas and terrorism. This paper finds out by using related statistical method relationship between terrorism threat and social inequality in society, level of citizen's education, standard of living, economic performance of state, unemployment, inflation, corruption, political instability, government ineffectiveness, criminality and war and violent conflict. According to results from this paper, it is possible to confirm conclusions of other authors described in this section.

2 METHODS

In the first stage, we established indicators and indexes, which expressed terrorism threat and individual social/economic/security-political factors (Table 1).

The dataset of these indexes and indicators comes from relevant sources and databases (Vision of Humanity, Social Progress Imperative, World Bank Open Data, Human Development Reports, The Global Economy and Transparency International). All these

Table 1: Indexes and indicators for individual factors. *(Source: Author's own construction.)*

FACTOR	INDEX INDICATOR
Terrorism threat	Global Terrorism Index
Social inequality in society	Social Progress Index
Level of citizen's education	Education Index
Standard of living	Gross National Product per capita (purchasing parity power)
Economic performance of state	Gross Domestic Product per capita
Unemployment	Unemployment rate
Inflation	Consumer Price Index
Corruption	Corruption Perceptions Index
Political instability	Political Stability Index
Government ineffectiveness	Government Effectiveness Index
Criminality	Criminality Index
War and violent conflict	Global Peace Index

indexes and indicators were considered in 162 countries from the year 2017 (more recent data is not available for all indexes and indicators). Based on these indexes and indicators we tested normality of the whole dataset for further statistical correlations. The normality of the dataset was not proved, so for the expression of correlations between related factors and terrorism threat the Spearman's correlation coefficient was selected. For the calculation of correlations and testing normality the IBM SPSS Statistics 25 [23] software was used. All correlations were determined using the 0.05 level of reliability (p-value ≤ 0.05) which means that the results were calculated with 95% probability of reliability.

3 RESULTS AND DISCUSSION

Statistical correlations in this section analyse link between related factors from social/economic/security-political areas and terrorism. Terrorist threat is expressed by Global Terrorism Index (GTI) [24], which provides a comprehensive summary of the key global trends and patterns in issue of terrorism. The overall score of GTI is quantified by a numeric value from 0 to 100 (the higher score, the higher terrorist threat is).

3.1 Social factors

Selected factors in this area: social inequality, citizen's standard of living and level of citizen's education.

3.1.1 Social inequality

Social inequality is expressed by Social Progress Index (SPI) [25], which measures the extent to which countries provide for the social and environmental needs of their citizens. Fifty-four indicators in the areas of basic human needs, foundations of well-being, and opportunity to progress show the relative performance of nations. The overall score of SPI is quantified by a numeric value from 0 to 100 (the higher score, the higher social inequality is). The result of correlation between terrorist threat and social inequality is described and explained in the following text, table and figures.

Null hypothesis (H_0): there is no correlation link between GTI and SPI.
Alternative hypothesis (H_1): there is correlation link between GTI and SPI.

According to the calculated correlation (H_0 is rejected, H_1 is accepted, p-value ≤ 0.05), there is a correlation link between GTI and SPI (Table 2) – the higher social inequality, the higher terrorist threat is (Fig. 1).

Table 2: Statistical correlation of GTI and SPI. *(Source: Author's own construction.)*

LEVEL OF RELIABILITY	CORRELATION COEFFICIENT	P-VALUE
0.05	0.186	0.030

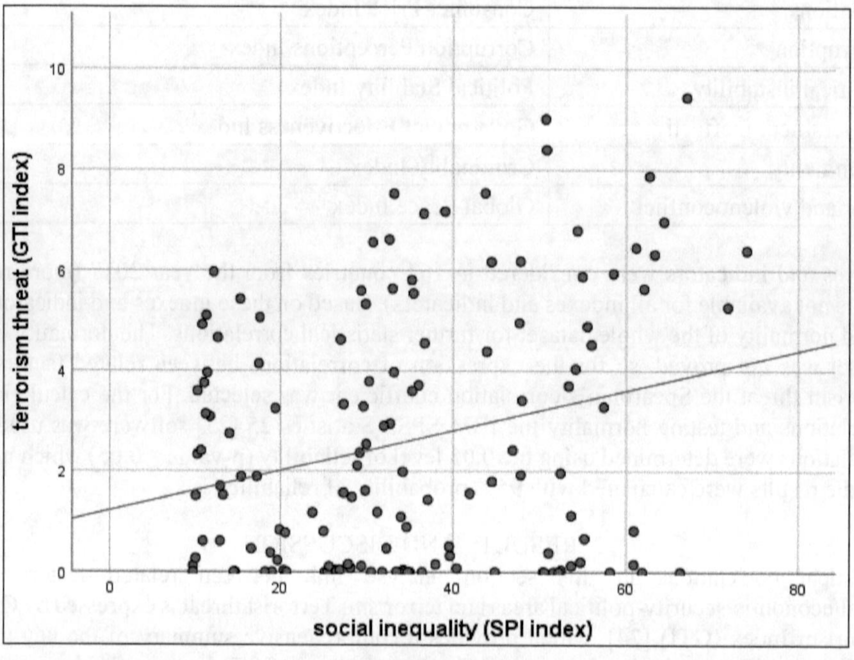

Figure 1: Statistical correlation of GTI and SPI. *(Source: Author's own construction.)*

3.1.2 Standard of living

Citizens standard of living is expressed by Gross National Income per capita at purchasing power parity (GNI per capita, PPP) [26]. GNI is the sum of value (in dollars) added by all resident producers plus any product taxes not included in the valuation of output plus net receipts of primary income from abroad. The result of correlation between terrorist threat and citizen's standard of living is described and explained in the following text and table.

H_0: there is no correlation link between GTI and GNI per capita, PPP.
H_1: there is correlation link between GTI and GNI per capita, PPP.

According to the calculated correlation (H_0 is accepted, H_1 is rejected, p-value ≥ 0.05), there is no correlation link between GTI and GNI per capita, PPP (Table 3).

Table 3: Statistical correlation of GTI and GNI per capita, PPP. *(Source: Author's own construction.)*

LEVEL OF RELIABILITY	CORRELATION COEFFICIENT	P-VALUE
0.05	-0.107	0.190

3.1.3 Level of citizen's education
Level of citizen's education is expressed by Education Index (EI) [27], which calculated years of schooling and expected years of schooling. The overall score of EI is quantified by a numeric value from 0 to 1 (the higher score, the higher level of citizen's education is). The result of correlation between terrorist threat and citizen's level of education is described and explained in the following text and table.

H_0: there is no correlation link between GTI and EI.
H_1: there is correlation link between GTI and EI.

According to the calculated correlation (H_0 is accepted, H_1 is rejected, p-value ≥ 0.05), there is no correlation link between GTI and EI (Table 4).

Table 4: Statistical correlation of GTI and EI. *(Source: Author's own construction.)*

LEVEL OF RELIABILITY	CORRELATION COEFFICIENT	P-VALUE
0.05	-0.130	0.105

3.2 Economic factors

Economic factors in this area: unemployment, economic performance of state and inflation.

3.2.1 Unemployment
Percentage of unemployed citizens in the country expresses factor of unemployment. Data about this percentage number comes from database The World Bank [28]. The result of correlation between terrorist threat and unemployment is described and explained in the following text and table.

H_0: there is no correlation link between GTI and unemployment.
H_1: there is correlation link between GTI and unemployment.

According to the calculated correlation (H_0 is accepted, H_1 is rejected, p-value ≥ 0.05), there is no correlation link between GTI and unemployment (Table 5).

Table 5: Statistical correlation of GTI and unemployment. *(Source: Author's own construction.)*

LEVEL OF RELIABILITY	CORRELATION COEFFICIENT	P-VALUE
0.05	0.067	0.403

3.2.2 Economic performance of state

Gross Domestic Product per capita (GDP per capita) [29] expresses economic performance of state. GDP per capita is a measure of a country's economic output that accounts for its number of people. The result of correlation between terrorist threat and economic performance of state is described and explained in the following text, table and figure.

H_0: there is no correlation link between GTI and economic performance of state.
H_1: there is correlation link between GTI and economic performance of state.

According to the calculated correlation (H_0 is rejected, H_1 is accepted, p-value ≤ 0.05), there is a correlation link between GTI and GDP per capita (Table 6) – the higher economic performance of state in the country, the lower terrorist threat is (Fig. 2).

Table 6: Statistical correlation of GTI and economic performance of state. *(Source: Author's own construction.)*

LEVEL OF RELIABILITY	CORRELATION COEFFICIENT	P-VALUE
0.05	-0.178	0.041

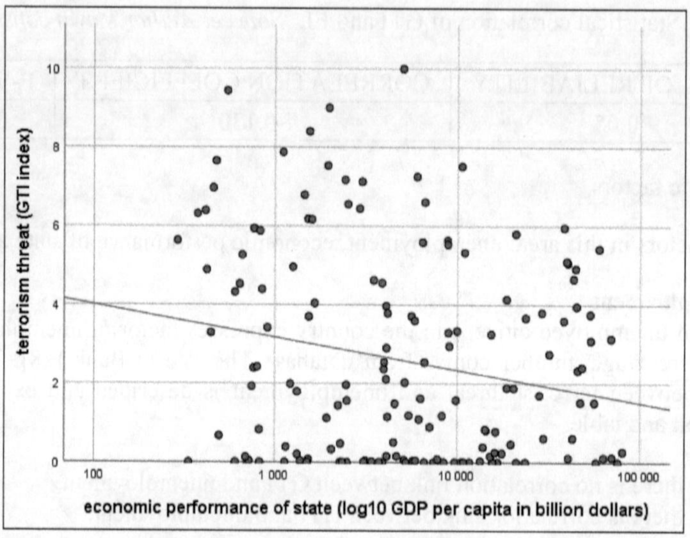

Figure 2: Statistical correlation of GTI and economic performance of state. *(Source: Author's own construction.)*

3.2.3 Inflation

Inflation rate is expressed by Customer Price Index (CPI) [30], which measures average change in prices over time that consumers pay for a basket of goods and services. The result of correlation between terrorist threat and inflation is described and explained in the following text and table.

H_0: there is no correlation link between GTI and CPI.
H_1: there is correlation link between GTI and CPI.

According to the calculated correlation (H_0 is accepted, H_1 is rejected, p-value ≥ 0.05), there is no correlation link between GTI and CPI (Table 7).

Table 7: Statistical correlation of GTI and CPI. *(Source: Author's own construction.)*

LEVEL OF RELIABILITY	CORRELATION COEFFICIENT	P-VALUE
0.05	0.145	0.084

3.3 Security: Political factors

Security: political factors in this area: war and violent conflict, criminality, political instability, government ineffectiveness and corruption.

3.3.1 War and violent conflict

Global Peace Index (GPI) [31] expresses factor of war and violent conflict. GPI measures the relative position of nations' and regions' peacefulness. The overall score of GPI is quantified by a numeric value from 0 to 5 (the higher score, the higher intensity of war and violent conflict is). The result of correlation between terrorist threat and war conflict is described and explained in the following text, table and figure.

H_0: there is no correlation link between GTI and GPI.
H_1: there is correlation link between GTI and GPI.

According to the calculated correlation (H_0 is rejected, H_1 is accepted, p-value ≤ 0.05), there is a correlation link between GTI and GPI (Table 8) – the higher intensity of war and violent conflict in the country, the higher terrorist threat is (Fig. 3).

Table 8: Statistical correlation of GTI and GPI. *(Source: Author's own construction.)*

LEVEL OF RELIABILITY	CORRELATION COEFFICIENT	P-VALUE
0.05	0.491	0.000

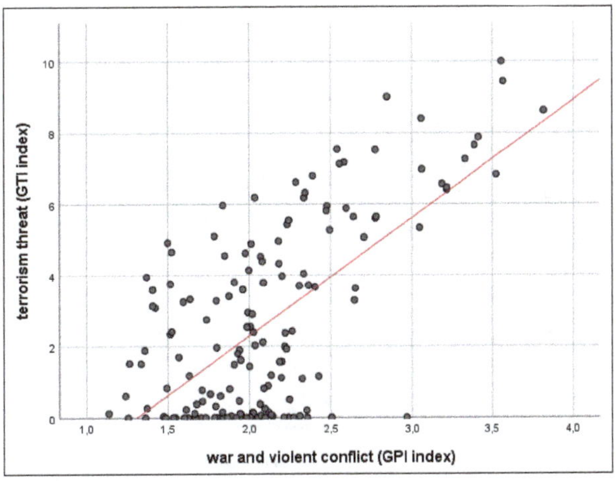

Figure 3: Statistical correlation of GTI and GPI. *(Source: Author's own construction.)*

3.3.2 Criminality

Crime index (CI) [32] expresses factor of national criminality. The overall score of GPI is quantified by a numeric value from 0 to 100 (the higher the score, the higher intensity criminality is). The result of correlation between terrorist threat and criminality is described and explained in the following text and table.

H_0: there is no correlation link between GTI and CI.
H_1: there is correlation link between GTI and CI.

According to the calculated correlation (H_0 is accepted, H_1 is rejected, p-value ≥ 0.05), there is no correlation link between GTI and CI (Table 9).

Table 9: Statistical correlation of GTI and CI. *(Source: Author's own construction.)*

LEVEL OF RELIABILITY	CORRELATION COEFFICIENT	P-VALUE
0.05	0.154	0.100

3.3.3 Political instability

Political Instability is expressed by Political Stability Index (PSI) [33]. The overall score of PSI is quantified by a numeric value from -3 to 3 (the higher score, the higher political stability is). The result of correlation between terrorist threat and political instability is described and explained in the following text, table and figure.

H_0: there is no correlation link between GTI and PSI.
H_1: there is correlation link between GTI and PSI.

According to the calculated correlation (H_0 is rejected, H_1 is accepted, p-value ≤ 0.05), there is a correlation link between GTI and PSI (Table 10) – the higher political instability in the country, the higher terrorist threat is (Fig. 4).

Table 10: Statistical correlation of GTI and PSI. *(Source: Author's own construction.)*

LEVEL OF RELIABILITY	CORRELATION COEFFICIENT	P-VALUE
0.05	-0.590	0.000

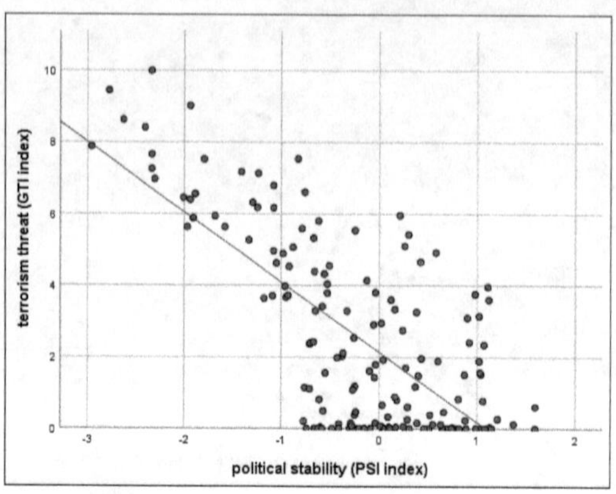

Figure 4: Statistical correlation of GTI and GPI. *(Source: Author's own construction.)*

3.3.4 Government ineffectiveness

Government Effectiveness Index (GEI) [34] expresses factor of government ineffectiveness. GEI captures perceptions of the quality of public services, the quality of the civil service and the degree of its independence from political pressure, the quality of policy formulation and implementation, and the credibility of the government's commitment to such policies. The overall score of GEI is quantified by a numeric value from -2.5 to 2.5 (the higher score, the higher government effectiveness is). The result of correlation between terrorist threat and government effectiveness is described and explained in the following text and table.

H_0: there is no correlation link between GTI and GEI.
H_1: there is correlation link between GTI and GEI.

According to the calculated correlation (H_0 is accepted, H_1 is rejected, p-value $\geq$ 0.05), there is no correlation link between GTI and GEI (Table 11).

Table 11: Statistical correlation of GTI and GEI. *(Source: Author's own construction.)*

LEVEL OF RELIABILITY	CORRELATION COEFFICIENT	P-VALUE
0.05	-0.066	0.410

3.3.5 Corruption

Factor of corruption is expressed by Corruption Perception Index (CPI) [35]. CPI ranks countries by their perceived levels of public sector corruption, as determined by expert assessments and opinion surveys. The overall score of CPI is quantified by a numeric value from 0 to 100 (the higher score, the higher corruption is). The result of correlation between terrorist threat and corruption is described and explained in the following text, table and figure.

H_0: there is no correlation link between GTI and CPI.
H_1: there is correlation link between GTI and CPI.

According to the calculated correlation (H_0 is rejected, H_1 is accepted, p-value $\leq$ 0.05), there is a correlation link between GTI and PSI (Table 12) – the higher corruption in the country, the higher terrorist threat is (Fig. 5).

Table 12: Statistical correlation of GTI and CPI. *(Source: Author's own construction.)*

LEVEL OF RELIABILITY	CORRELATION COEFFICIENT	P-VALUE
0.05	0.165	0.041

4 CONCLUSION

Based on our results, there are correlations link between terrorism and some factors from social/economical/security-political areas in 162 countries in the year 2017. Social inequality in society, economic performance of state, war and violent conflict, corruption in state and state's political instability have influenced terrorism. The results have been confirmed with 95% probability of reliability.

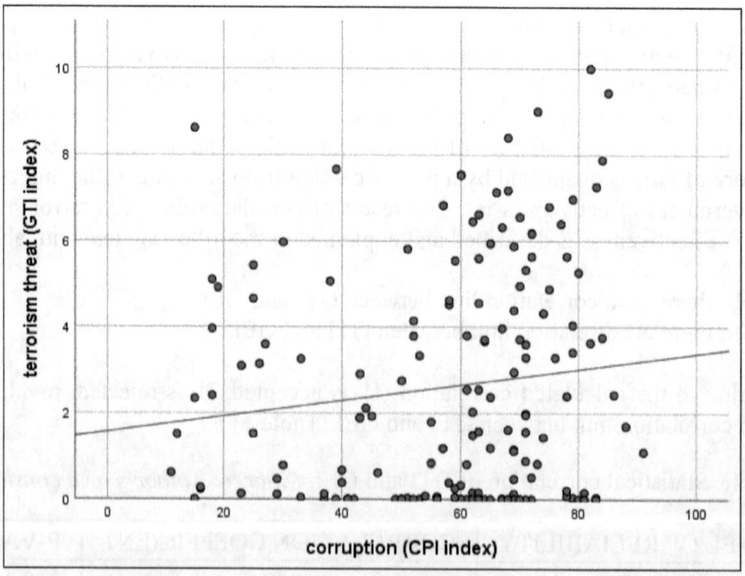

Figure 5: Statistical correlation of GTI and CPI. *(Source: Author's own construction.)*

Terrorist attacks are different and each of them is characterized by individual and specific form, type and motivational character of the realization. These aspects of terrorism are extensive and complex issue of modern society.

ACKNOWLEDGEMENT

This paper was supported by the Ministry of Education, Youth and Sports of the Czech Republic (SV18-FVL-K106-BŘE).

REFERENCES

[1] Ola, T., Re-thinking poverty, inequality and their relationship to terrorism. *Journal of Sciences: Basic and Applied Research*, **21**(2), pp. 264–292, 2018.

[2] Lai, B., Draining the swamp: An empirical examination of the production of international terrorism. *Conflict Management and Peace Science*, **24**(4), pp. 297–310, 2016.

[3] Azam, J.P. & Thelen, V., The roles of foreign aid and education in the war on terror. *Public Choice*, **135**(3–4), pp. 375–397, 2008.

[4] Drakos, K. & Gofas, A., In search of the average transtational terrorist attack venue. *Defence and Peace Economics,* **17**(2), pp. 73–93, 2006.

[5] Kurrild-Klitgaard, P., Justesen, M.K. & Klemmensen, R., The political economy of freedom, democracy and transnational terrorism. *Public Choice*, **128**(1/2), pp. 289–315, 2006.

[6] Krueger, A.B. & Maleckova, J., Education, poverty and terrorism: Is there a causal connection? *Journal of Economic Perspectives,* **17**(4), pp. 119–144, 2003.

[7] Piazza, J.A., Poverty, minority economic discrimination, and domestic terrorism. *Journal of Peace Research,* **48**(3), pp. 339–353, 2011.

[8] Azam, J.-P. & Delacroix, A., Aid and the delegated fight against terrorism. *Review of Development Economic*, **10**(2), pp. 330–344, 2006.

[9] Blomberg, S.B. & Hess, G.D., From (no) butter to guns? Understanding the economic role in transnational terrorism. *SSRN Electronic Journal,* 2006.

[10] Krueger, A.B. & Laitin, D., Kto Kogo? A cross-country study of the origins and targets of terrorism. *Terrorism, Economic Development, and Political Openness*, pp. 148–173, 2008.

[11] Goldstein, K., Unemployment, inequality and terrorism: another look at the relationship between economics and terrorism. *Undergraduate Economic Review,* **1**(1), 2003.

[12] Piazza, J., The cost of living and terror: Does consumer price volatility fuel terrorism? *Southern Economic Journal,* **79**(4), pp. 812–231, 2013.

[13] Campos, N. & Gassebner, M., International terrorism, domestic political instability, and the escalation effect. *Economics & Politics*, **25**(1), pp. 27–47, 2013.

[14] Dural, B.Y. & Jahangir, S.M.R., Relationship between terrorism and macroeconomic variables: Especially import of crude oil and natural gas in Turkey. *Ulakbilge*, **5**(14), pp. 1373–1394, 2009.

[15] Boussiga, N. & Ghdamsi, M., The corruption-terrorism nexus: A panel data approach. *International Journal of Economics and Finance*, **8**(11), pp. 111–117, 2016.

[16] Simpson, M., Terrorism and corruption. *International Journal of Sociology*, **44**(2), pp. 87–104, 2014.

[17] Odehnal, J. & Sedlacik, M., Political stability as determinant of terrorist attacks in developed and developing countries: An empirical multivariate classification analysis. *AIP Conference Proceedings,* 2018.

[18] Li, Q., Does democracy promote or reduce transnational terrorist incidents? *Journal of Conflict Resolution,* **49**(2), pp. 278–297, 2016.

[19] Asongu, S., Tchamyou, V., Asongu, N. & Tchamynou, N., Fighting terrorism in Africa: Evidence from bundling and unbundling institutions. *Empirical Economics,* **56**(3), pp. 883–933, 2019.

[20] Freytag, A., Krueger, J.J. & Meierreieks, D., The origins of terrorism: cross-country estimates on socio-economic determinants of terrorism. Economics of Security Working Paper 27, 2010.

[21] Stanojoska, A., The connection between terrorism and organized crime: Narcoterrosism and the other hybrids. *Combating Terrorism: International Standards and Legislation Conference Proceedings*, 2011.

[22] Plamper, T. & Neumayer, T., The friend of my enemy is my enemy: International alliances and international terrorism. *European Journal of Political Research,* **49**(1), pp. 75–96, 2010.

[23] IBM Corp., IBM SPSS Statistics for Windows, Version 25.0, Released 2017. Armonk, NY: IBM Corp.

[24] Vision of Humanity, Global Terrorism Index 2017. http://visionofhumanity.org/app/uploads/2017/11/Global-Terrorism-Index-2017.pdf. Accessed on: 7 Aug. 2019.

[25] Social Progress Imperative, 2017 Social Progress Index. www.socialprogress.org/. Accessed on: 7 Aug. 2019.

[26] The World Bank, GNI per capita, PPP (current international dollars). https://data.worldbank.org/indicator/ny.gnp.pcap.pp.cd. Accessed on: 7 Aug. 2019.

[27] Human Development Report, Education Index. http://hdr.undp.org/en/content/education-index. Accessed on: 7 Aug. 2019.

[28] The World Bank, Unemployment, total (% of total labour force). https://data.worldbank.org/indicator/SL.UEM.TOTL.ZS. Accessed on: 8 Aug. 2019.

[29] The World Bank, GDP per capita (current US dollars).

https://data.worldbank.org/indicator/ny.gdp.pcap.cd. Accessed on: 8 Aug. 2019.
[30] The World Bank, Inflation, consumer prices (annual %). https://data.worldbank.org/indicator/FP.CPI.TOTL.ZG. Accessed on: 8 Aug. 2019.
[31] Vision of Humanity, Global Peace Index 2017. https://reliefweb.int/sites/reliefweb.int/files/resources/GPI-2017-Report-1.pdf. Accessed on: 8 Aug. 2019.
[32] Numbeo Database, Crime Index for Country 2017. www.numbeo.com/crime/rankings_by_country.jsp?title=2017. Accessed on: 8 Aug. 2019.
[33] The Global Economy, Political stability – Country rankings. www.theglobaleconomy.com/rankings/wb_political_stability/. Accessed on: 8 Aug. 2019.
[34] The World Bank, Government Effectiveness. https://tcdata360.worldbank.org/indicators/h1c9d2797?country=BRA&indicator=388&viz=line_chart&years=1996,2017. Accessed on: 8 Aug. 2019.
[35] Transparency International, Index 2017. www.transparency.org/news/feature/corruption_perceptions_index_2017. Accessed on: 8 Aug. 2019.

QUANTIFYING PHYSICAL AND PSYCHOLOGICAL IMPACTS OF EXPLOSIVE ATTACKS ON BUILDING OCCUPANTS

STEVEN SCHULDT[1], AHMET SOYLEMEZOGLU[2], NOAH GARFINKLE[2] & KHALED EL-RAYES[3]
[1]Department of Systems Engineering and Management, Air Force Institute of Technology, USA
[2]US Army Corps of Engineers, Engineer Research and Development Center, Construction Engineering Research Laboratory, USA
[3]Department of Civil and Environmental Engineering, University of Illinois at Urbana-Champaign, USA

ABSTRACT

Personnel suffer devastating physical and psychological impacts from explosive terrorist attacks targeting buildings. Explosive attacks produced 42,972 casualties in 2017 alone and survivors of terrorist attacks experience post-traumatic stress disorder (PTSD) at rates as high as 40%. Designers use three primary strategies to protect buildings and their occupants against explosive terrorist attacks: (1) maximize the distance between a building and where an explosive can be easily placed; (2) construct perimeter blast walls; and (3) employ blast-resistant building materials. This paper presents a personnel impact assessment model capable of efficiently quantifying physical and psychological impacts experienced by the occupants of buildings damaged by explosive attacks. The model provides a comprehensive analysis of significant personnel impacts, including fatalities, serious injuries, minor injuries, and occurrences of PTSD. Model performance was evaluated using case studies of single and multi-building sites, and the results illustrated the model's expediency and flexibility. These capabilities are expected to assist building designers in their critical task of analyzing and selecting the design strategy that minimizes the security risks to site personnel from the threat of explosive terrorist attacks.
Keywords: blast effects, consequence, post-traumatic stress disorder, injury, terrorism.

1 INTRODUCTION

Personnel suffer devastating physical and psychological impacts from explosive terrorist attacks targeting buildings. In 2017 alone, explosive attacks resulted in 42,972 casualties worldwide, 74% of which were civilians [1]. The survivors of these terrorist attacks experience emotional and psychological disorders, including post-traumatic stress disorder, at rates as high as 40% [2], [3]. Building designers can significantly reduce facility damage and the likelihood of occupant casualties caused by an explosive attack by incorporating three main design strategies. The most effective design strategy is maximizing the standoff distance between a building and the likely location of an explosive. If additional space is not available, perimeter blast walls can be constructed to reduce blast loads on the building and provide fragmentation protection. The final design strategy is building hardening [4]. Building designers require a method to accurately and efficiently evaluate all feasible design alternatives in order to select the design configuration that minimizes the security risks to building occupants from the threat of explosive terrorist attacks.

Numerous research studies have analyzed the frequency and severity of fatalities, injuries, and psychological impacts from recent historical terrorist attacks, including the 1995 Oklahoma City bombing [5], [6]; the 1998 US Embassy bombing in Nairobi, Kenya [7], [8]; the September 11th attack on New York City, 2001 [9], [10]; and the 2004 Madrid, Spain train bombing [11], [12]. Victims of explosive attacks experience fatalities and several common injury types, including severe head trauma [13]; lung [14], ear [15], and eye [16] damage, as well as lacerations and other injuries caused by flying glass debris [17]. Additionally, victims and bystanders of these attacks were diagnosed with myriad emotional

www.witpress.com, ISSN 1743-3509 (on-line)
doi:10.2495/DMAN190171

and psychological disorders, including PTSD, major depression, panic disorder, agoraphobia, generalized anxiety disorder, and alcohol use disorder.

Several other studies produced models that optimize site layout planning in order to protect buildings and increase site security [18]–[20]. Notably, Schuldt and El-Rayes (2018) developed a multi-objective optimization model that selects the site layout, blast wall type, and building material that presents the optimal trade-off between minimizing building destruction levels and minimizing site construction costs [21]. Despite their significant contributions, these studies do not: (1) efficiently quantify the expected number of fatalities and injuries suffered by building occupants from an explosive attack; and (2) predict the extent of psychological impacts among explosive attack survivors. Accordingly, this paper presents the development of a personnel impact assessment model capable of efficiently quantifying physical and psychological impacts experienced by the occupants of buildings damaged by explosive attacks.

2 PERSONNEL IMPACT ASSESSMENT MODEL FORMULATION

This section presents the formulation of a personnel impact assessment model. Model development is accomplished in the following three steps: (1) identifying model input parameters; (2) quantify physical impacts, including fatalities, serious, and minor injuries on building occupants; and (3) calculating psychological impacts on attack survivors.

2.1 Input parameters

In order to quantify the effects of explosive attacks on building occupants, the model must first calculate blast damage levels of buildings and account for changes in the three aforementioned protection strategies. Accordingly, the model utilizes three main types of input parameters: (1) explosive parameters – blast charge weight (kg) and location of the explosive; (2) blast wall parameters – location of the blast wall, blast wall material, and blast wall height (m); and (3) building parameters – number of building occupants, building material, building geometry, location of the building and its orientation as shown in Fig. 1.

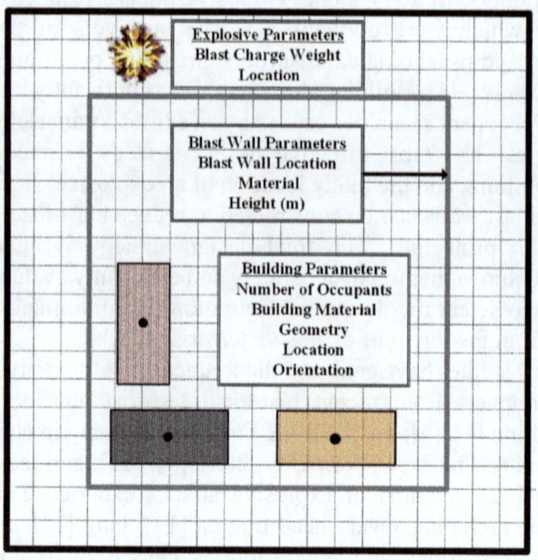

Figure 1: Model input parameters.

The model uses a grid system with a user-defined grid interval to specify explosive, blast wall, and building locations. Buildings locations are established by the placement of their centroid on the grid system and building orientation is the degree of rotation about the centroid. Building occupants are assumed to be uniformly distributed within each building. Furthermore, occupants are assigned to a building based upon the prorated amount of time they spend within a building each day. For example, if an individual was assigned to a site where they both lived and worked, a typical work day may be allotted as follows: 12 hours in their residence, 8 hours in their office building, 2 hours in a dining facility, 1 hour in a fitness center, and 1 hour commuting, corresponding to a prorated occupancy of 0.5, 0.33, 0.08, 0.04, and 0.04, respectively.

The present model utilizes a recently developed method for quantifying blast effects on buildings behind blast walls in order to compute the percentage of a building within five specified damage levels: minimal, minor, moderate, heavy, and severe, and to calculate the total percent building destruction [22]. The present model uses these percentages to quantify the physical and psychological impacts on building occupants.

2.2 Quantify physical impacts

Physical impacts of explosive attacks include fatalities, serious injuries, and minor injuries. The prevalence of each injury type is quantified by multiplying the aforementioned percentage of a building within the five specified damage levels (BA_l) by the number of building occupants and the appropriate injury ratio, which is the percentage of occupants expected to suffer each injury type within each damage level (P_l^F, P_l^{SI}, and P_l^{MI} for fatalities, serious injuries, and minor injuries, respectively), as shown in eqns (1)–(3).

$$F = \sum_{l=1}^{5} BA_l \times O \times P_l^F, \tag{1}$$

$$SI = \sum_{l=1}^{5} BA_l \times O \times P_l^{SI}, \tag{2}$$

$$MI = \sum_{l=1}^{5} BA_l \times O \times P_l^{MI}, \tag{3}$$

where,
F = number of expected building occupant fatalities;
l = facility damage level, where l = 1,2,3,4,5 represents minimal, minor, moderate, heavy, and severe damage, respectively;
BA_l = percent building area within damage level (l);
O = prorated number of building occupants;
P_l^F = percentage of occupant fatalities expected within damage level (l);
SI = number of building occupants expected to suffer serious injuries;
P_l^{SI} = percentage of occupants expected to suffer serious injuries within damage level (l);
SI = number of building occupants expected to experience minor injuries; and
P_l^{MI} = percentage of occupants expected to suffer serious injuries within damage level (l).

The five damage levels are represented as concentric rings, centered at the explosion, with radii equal to the standoff distance associated with each damage level. These blast damage level radii are a function of the blast charge weight; explosive location; blast wall type, height and location; and the building location, geometry and building material. The injury ratio represents the upper limit of reported injury levels within each blast damage level from existing design manuals [23].

2.3 Calculate psychological impacts

Survivors of explosive attacks experience a wide range of emotional and psychological disorders. Post-traumatic stress disorder (PTSD) is the best-defined and most studied psychological disorder following terrorist events. Additionally, PTSD is one of the most frequent and debilitating psychological disorders experienced by explosive attack victims [2], [3]. For these reasons, the present model calculates psychological impact as the likelihood that an individual will be diagnosed with PTSD.

The prevalence of PTSD among explosive attack survivors varies by both the individual's degree and type of exposure. Injured survivors, rescue workers, and uninjured bystanders experience PTSD between 30–40%, 10–20%, and 5–10% respectively [2]. The present model uses the upper limit of the reported ranges to calculate the total expected prevalence of PTSD (PTSD), as shown in eqn (4).

The number of injured personnel (I) is equal to the sum of personnel with serious (SI) and minor injuries (MI), as shown in eqn (5). The number of uninjured bystanders (U) is then computed as the number of assigned building occupants (O) minus the number of personnel fatalities and injuries, as shown in eqn (6). The number of rescue workers is a model input based primarily on the attack severity and response capability of the surrounding site or community.

$$PTSD = \lceil 0.4I + 0.2RW + 0.1U \rceil, \tag{1}$$

$$I = SI + MI, \tag{2}$$

$$U = O - (F + I), \tag{3}$$

where,
$PTSD$ = number of building occupants expected to be diagnosed with PTSD;
I = number of injured building occupants;
RW = number of rescue workers that respond to the explosive attack; and
U = number of uninjured building occupants.

3 CASE STUDIES

This section analyzes four case studies to evaluate the performance of the developed model and demonstrate its distinctive capability to efficiently quantify the physical and psychological impacts of explosive attacks on building occupants.

The selected case studies are intended to highlight the effectiveness of the three aforementioned protection strategies. All four case studies analyze two 80 m x 40 m, two-story office buildings subjected to a 454.5 kg blast charge weight, which is the design blast charge weight carried in a full-size van [24]. The two office buildings are 40 m and 80 m from the explosion, respectively, as shown in Fig. 2 and Fig. 3. Both office buildings are assigned 400 occupants.

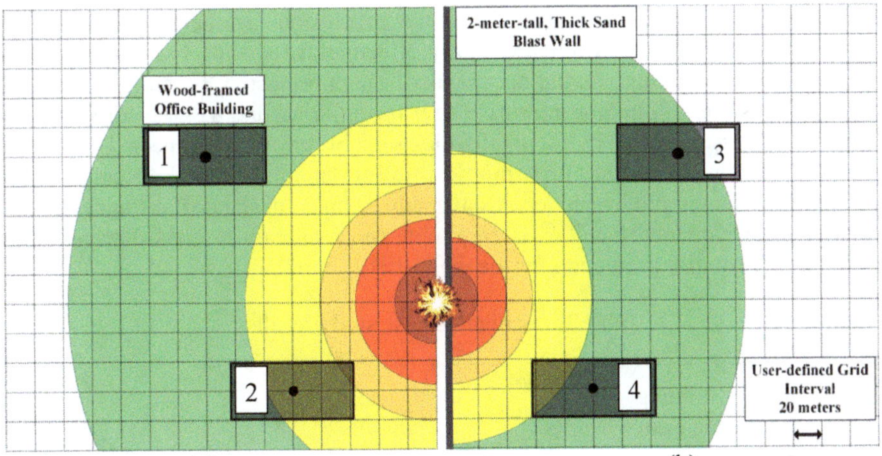

(a) (b)

Figure 2: Damage visualizations for wood-framed office buildings exposed to 454.5 kg explosive attack. (a) No blast wall; (b) 2 m tall, thick sand blast wall.

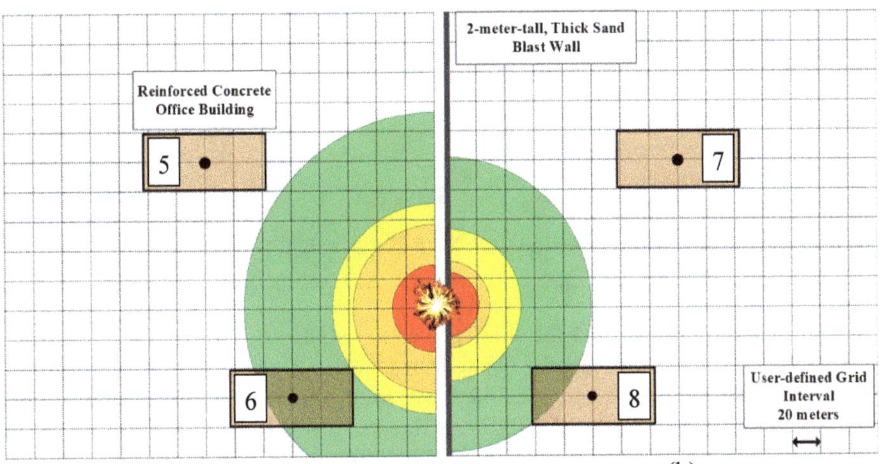

(a) (b)

Figure 3: Damage visualizations for reinforced concrete office buildings exposed to 454.5 kg explosive attack. (a) No blast wall; (b) 2 m tall, thick sand blast wall.

A summary of the generated case study data is recorded in Table 1. Case study one analyzed wood-framed office buildings with no blast wall protection. At a 40 m standoff distance (Building 2), 237 minor injuries, 29 serious injuries, one fatality, and 127 PTSD diagnoses are expected. Doubling the standoff distance to 80 m (Building 1), without making any other design changes, significantly reduced the number of expected physical and psychological impacts. This scenario resulted in 40 minor injuries, zero serious injuries and fatalities, and only 52 cases of PTSD, mostly suffered by uninjured building occupants.

Case studies two and four evaluated the reduction in expected personal and psychological impacts from constructing a perimeter blast wall to protect wood-frame and reinforced concrete (RC) buildings, respectively. Two main conclusions can be drawn from the table results. First, perimeter blast walls are highly effective at reducing blast consequences at close-in distances. For example, the occupants of the unprotected RC building (6) at 40 m are expected to suffer 128 minor injuries, 11 serious injuries, and 82 cases of PTSD. When the same building is protected by a 2 m tall, thick sand blast wall, the expected consequences plummet to just nine expected minor injuries, no serious injuries, and 43 cases of PTSD, which are mostly uninjured bystanders. Conversely, at an 80 m standoff distances, blast wall effectiveness for hardened facilities is negligible (no reduction in consequences), but the wall does provide minor protection for the wood-frame building.

Table 1: Generated case study results.

Building no.	Building material	Standoff distance (m)	Blast wall type	MI	SI	F	PTSD
1	Wood	80	–	40	–	–	52
2	Wood	40	–	257	29	1	127
3	Wood	80	2 m sand	30	–	–	49
4	Wood	40	2 m sand	109	9	–	73
5	Reinforced concrete	80	–	–	–	–	40
6	Reinforced concrete	40	–	128	11	–	82
7	Reinforced concrete	80	2 m sand	–	–	–	40
8	Reinforced concrete	40	2 m sand	9	–	–	43

Case study three investigated the third protection strategy – hardening buildings – by comparing the relatively weak wood-frame construction to the more robust RC. At 40 m, the hardened building is expected to have 148 fewer minor injuries, 20 fewer serious injuries, no fatalities, and 54 fewer cases of PTSD. As the standoff distances doubles, the hardened facility loses its clear advantage, resulting in only 10 fewer minor injuries and 3 fewer cases of PTSD. The present model is implemented in Python and all case studies were analyzed using a 2.0 GHz quad-core Intel Core i7 processor with 6 MB of cache memory and 16 GB of synchronous-dynamic random-access memory (SDRAM). The model required an average completion time of 0.23 seconds per case study.

4 SUMMARY AND CONCLUSIONS

This paper presented the development of an innovative personnel impact assessment model capable of efficiently quantifying physical and psychological impacts experienced by the occupants of buildings damaged by explosive attacks. The model was developed in three main steps. First, explosive, blast wall, and building inputs parameters were identified and defined. Second, physical impacts, including fatalities, serious injuries, and minor injuries suffered by building occupants were quantified. Third, psychological impacts, measured as expected number of personnel to be diagnosed with PTSD, were calculated for attack survivors.

Four case studies were analyzed to demonstrate the efficiency of the model and its unique capabilities. The selected case studies highlighted the effectiveness of the three primary blast design protection strategies: (1) maximize the distance between a building and where an explosive can be easily placed; (2) construct perimeter blast walls; and (3) employ blast-resistant building materials. The model was able to quantify the expected physical and psychological impacts resulting from a 454.5 kg explosive attack – the design blast charge weight carried in a full-size van – in an average of 0.23 seconds per case study. Case study results confirm that increasing standoff distance is typically the most effective blast design strategy. Doubling standoff distance decreased the expected number of injured personnel in the wood-frame office building by 86% and completely eliminated injuries in the reinforced concrete building. Additionally, the increased standoff distance reduced the expected number of PTSD diagnoses in the wood-frame and reinforced concrete office building by 59% and 51%, respectively. The case studies also verify that blast walls effectiveness increases as the standoff distance decreases. For example, a 2 m tall, thick sand blast wall decreased the expected number of injured personnel in the wood-frame building by 59% at a standoff distance of 40 m compared to a 25% reduction at 80 m.

The primary contribution of this research is the development of an innovative model that enables designers to efficiently quantify the expected number of fatalities and injuries suffered by building occupants from an explosive attack and predict the extent of psychological impacts among explosive attack survivors. The scope of the developed model can be expanded in future research studies that consider and evaluate additional blast consequences, including economic losses and operational impacts. This model should prove useful to building designers, allowing them to accurately and efficiently evaluate all feasible design alternatives in order to select the design configuration that minimizes the physical and psychological impacts of explosive attacks on building occupants.

ACKNOWLEDGEMENT

The views expressed in this paper are those of the authors and do not reflect the official policy or position of the United States Air Force, Department of Defense, or the United States government.

REFERENCES

[1] Dathan, J. & Kearney, J., Burden of Harm: Monitoring Explosive Violence in 2017. Action on Armed Violence 2018. https://aoav.org.uk/2018/2017-saw-38-increase-civilian-deaths-explosive-violence-new-report-finds/. Accessed on: 21 Jun. 2019.

[2] Neria, Y., Nandi, A. & Galea, S., Post-traumatic stress disorder following disasters: a systematic review. *Psychological Medicine*, **38**, 2008.

[3] Paz García-Vera, M., Sanz, J. & Gutiérrez, S., A systematic review of the literature on posttraumatic stress disorder in victims of terrorist attacks. *Psychological Reports*, **119**, pp. 328–359, 2016.

[4] Longinow, A. & Mniszewski, K.R., Protecting buildings against vehicle bomb attacks. *Practice Periodical on Structural Design and Construction*, **1**, pp. 51–54, 1996.

[5] North, C.S. et al., Psychiatric disorders among survivors of the Oklahoma City bombing. *JAMA*, **282**, pp. 755–762, 1999.

[6] North, C.S. et al., Psychiatric disorders in rescue workers after the Oklahoma City bombing. *AJP*, **159**, pp. 857–859, 2002.

[7] North, C.S. et al., Comparison of post-disaster psychiatric disorders after terrorist bombings in Nairobi and Oklahoma City. *The British Journal of Psychiatry*, **186**, pp. 487–493, 2005.

[8] Zhang, G., Pfefferbaum, B., Narayanan, P., Lee, S., Thielman, S. & North, C.S., Psychiatric disorders after terrorist bombings among rescue workers and bombing survivors in Nairobi and rescue workers in Oklahoma City. *Annals of Clinical Psychiatry*, **28**, pp. 22–30, 2016.

[9] Galea, S. et al., Psychological sequelae of the September 11 terrorist attacks in New York City. *New England Journal of Medicine*, **346**, pp. 982–987, 2002.

[10] Schlenger, W.E. et al., Psychological reactions to terrorist attacks: Findings from the national study of Americans' reactions to September 11. *JAMA*, **288**, pp. 581–588, 2002.

[11] Gabriel, R. et al., Psychopathological consequences after a terrorist attack: An epidemiological study among victims, the general population, and police officers. *European Psychiatry*, **22**, pp. 339–346, 2007.

[12] Vázquez, C., Hervás, G. & Pérez-Sales, P., Chronic thought suppression and posttraumatic symptoms: Data from the Madrid March 11, 2004 terrorist attack. *Journal of Anxiety Disorders*, **22**, pp. 1326–1336, 2008.

[13] Mallonee, S., Shariat, S., Stennies, G., Waxweiler, R., Hogan, D. & Jordan, F., Physical injuries and fatalities resulting from the Oklahoma City Bombing. *JAMA*, **276**, pp. 382–387, 1996.

[14] Sasser, S.M., Sattin, R.W., Hunt, R.C. & Krohmer, J., Blast lung injury. *Prehospital Emergency Care*, **10**, pp. 165–172, 2006.

[15] Cave, K.M., Cornish, E.M. & Chandler, D.W., Blast injury of the ear: Clinical update from the global War on Terror. *Military Medicine*, **172**, pp. 726–730, 2007.

[16] Morley, M.G., Nguyen, J.K., Heier, J.S., Shingleton, B.J., Pasternak, J.F. & Bower, K.S., Blast eye injuries: A review for first responders. *Disaster Medicine and Public Health Preparedness*, **4**, pp. 154–60, 2010.

[17] Ataei, H. & Anderson, J.C., Mitigating the injuries from flying glass due to air blast. *Sixth Forensic Engineering*, pp. 133–142, 2012.

[18] Khalafallah, A. & El-Rayes, K., Minimizing construction-related security risks during airport expansion projects. *Journal of Construction Engineering and Management*, **134**, pp. 40–48, 2008.

[19] Said, H. & El-Rayes, K., Optimizing the planning of construction site security for critical infrastructure projects. *Automation in Construction*, **19**, pp. 221–234, 2010.

[20] Li, Z., Shen, W., Xu, J. & Lev, B., Bilevel and multi-objective dynamic construction site layout and security planning. *Automation in Construction*, **57**, pp. 1–16, 2015.

[21] Schuldt, S. & El-Rayes, K., Optimizing the planning of remote construction sites to minimize facility destruction from explosive attacks. *Journal of Construction Engineering and Management*, **144**, p. 04018020, 2018.

[22] Schuldt, S. & El-Rayes, K., Quantifying blast effects on constructed facilities behind blast walls. *Journal of Performance of Constructed Facilities*, **31**, p. 04017027, 2017.

[23] Department of Defense (DoD), DoD minimum antiterrorism standards for buildings. UFC 4-010-01, Washington, DC, 2012.

[24] Federal Emergency Management Agency (FEMA), Reference manual to mitigate potential terrorist attacks against buildings. FEMA-426/BIPS-06 Edition 2, Washington, DC, 2011.

Author index

Safety and Security Engineering VIII

Edited by: ***G. PASSERINI****, Marche Polytechnic University, Italy,* **F. GARZIA**, *University of Rome "La Sapienza", Italy and* ***M. LOMBARDI****, University of Rome "La Sapienza", Italy*

In its 8th edition the SAFE conference continues to publish important research contributing to the development of the field. The papers included in this volume are the work of engineers, scientists, field researchers, managers and other specialists involved in one or more of the theoretical and practical aspects of safety and security.

Safety and Security Engineering, due to its special nature, is an interdisciplinary area of research and application that brings together in a systematic way, many disciplines of engineering, from the traditional to the most technologically advanced. This volume covers topics such as crisis management, security engineering, natural and man-made disasters and emergencies, risk management, and control, protection and mitigation issues.

Specific themes include: Risk analysis, assessment and management; System safety engineering; Incident monitoring; Information and communication security; Disaster management; Emergency response; Critical infrastructure protection; Counter terrorism issues; Human factors; Transportation safety and security; Modelling and experiments; Security surveillance systems; Loss prevention; BIM in Safety and Security.

ISBN: 978-1-78466-351-3 **eISBN: 978-1-78466-352-0**
Published 2019 / 162pp

www.ingramcontent.com/pod-product-compliance
Lightning Source LLC
LaVergne TN
LVHW062238200926
848484LV00006B/1567